MINIMAL RESIDUAL DISEASE IN ACUTE LEUKEMIA

DEVELOPMENTS IN ONCOLOGY

F.J. Cleton and J.W.I.M. Simons, eds., Genetic Origins of Tumour Cells
ISBN 90-247-2272-1

J. Aisner and P. Chang, eds., Cancer Treatment Research
ISBN 90-247-2358-2

B.W. Ongerboer de Visser, D.A. Bosch and W.M.H. van Woerkom-Eykenboom, eds.,
Neuro-oncology: Clinical and Experimental Aspects
ISBN 90-247-2421-X

K. Hellmann, P. Hilgard and S. Eccles, eds., Metastasis: Clinical and Experimental Aspects
ISBN 90-247-2424-4

H.F. Seigler, ed., Clinical Management of Melanoma
ISBN 90-247-2584-4

P. Correa and W. Haenszel, eds., Epidemiology of Cancer of the Digestive Tract
ISBN 90-247-2601-8

L.A. Liotta and I.R. Hart, eds., Tumour Invasion and Metastasis
ISBN 90-247-2611-5

J. Bánóczy, ed., Oral Leukoplakia
ISBN 90-247-2655-7

C. Tijssen, M. Halprin and L. Endtz, eds., Familial Brain Tumours
ISBN 90-247-2691-3

F.M. Muggia, C.W. Young and S.K. Carter, eds., Anthracycline Antibiotics in Cancer
ISBN 90-247-2711-1

B.W. Hancock, ed., Assessment of Tumour Response
ISBN 90-247-2712-X

D.E. Peterson, ed., Oral Complications of Cancer Chemotherapy
ISBN 0-89838-563-6

R. Mastrangelo, D.G. Poplack and R. Riccardi, eds., Central Nervous System Leukemia.
Prevention and Treatment
ISBN 0-89838-570-9

A. Polliack, ed., Human Leukemias. Cytochemical and Ultrastructural Techniques in
Diagnosis and Research
ISBN 0-89838-585-7

W. Davis, C. Maltoni and S. Tanneberger, eds., The Control of Tumor Growth and its
Biological Bases
ISBN 0-89838-603-9

A.P.M. Heintz, C.Th. Griffiths and J.B. Trimbos, eds., Surgery in Gynecological Oncology
ISBN 0-89838-604-7

M.P. Hacker, E.B. Double and I. Krakoff, eds., Platinum Coordination Complexes in
Cancer Chemotherapy
ISBN 0-89838-619-5

M.J. van Zwieten, The Rat as Animal Model in Breast Cancer Research: A Histopathological Study of Radiation- and Hormone-Induced Rat Mammary Tumors
ISBN 0-89838-624-1

MINIMAL RESIDUAL DISEASE IN ACUTE LEUKEMIA

edited by

B. LÖWENBERG, MD, PhD
A. HAGENBEEK, MD, PhD

The Dr Daniël den Hoed Cancer Center and

Rotterdam Radio-Therapeutic Institute,

Rotterdam, The Netherlands

1984 **MARTINUS NIJHOFF PUBLISHERS**
a member of the KLUWER ACADEMIC PUBLISHERS GROUP
BOSTON / THE HAGUE / DORDRECHT / LANCASTER

Distributors

for the United States and Canada: Kluwer Boston, Inc., 190 Old Derby Street, Hingham, MA 02043, USA
for all other countries: Kluwer Academic Publishers Group, Distribution Center, P.O.Box 322, 3300 AH Dordrecht, The Netherlands

Library of Congress Catalog Card Number 83-27562

ISBN-13: 978-94-010-9002-5   e-ISBN-13: 978-94-009-5670-4
DOI: 10.1007/978-94-009-5670-4

Preface

The objective of the treatment of acute leukemia involves the eradication of all neoplastic cells, including the last one. Ideally, treatment should be controlled by monitoring cell kill. If the last cells could be discovered and their biological properties be determined, the qualitative and quantitative effects of treatment should be directly evaluable. This should ultimately permit a calculated tumor cell reduction thereby avoiding overtreatment and excessive toxicity and thus providing a basis for individualized antileukemic treatment.

In recent years several new developments have contributed to the selective discovery of minimal numbers of leukemic cells which are hidden among the normal cells in the marrow cavities. These methods are the first steps to the realization of the therapeutic goals indicated above. They include the production and application of monoclonal antibodies against differentiation antigens on the cell surface, the use of pulse cytophotometry – and cell sorter techniques, the employment of cytogenetics, the development of culture techniques for selective growth of precursor cells and several others. These methodologies offer prospects for refined diagnosis and, as far as the elimination of leukemic cells is concerned, the further development of autologous bone marrow transplantation. Eliminating tumor cells from autologous grafts requires the detailed knowledge of the cellular inter-relationships within the neoplasm so that the neoplastic cells responsible for tumor propagation are specifically removed. Recognition and characterization of the clonogenic cells of the neoplasm should then lead to determining their sensitivity to the therapeutic agents which are clinically applied.

New therapeutic principles involve intensive treatment of minimal residual disease. During complete remission, small numbers of tumor cells persist and are responsible for ultimate relapse and mortality. Allogeneic and autologous bone marrow transplantation as well as sequential and intensive chemotherapy have produced promising results recently and their comparative merits are only now becoming evaluable. While the treatment of ALL in children has enjoyed a high rate of curability for several years as a result of continued treatment of minimal residual disease throughout remission, promising results in young adults with ALL and AML are presently attained too.

This monograph summarizes the recent achievements in this rapidly evolving area in which laboratory and clinical developments go hand in hand. Many of the leading groups have added contributions and have furnished a picture of the technical advancements and clinical applications in the field. The current experiences in leukemia disclose new principles which will probably have a wide impact on the development of new diagnostic and therapeutic strategies in patients with other cancers as well.

BOB LÖWENBERG and ANTON HAGENBEEK
Rotterdam, October 12, 1983

Contents

List of First Authors with Co-Authors

BARLOGIE, B., The University of Texas System Cancer Center, M.D. Anderson Hospital and Tumor Institute, Dept. of Developmental Therapeutics, Houston TX 77030, USA
Co-authors: W.N. Hittelman, F.M. Davis, H. Katarjian

BEKKUM, D.W. VAN, Radiobiological Institute TNO, Lange Kleiweg 151, P.O. Box 5815, 2280 HV Rijswijk, The Netherlands

BUCHANAN, G.R., University of Texas Health Science Center, Dallas TX 75235, USA
Co-author: R. Graham Smith

BURKE, P.J., The Johns Hopkins Oncology Center, Baltimore MD 21205, USA

BURNETT, A.K., Glasgow Royal Infirmary, Dept. of Haematology, Glasgow G4 0SF, United Kingdom
Co-authors: P. Tansey, M. Alcorn, C.R.J. Singer, G.A. McDonald, A.G. Robertson (The Institute of Radiotherapeutics, Glasgow G11 6NT, United Kingdom)

DICKE, K.A., The University of Texas System Cancer Center, M.D. Anderson Hospital and Tumor Institute, Dept. of Developmental Therapeutics, Houston TX 77030, USA
Co-authors: C.H. Poynton, C.L. Reading

DONGEN, J.J.M. VAN, Erasmus University, Dept. of Cell Biology and Genetics, P.O. Box 1738, 3000 DR Rotterdam, The Netherlands
Co-authors: H. Hooykaas, K. Hählen, K. Benne, W.M. Bitter, A.A. van der Linde-Preesman, I.L.M. Tettero, M. van de Rijn, J. Hilgers, G.E. van Zanen, A. Hagemeijer

GOLDSTONE, A.H., University College Hospital, Dept. of Haematology, London WC 1E 6AU, United Kingdom
Co-authors: D.C. Linch, C.C. Anderson, M. Jones, S.P. Closs, J.C. Cawley, J.D.M. Richards

HAGENBEEK, A., Dr. Daniël den Hoed Cancer Center, Groene Hilledijk 301, 3075 EA Rotterdam, The Netherlands and Radiobiological Institute TNO, Lange Kleiweg 152, P.O. Box 5815, 2280 HV Rijswijk, The Netherlands
Co-author: A.C.M. Martens

KEATING, M.J., The University of Texas System Cancer Center, M.D. Anderson Hospital and Tumor Institute, Dept. of Developmental Therapeutics, Houston TX 77030, USA

KERSEY, J.H., Bone Marrow Transplantation Program, and Departments of Pediatrics, Laboratory Medicine and Pathology, University of Minnesota, Minneapolis, USA
Co-authors: D. Vallera, N. Ramsay, L.F. Filipovich, R. Stong, T. LeBien, R. Youle, D. Neville (National Institute of Mental Health, Bethesda, MD, USA), P. Beverley (University College Hospital, London)

LANGE, B., The Wistar Institute, Philadelphia PA 19104, USA
Co-authors: D. Ferrero, S. Pessano, H. Hubbell, A. Palumbo, S.K. Lai, G. Rovera

LISTER, T.A., St. Bartholomew's Hospital, Dept. of Medical Oncology, London EC1A 7BE, United Kingdom
Co-authors: W. Gregory, A.Z.S. Rohatiner, B. Birkhead, R. Biruls, M. Barnett, H.S. Dhaliwal, M.L. Slevin, J.A.L. Amess

LÖWENBERG, B., Dr. Daniël den Hoed Cancer Center, Groene Hilledijk 301, 3075 EA Rotterdam, The Netherlands
Co-authors: J. Bauman, J. Abels (Institute of Hematology, University Hospital Dijkzigt, Rotterdam), G. Dzoljic (Dept. of Bacteriology, University Hospital Dijkzigt, Rotterdam), W.D.H. Hendriks, J. van de Poel, W. Sizoo, K. Sintnicolaas and G. Wagemaker (Radiobiological Institute TNO, Rijswijk, The Netherlands)

PREISLER, H.D., Roswell Park Memorial Institute, Dept. of Medical Oncology, Buffalo NY 14263, USA
Co-authors: A. Raza, N. Azarnia, G. Browman

SALLAN, S.E., Dana Farber Cancer Institute, Div. of Tumor Immunology, Boston MA 02115, USA
Co-authors: R.C. Bast jr., J.M. Lipton, J. Ritz

SANTOS, G.W., The Johns Hopkins Oncology Center, Baltimore MD 21205, USA
Co-author: H. Kaizer

SPECK, B., Kantonsspital Basel, Dept. of Hematology, Basle CH-4000, Switzerland
Co-author: A. Gratwohl

STIFF, P.J., Southern Illinois University, School of Medicine, Springfield IL 62708, USA
Co-authors: T.P.U. Wustrov, A.R. Koester, M.F. Derisi, B.D. Clarkson

THIERFELDER, S., Institut für Hämatologie, D-8000 Munich-2, BRD
Co-authors: B. Netzel, G. Hoffmann-Fezer, B. Kranz, J. Haas

THOMAS, E.D., Fred Hutchinson Cancer Research Center, Seattle WA 98104, USA

VISSER, J.M.W., Radiobiological Institute TNO, Lange Kleiweg 151, P.O. Box 5815, 2280 HV Rijswijk, The Netherlands

VITETTA, E.S., University of Texas, Dept. of Microbiology, Southwestern Medical School, Dallas TX 75235, USA
Co-author: J.W. Uhr

VOSSEN, J.M.J.J., Academic Hospital, Dept. of Pediatrics, Rijnsburgerweg 10, 2333 AA Leiden, The Netherlands

WEINER, R.S., The J. Hillis Miller Health Center, University of Florida, Div. of Medical Oncology, Gainesville FL 32610, USA

WEINSTEIN, H.J., Dana Farber Cancer Institute, Div. of Pediatric Oncology, Boston MA 02115, USA
    Co-authors: R.J. Mayer, F.S. Coral, H.E. Grier, R.D. Gelber, D.S. Rosenthal, B.M. Camitta, E. Frei III

ZITTOUN, R., Service d'Hématologie, Hôtel-Dieu, 75181 Paris Cedex 04, France
    Co-author: J.P. Marie

ZWAAN, F.E., Academic Hospital, Bone Marrow Transplant Unit, Rijnsburgerweg 10, 2333 AA Leiden, The Netherlands
    Co-author: J. Hermans (Medical Statistics, University Medical Center, Leiden, The Netherlands)

NUCLEIC ACID CYTOMETRY, INTERPHASE CHROMOSOMES AND NUCLEOLAR ANTIGEN IN THE DETECTION OF RESIDUAL LEUKEMIA IN MORPHOLOGIC REMISSION

B. Barlogie, W. N. Hittelman, F. M. Davis, H. Kantarjian

INTRODUCTION

Currently available combination chemotherapy for acute leukemia in adults produces complete hematologic normalization, commonly referred to as complete remission, in approximately 65% of patients (1,2,3). Although marrow from these patients is indistinguishable by standard morphologic criteria from the marrow of normal individuals, at least 80% of such patients will eventually relapse, with a median time to leukemic recurrence of 12 to 14 months (1,4). Efforts to improve the duration of disease control, and thus increase the proportion of patients potentially cured of their disease, include the use of cytotoxic chemotherapy in remission, using either conventional or high dose schedules, with or without bone marrow transplantation. The notion of a finite cure rate in adult acute leukemia emphasizes the principal usefulness of today's chemotherapeutic armamentarium and points to the remarkable disease heterogeneity among different patients. The prospect of long term disease control, even with less intensive therapy during the past 2 decades, underscores the need for reliable prognostic factors to judge an individual patient's risk of recurrence.

In our experience, using standard clinical and laboratory parameters, the duration of complete remission is affected by cytogenetics, the degree of leukemic differentiation and the speed of initial cytoreduction (5). Thus, the durability of response, at least for the first year, is predominantly determined by disease rather than host factors. Biologically, one would expect the duration of remission to be a function of the degree of leukemic cytoreduction, which is a function of drug sensitivity, and tumor regrowth characteristics. The latter has indeed been shown to affect the time to recurrence, which is shorter when the proportion of leukemic cells in S phase measured prior to therapy is high (6). Cytoreduction during induction therapy has been assessed using changes in marrow biopsy cellularity and combined cytokinetics and hematocrit information on marrow and peripheral blood (7,8). In this report, we will focus on the leukemic burden present at the onset of complete remission as a first step to detect residual leukemia in morphologically normal marrow. The tumor load early in remission is determined by the initial tumor burden at diagnosis and the relative drug sensitivity of leukemic cells during an intensive phase of therapy. The degree of residual leukemia at the onset of complete remission might therefore be representative of the ultimate degree of tumor cell kill achieved and hence be useful, along with information on leukemia regrowth kinetics, for the prediction of remission duration.

A number of approaches have been employed to detect residual leukemia in remission, including cytogenetics, biophysical and biochemical assays, immunologic tests, and in vitro growth characteristics. These assays either assess rare tumor cells directly or indirectly by examining the interaction between leukemic and normal hemopoiesis.

Our laboratories have previously reported that abnormal DNA content, as assessed by flow cytometry (FCM) of cells stained with a DNA-specific fluorochrome, is an exquisite stigma of neoplastic disease that can be detected at a low frequency because of its distinct expression (9). Unfortunately, however, aneuploid DNA stemlines are encountered in only 20-25% of adult patients with acute leukemia (10,11). Therefore, alternative neoplastic markers have been sought. The human malignancy associated nucleolar antigen (HMNA) is highly sensitive and specific for human tumor cells including various forms of human leukemia (12,13). It is recognized by indirect immunofluorescence using heterologous antisera against HeLa cell nucleoli. Possibly related to the expression of HMNA because of its frequent nucleolar localization is double-stranded RNA (ds-RNA), as evaluated by FCM of propidium iodide stained cells after DNase treatment (14). We have noted a 2-3 fold excess in ds-RNA content particularly in myeloblastic leukemia compared to normal marrow, concomitant with an elevation of total RNA content.

In addition to these direct means of tumor cell detection, we have also conducted cytokinetic studies to determine whether residual leukemia can be detected on the basis of inhibition of normal hemopoietic proliferation via leukemic inhibitory activity (LIA) using DNA FCM (15). Finally, the technique of premature chromosome condensation (PCC) has shown differences in condensation patterns of cells in G_1 phase for normal and malignant cells including leukemic cells (16,17). The latter are characterized by a higher proportion of cells with decondensed chromatin, indicative of arrest in late G_1 phase. Such predominance of late G_1PCC was also noted in patients during morphologic remission antedating relapse (18). This may reflect the presence of differentiated leukemic cells or may be linked to LIA release inducing arrest of normal hemopoietic cells in late rather than in early G_1 phase.

In this communication, we will present our experience with nucleic acid FCM (DNA, RNA, ds-RNA), HMNA and PCC parameters, all of which demonstrate marked abnormalities in overt leukemia, to detect residual disease early in morphologic remission and, where available, report on the time course of these parameters towards morphologic relapse.

MATERIALS AND METHODS

Investigative laboratory procedures reported here were conducted as part of a comprehensive Leukemia Research Center Program during all stages of leukemic disease. In this report, we will focus on studies early in remission ($\leq$ 2 months), as they pertain to the detection of residual leukemia.

For analysis of DNA and RNA content, marrow cells were stained with acridine orange according to the 2-step procedure reported by Traganos et al (19). High resolution DNA content analysis was conducted with the highly DNA-specific dye mixture of mithramycin and ethidium bromide employing energy transfer between these two dyes (20). Ds-RNA was measured with propidium iodide after prior DNA digestion with DN'ase (14). Stained cells were measured in an ICP 22 mercury arc flow cytometer (acridine orange, mithramycin-ethidium bromide) or in an EPICS V flow sorter (propidium iodide). The derived parameters include the DNA index, representing the ratio of modal channel numbers of tumor vs normal G_1 cells (10); RNA index, representing the ratio of mean RNA content of target cells vs median RNA content of lymphocyte controls (21); cell cycle distribution in G_1 and in $(S+G_2M)$, using previously published gating procedures (22); and ds-RNA excess, by subtracting from each experimental curve a histogram of lymphocyte controls, using the EASY system (Coulter) (23).

The PCC technique involves fusion of mitotic inducer cells with bone marrow mononuclear cells, resulting in the induction of premature condensation of the interphase chromatin. A detailed description of this methodology is presented elsewhere (24). The morphology of the PCC indicates the cell cycle phase of the interphase cells at the time of fusion, i.e. G_1, S or G_2 phase. Moreover, earlier studies have shown that the conformation of the PCC also reflects a condensation cycle: mitotic chromosomes represent the most condensed state of chromatin and early S phase chromosomes have the least condensed chromatin. Early G_1 cells give rise to highly condensed G_1 PCC, whereas late G_1 cells yield highly extended G_1 PCC. Similarly, unstimulated normal human peripheral blood lymphocytes give rise to condensed G_1 PCC, whereas after mitogenic stimulation (but prior to entry into S phase), the G_1 PCC appear highly elongated. For purposes of quantitation, G_1 PCC are evaluated on a scale of 1 to 6 with a value of 1 representing the most condensed G_1 PCC state and a value of 6 representing the most elongated G_1 PCC state. Since mitogenic stimulation of lymphocytes resulted in an increased fraction of cells in late G_1, the Proliferative Potential Index (PPI) was defined as the fraction of G_1 cells in late G_1 (i.e. the fraction of G_1 PCC with condensation values of 4,5, and 6). Thus, a cell population with a high frequency of late G_1 cells would have a high PPI value, regardless of the number of cells in S or G_2 phase.

Human malignancy-associated nucleolar antigen (HMNA) studies employ rabbit antiserum raised against the nucleoli of HeLa cells. Antibodies to normal nucleolar antigens are removed by absorption with human placental nucleoli, normal peripheral blood lymphocytes and serum. The presence of HMNA is then detected by indirect immunofluorescence staining of methanol-fixed cytocentrifuge preparations using fluorescein-conjugated goat anti-rabbit immunoglobulin as the indicator antibody (12). Some slides were stained with Wright-Giemsa (Harleco, Gibbstown, N.J.) after observation for fluorescence. Stained cells were examined using a Nikon Optiphot microscope. For each determination 200 cells were counted.

RESULTS

DNA Index:

Abnormal DNA stemlines were noted in 27% of 175 patients at diagnosis. Of 23 patients with DNA-aneuploidy studied serially at diagnosis and in complete remission, only 2 of 6 patients with ALL demonstrated persistence of an abnormal DNA stemline in remission involving 6 and 12% of marrow cells, respectively. These 2 individuals had biclonal abnormalities at diagnosis with both hypo- and hyperdiploid stemlines, and only the hyperdiploid abnormality persisted in remission, lasting 3 and 7 months, respectively.

Cell Cycle Distribution:

We have previously reported that the proliferative activity as measured by the proportion of cells with $(S+G_2M)$ DNA content is lower during active disease, i.e. at diagnosis and at relapse (median 12%), than in remission (median, 19%). There was considerable spread in $(S+G_2M)$ values in remission both for patients with AML and ALL (4-33%). The 37 patients with values of $(S+G_2M) >22\%$ showed a longer remission duration with a median of 72 weeks compared to 42 weeks for the 28 patients with lower values (Figure 1).

Further follow-up of $(S+G_2M)$ compartment size during remission until relapse revealed a decline by ca. 30% beyond one half year in remission.

Relapsing patients did not diverge from this general pattern; i.e. patients relapsing within 6 months generally displayed higher (S+G₂M) values than those with recurrences at later time intervals.

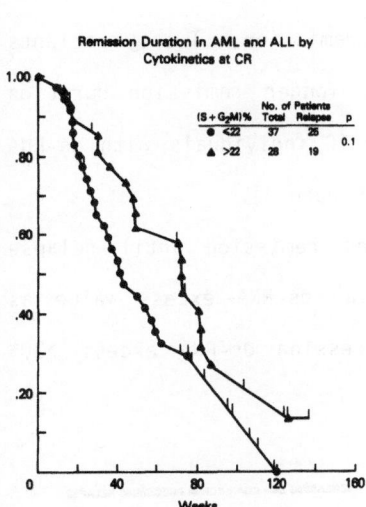

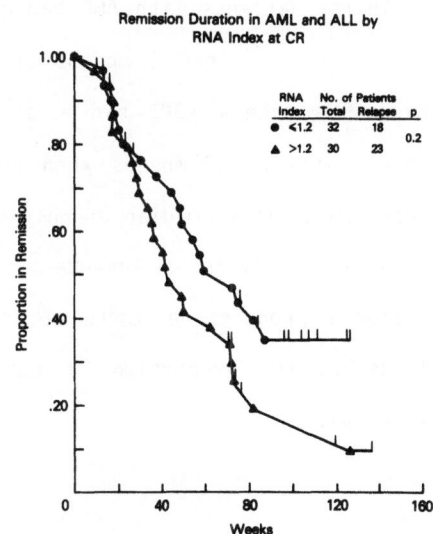

FIGURE 1 Remission duration by cytokinetics at the onset of complete remission. Patients with a higher proportion of cells in (S+G₂M) tend to have longer remissions than those with values ≤22%.

FIGURE 2 Remission duration by RNA index at the onset of complete remission. Low values ≤1.2 (within normal marrow range) are associated with longer remissions than higher values.

Total RNA Content (RNA Index):

At the time of attainment of complete remission, the RNA index generally declined towards values noted for normal bone marrow. As in the case of (S+G₂M)%, there was considerable variation also in RNA index values

8

among different patients (0.6-3.6, median 1.3). Thirty patients with RNA index > 1.2 tended to have shorter remissions (median of 42 weeks) than 32 individuals with lower values (median of 62 weeks)(Figure 2).

Ds-RNA Content:

Thirty patients with AML had determinations performed of ds-RNA excess during the first 2 months of complete remission. Twenty patients with ds-RNA excess <30% had a significantly longer remission duration with a median of 22 months when compared to 10 individuals with ds-RNA excess >30%, with a median of only 6 months (Figure 3).

Serial analysis of ds-RNA excess during remission until relapse revealed a progressive increase in the median ds-RNA excess value as well as in the proportion of patients expressing ds-RNA excess >30% (Figure 4).

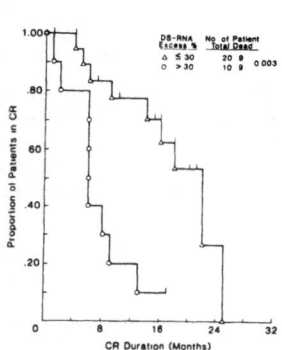

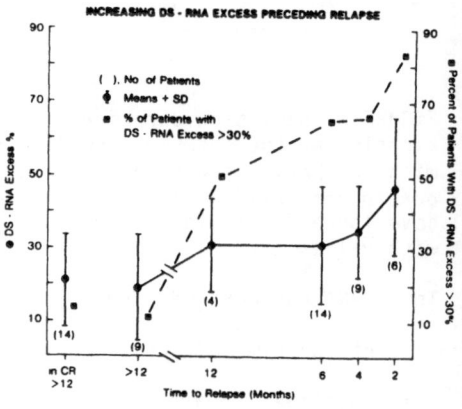

FIGURE 3 Remission duration in AML by ds-RNA excess at the onset of complete remission. Patients with ds-RNA excess within normal marrow range (<30%) display significantly longer remissions than individuals with higher values.

FIGURE 4 Serial ds-RNA excess analys during remission until relapse in AM The proportion of patients with ds-F excess values >30% progressively increases during the 12 mos preceeding relapse. Likewise, the average ds-RN excess (in relationship to lymphocytes) increases particularly during the 6 mos prior to relapse.

Proliferative Potential Index (PPI):

Twenty-five patients had PCC analysis during the first 2 months of complete remission. Seven of 9 patients with PPI >35% have already relapsed with a median time from sampling to relapse of 13 weeks, compared to 4 relapses in 16 patients in the low PPI group, where the median time to relapse has not yet been reached (Figure 5).

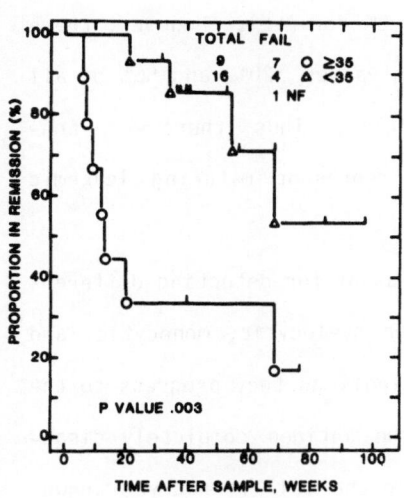

FIGURE 5 Remission duration by PPI values obtained during the first 2 mos of remission. Patients expressing low values (<35%) have significantly longer remissions than individuals with high values.

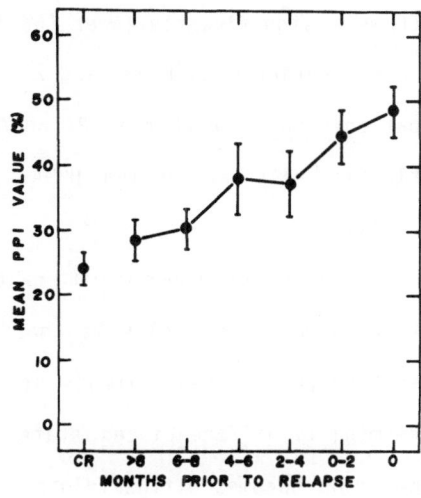

Figure 6 Progressive increase in PPI values during the 8 mos prior to relapse.

Nineteen separate patients were studied serially during remission. PPI values > 35% developed in 11 of 14 relapsing patients. The median time from PPI elevation to morphologic relapse was 3.5 months. Figure 6 illustrates the progressive increase in mean PPI score for relapsing patients as a function of time prior to relapse.

HMNA Expression:

Figure 7 shows the percentage of HMNA-positive cells in the bone marrow of normal donors, patients with solid tumors without marrow involvement and of patients with various leukemic conditions, both during phases of active disease and in remission. All 31 non-leukemic individuals had HMNA levels <2%, whereas all 72 patients with active leukemia had >2% HMNA-positive cells. Median HMNA values for patients with active leukemia were 70% for AML and 90% for ALL. The corresponding values in CR were significantly lower (6% for AML and 2% for ALL). However, there were 6 patients with AML and 2 with ALL with values >20%, and 56% of all patients in CR harbored >2% HMNA-positive cells. Thus, there were non-blastic cells expressing HMNA, which may represent maturing leukemic cells.

One of the problems with using the HMNA assay for detecting differentiating malignant cells is that cells of the myelocytic, monocytic, and erythrocytic series normally lose their nucleoli as they progress to the terminally differentiated state. Whether the antigen completely disappears or becomes diffusely distributed within the cell is not yet known. However, in a number of patients, we have been able to detect residual HMNA positivity in morphologically differentiated cells (Figure 8). This has been observed in several clinical situations, including the smoldering leukemic phase, acute phase prior to therapy, early during remission induction therapy when the fraction of differentiated cells in the blood rises quickly as the blast count falls, and during complete remission.

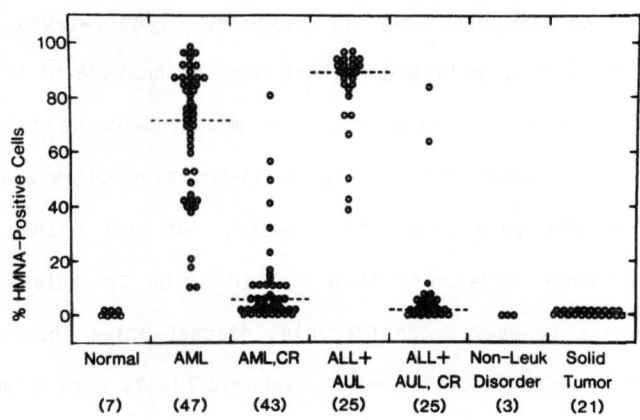

FIGURE 7 HMNA expression in the bone marrow of patients with various forms of leukemia during different phases of their diseases and in morphologically normal marrow from normal volunteers and patients with non-leukemic conditions. More than 2% HMNA-positive cells are found in all patients with active phaes of AML or ALL/AUL, contrasting with negative findings in all individuals with non-leukemic conditions. In complete remission, high values of HMNA >20% are rare.

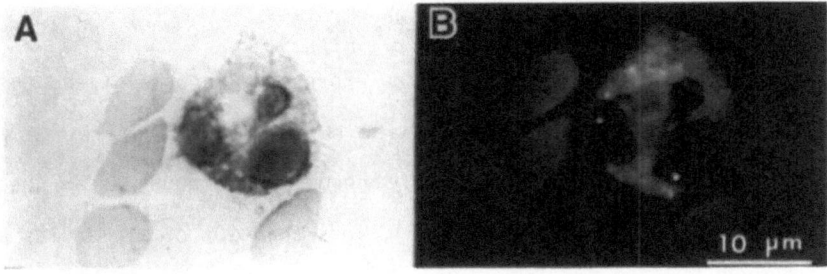

Figure 8 Photomicrographs of mature granulocyte expressing distinct HMNA positivity.

HMNA studies within the first 2 months of remission were available in 10 individuals, 5 of whom had values ≥5% and 2 had values above 5% (15 and 24%). For this small patient sample, trends for remission duration are not yet apparent.

It was of interest to determine if the percentage of HMNA-positive cells was related to the proximity of relapse. Twenty-seven of the patients in this study have relapsed and the mean percentage of HMNA-positive cells as a function of time from the measurement to relapse is shown in Figure 9. The mean percentage of HMNA-positive cells was higher than normal during the year prior to relapse, but was within normal limits for measurements made more than 1 year prior to relapse. For individual patients, however, considerable discrepancies between the proportions of HMNA-positive cells and of leukemic blasts were seen. Such extreme examples are illustated in Figure 10, where in one case HMNA-positivity >50% was observed 50 weeks prior to relapse, whereas HMNA-positive cells and blasts emerged concurrently in the other case.

DISCUSSION

While standard morphologic criteria of complete remission applied to all patients of this study, there was considerable variation in the research parameters under investigation. In comparison to normal marrow, approximately half of the patients expressed abnormalities, usually associated with overt leukemia, in all but DNA index parameters at the onset of remission. If one accepts abnormal DNA content as an unequivocal stigma of neoplastic disease (25), less than 10% of all adults and so far no patient with AML presenting with this abnormality express this feature in a detectable proportion in remission. The high incidence and degree of aberration of the remaining parameters therefore suggest that they are predominantly not related to leukemic cells but probably originate from normal cells in the presence of residual leukemia. Thus, similar abnormalities particularly in ds-RNA excess, PPI and $(S+G_2M)$ seem to be associated both with normal hemopoiesis under the influence of residual leukemia in remission and with overt disease. Regardless of cellular origin, these abnormalities, typical for overt leukemia, adversely affect remission duration when present at the onset of complete remission.

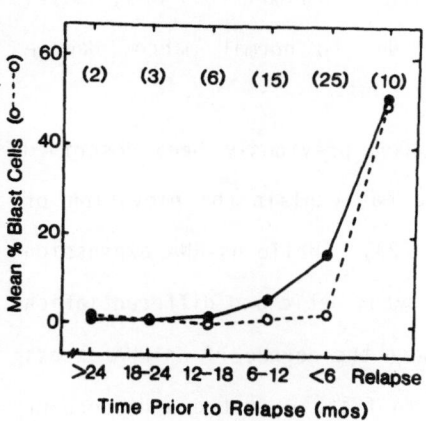

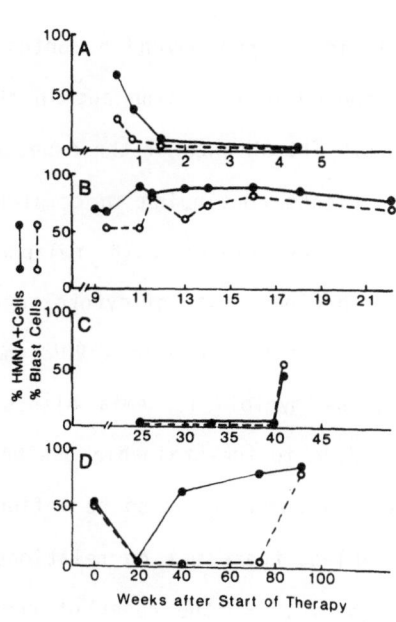

FIGURE 9 Time course of the proportion of leukemic blast cells and HMNA-positive cells during remission until relapse. Already during the interval of 6 to 12 mos prior to relapse, some patients demonstrate an increased proportion of HMNA-positive cells. During the 6 mos immediately preceeding relapse, the average proportion of HMNA-positive cells rises to 15% and reaches 50% at the time of relapse.

FIGURE 10 Time course of blast percent and proportion of HMNA-positive cells in 4 separate patients with AML. A concordant behavior is noted in cases A, B and C during the various phases of the disease. Panel D demonstrates an example of marked elevation of HMNA expression, antedating morphologic relapse by almost one year.

Abnormal cytokinetic features (low S+G$_2$M% and high PPI values) in remission can be explained on the basis of humoral inhibitory activity such as LIA elaborated by leukemic cells, leading to a late G$_1$ phase arrest with subsequent diminution of the (S+G$_2$M) compartment of normal hemopoietic cells. There was, however, a decline in the proportion of cells in (S+G$_2$M) beyond 6 months of complete remission both in patients continuing in remission and in those relapsing during various time segments. The absence of the expected sustained high proliferative activity in patients continuing in complete remission as opposed to a progressive decrease associated with relapse may be due to normal marrow damage after prolonged use of cytotoxic therapy.

"Giant heterogeneous RNA" molecules have previously been described in acute myeloid leukemia blasts (26) and may explain the elevation of propidium iodide-stainable ds-RNA content (23). While ds-RNA expression has been shown by us to be influenced by cytokinetic and differentiation variables, there was no relationship between the degree of ds-RNA excess and (S+G$_2$M)% at the onset of remission. In fact, we noted a discordant prognostic impact of these 2 variables. It is possible that the presumed elevation of ds-RNA content in normal hemopoietic cells in remission is associated with cell cycle arrest in late G$_1$ phase. While total RNA content has previously been shown to distinguish myeloblastic from lymphoblastic leukemias, total RNA appeared inferior to ds-RNA content in assessing the risk of recurrence.

The origin of HMNA-positive cells in remission is equally obscure. Both possibilities of leukemic cell differentiation (see "Results") and HMNA-positive normal hemopoietic cells in the presence of subclinical leukemia have to be considered. In vitro cloning assays and combined phenotypic (ds-RNA, HMNA) and cytogenetic examinations of individual colonies may help to elucidate the nature of leukemic marker expression in seemingly normal marrow cells.

In summary, during the early phase of hemopoietic normalization, persistence of an appreciable fraction of cells with aneuploid DNA content is a rare event, suggesting that leukemic cell differentiation is uncommon or limited to a small proportion of cells, using current cyto-toxic therapy. This consideration is based on the assumption of geno-typic stability of DNA content abnormalities without reversal to diploidy in case of terminal tumor cell differentiation. Although relatively rare, aneuploid leukemias represent an important research resource to examine the biology of tumor cell differentiation in vivo and in vitro, if indeed aneuploidy is maintained. The detection rate of rare DNA-aneu-ploid cells can possibly be enhanced by the use of the recently introduc-ed BUdR antibody immunofluorescence assay, whereby normal cells in S phase can be distinguished from aneuploid G_1 cells that are not labeled (27).

Rather than representing residual tumor burden directly, abnormali-ties in ds-RNA excess, PPI and (S+G_2M)% in remission seem to result from an indirect effect of subclinical leukemia on normal hemopoiesis, signifying earlier relapse. We are currently investigating whether the combined use of marrow cellular parameters early in remission and at diagnosis (e.g. (S+G_2M)% as a parameter of leukemia regrowth kinetics) may help refine the risk assessment of relapse from acute leukemia. These parameters could then be utilized prospectively for clinical trial designs that gauge the intensity of therapy according to individual patients' risk factors. If, in addition, parameters could be identified later in remission that sufficiently antecede morphologic relapse (e.g. HMNA, PPI and ds-RNA), the value of early re-intensification therapy as opposed to standard reinduction treatment can be assessed.

REFERENCES

1. Keating, M., Smith, T., McCredie, K., Hersh, E., Gutterman, J., Gehan, E. and Freireich, E.: A four year experience with anthracycline, cytosine arabinoside, vincristine ad prednisone combination chemotherapy in 325 adults with acute leukemia. Cancer 47:2779-2788, 1981.

2. Weinstein, H.J., Mayer, R.J., Rosenthal, D.S., Camitta, B.M., Caroll, F.S., Nathan, D.G., Frei, E.: Treatment of acute myelogenous leukemia in children and adults. N.E.J.M. 303:473-478, 1980.

3. Gale, R.P., Foon, D.A., Cline, M.J., Zighelboim, J. and the UCLA Acute Leukemia Study Group: Intensive chemotherapy for acute myelogenous leukemia. Ann. Intern. Med. 94:753-757, 1981.

4. Peterson, B.A. and Bloomfield, C.D.: Long-term disease-free survival in acute nonlymphocytic leukemia. Blood 57:1144-1147, 1981.

5. Keating, M., Smith, T., Gehan, E., McCredie, K., Bodey, G.P., Spitzer, G., Hersh, E., Gutterman, J.U. and Freireich, E.J: Factors related to length of complete remission in adult acute leukemia. Cancer 45:2017-2019, 1980.

6. Dosik, G., Barlogie, B., Smith, T., Gehan, E., Keating, M. and Freireich, E.J: Pre-treatment flow cytometry of DNA content in adult acute leukemia. Blood 55:474-482, 1980.

7. Blumenreich, M.S., Strife, A. and Clarkson, B.: Techniques to quantify cytoreduction in bone marrow induced by cytotoxic chemotherapy. J.C.O., in press, 1983.

8. Hiddemann, W., Buchner, T., Andreeff, M., Wormann, B., Melamed, M.R. and Clarkson, B.: Cell kinetics in acute leukemia: A critical re-evaluation based on new data. Cancer 50:250-258, 1982.

9. Barlogie, B., Drewinko, B., Schumann, J., Godhe, W., Dosik, G., Johnston, D. and Freireich, E: Cellular DNA content as a marker of neoplasia in man. Am. J. Med. 69:195-203, 1980.

10. Barlogie, B., Hittelmann, W., Spitzer, G., Hart, J., Trujillo, J., Smallwood, L. and Drewinko, B.: Correlation of DNA distribution abnormalities with cytogenetic findings in human adult leukemia and lymphoma. Cancer Res. 37:4400-4407, 1977.

11. Barlogie, B., Maddox, A., Johnston, D., Raber, M., Drewinko, B., Keating, M. and Freireich, E.: Quantitative cytology in leukemia research. Blood Cells 9:35-55, 1983.

12. Davis, F., Gyorkey, F., Busch, R.K., Busch, H.: Nucleolar antigen found in several human tumors but not in the nontumor tissues studied. Proc. Natl. Acad. Sci. U.S.A. 76:892-896, 1979.

13. Davis, F., Hittelman, W.N., McCredie, K.B. and Rao, P.N.: Estimation of tumor burden in leukemic patients using antibodies to neoplastic nucleoli. Proc. AACR Cancer Res. 21:229, 1980.

14. Frankfurt, O.: Flow cytometric analysis of double-stranded RNA content distributions. J. Histochem. Cytochem. 28:663-669, 1980.

15. Broxmeyer, H.E., Grossbard, E., Jacobson, N. and Moore, M.A.S.: Persistence of inhibitory activity against normal bone marrow cells during remission of acute leukemia. N.E.J.M. 30:346-351, 1979.

16. Johnson, R. and Rao, P.N.: Mammalian cell fusion: Induction of premature chromosome condensation in interphase nuclei. Nature 226: 717-722, 1970.

17. Hittelman, W.N., Broussard, L.C. and McCredie, K.: Premature chromosome condensation studies in human leukemia. I. Pretreatment Characteristics. Blood 54:1001-1014, 1979.

18. Hittelman, W.N., Broussard, L.C., Dosik, G. and McCredie, K.: Predicting relapse of human leukemia by means of premature chromosome condensation. N.E.J.M. 303:479-484, 1980.

19. Traganos, F., Darzynkiewicz, Z., Sharpless, T., Melamed, M.R.: Simultaneous staining of ribonucleic and deoxyribonucleic acid on unfixed cells using acridine orange in a flow cytofluorometric system. J. Histochem. Cytochem. 25:46-56, 1977.

20. Barlogie, B., Spitzer, G., Hart, J., Johnston, D., Buchner, T., Schumann, J. and Drewinko, B.: DNA-histogram analysis of human hemopoietic cells. Blood 48:245-258, 1976.

21. Andreeff, M., Darzynkiewicz, Z., Sharpless, T., Clarkson, B., Melamed, M.R.: Discrimination of human leukemia subtypes by flow cytometric analysis of cellular DNA and RNA. Blood 55:282-293, 1980.

22. Barlogie, B., Latreille, J., Swartzendruber, D., Smallwood, L., Maddox, A., Raber, M., Drewinko, B. and Alexanian, R.: Quantitative cytology in myeloma research. In: Clinics in Haematology. William R. Schmidt. (ed), W.B. Saunders Co., Ltd., 1982, pp. 19-45.

23. Kantarjian, H., Barlogie, B. and Stroehlein, J.: Preferential expression of double-stranded (DS)-RNA in tumor vs normal cells. ASCO, Abstract, 1983.

24. Hittelman, W.M.: Applications in basic and clinical research. In: Premature Chromosome Condensation. Johnson, R., Rao, P.N., Sperling, K. (ed), Academic Press, New York, pp. 309-358, 1982.

25. Barlogie, B., Raber, M., Schumann, J., Freireich, E., Drewinko, B., Swartzendruber, D., Gohde, W. and Andreeff, M.: Perspectives in Cancer Research: Flow cytometry in clinical cancer research. Cancer Res. 43:3982-3997, 1983.

26. Torelli, U., Torelli, G., Cadossi, R., Farrari, S., Farrari, S., Narni, F. and Montagnani, G.: Accumulation of giant heterogenous RNA molecules in acute myeloid leukemia blasts. Cancer Res. 36:4631-4638, 1976.

27. Gratzner, H.G.: Monoclonal antibody to 5-bromo- and 5-iododeoxyuridine: A new reagent for detection of DNA replication. Science 218:474-475, 1982.

AUTOMATED DETECTION OF RARE HEMOPOIETIC CELL TYPES BY FLOW CYTOMETRY AND
IMAGE ANALYSIS

J.W.M. Visser

INTRODUCTION

The first attempts at automated counting and analysis of mammalian
cells and also the first large scale applications of automated detection
devices concerned the blood cells (1, 5, 10, 23, 24, 30, 37, 38, 47,
52). The development of automated devices is directed towards the analysis of mature blood cells. The dynamics of the hemopoietic system, the
release and loss of mature cells and the replacement by precursor cells
is generally not monitored.

Automated analysis of the precursor cell types is difficult for
several reasons. Firstly, the production of mature blood cells occurs by
multiple divisions of the precursor cells (Fig. 1) and, consequently,
the incidence of the earliest precursor cell types is the lowest. These
early cells, however, play the dominant roles in the regulation of hemopoiesis; errors in the first divisions are amplified one thousandfold
due to the multiplication process. The earliest cells in hemopoiesis are
the pluripotent hemopoietic stem cells (PHSC). These cells are capable
of both self-renewal and differentiation into precursor cells which are
committed to the erythroid, myeloid, lymphoid or megakaryocytic series.
Most of the PHSC and committed progenitor cells normally reside in the
bone marrow. The incidence of PHSC in bone marrow can be estimated to be
between 0.1 and 1% of the nucleated cells. Therefore, accurate counting
of the PHSC in a bone marrow cell suspension requires the analysis of at
least between 10^4 and 10^5 bone marrow cells. A second difficulty in
automated stem cell counting is that no specific cytochemical marker is
known for this cell type at present. The same holds true for most of the
other hemopoietic precursor cells. The third difficulty in differentiated analysis of the early cells of the hemopoietic system is the con-

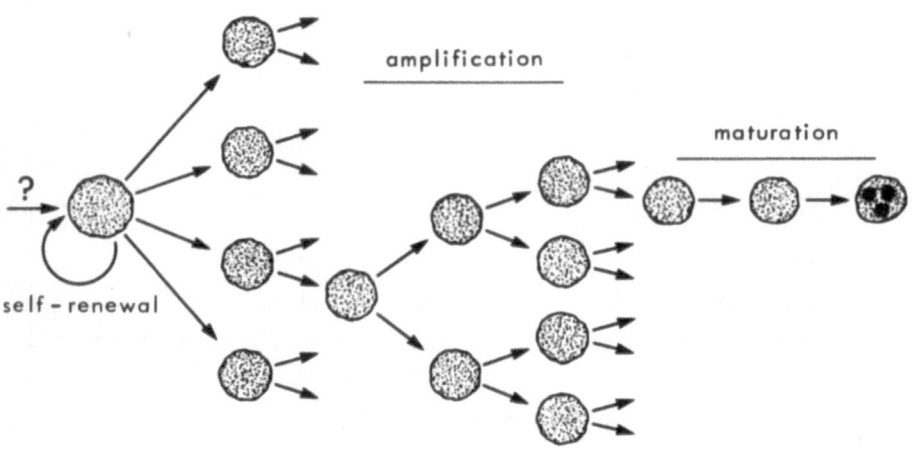

FIGURE 1: Schematic outline of self-renewal, differentiation and maturation in hematopoiesis.

tamination of bone marrow punctures with peripheral blood (29). Fewer blood cells are found in bone marrow biopsies; however, these are more difficult to suspend as single cells (48).

The problems encountered in the development of the automated detection of rare hemopoietic cells strongly resemble those of screening cervical specimens for abnormal cell types. Solutions for the problems in that field come from three research areas: 1) instrumentation; 2) specimen preparation and labeling; 3) data analysis. This paper discusses these topics with respect to the detection of rare hemopoietic cells. The analysis of abnormal hemopoietic cells such as leukemias and cells belonging to the immune system will be described by other contributors to this volume.

GENERAL CONSIDERATIONS

Fig. 2 shows an idealized frequency distribution of the fluorescence intensities of bone marrow cells which are labelled with a fluorescent marker which is specific for one of the subpopulations. The analysis is performed by taking a random sample. The marker is highly

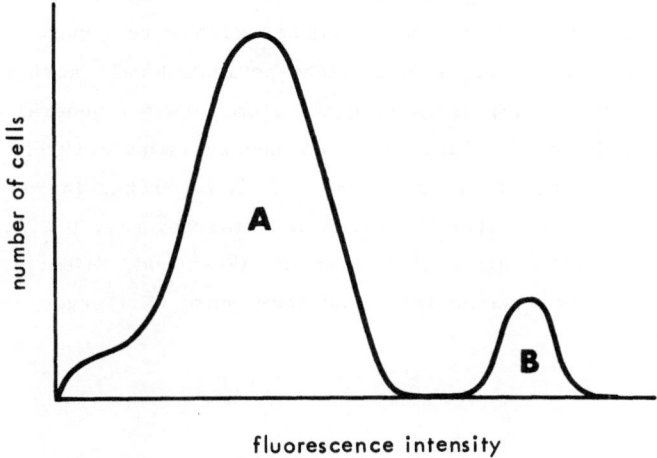

FIGURE 2: Idealized fluorescence histogram of a cell suspension containing a positively labeled subpopulation.

specific and the instrument contributes negligible noise to the measurement. Briefly, in this idealized situation for enumerating the subpopulation, we only have to count the cells of peak B in relation to all cells analyzed. In practice, however, histograms tend to look different from this example. The specificity of the marker is generally less pronounced and, as a consequence, either peak B partially overlaps with peak A or the valley between the peaks is filled with other cells. The labeling procedure itself may introduce errors such as the unwanted labeling of B lymphocytes by fluoresceinated anti-immunoglobulin in the indirect immunofluorescence assay. If subpopulation B is of low incidence, then other problems and limits have to be dealt with. Accurate determination of rare events requires analysis of large samples. In practice, sample sizes are limited and so is the speed of the analyzing equipment. Table 1 gives an indication of the speed of commercially available devices which can be used for differentiation of hemopoietic cells. The number of samples processed per hour in such instruments is mainly determined by sample loading and preparation and the rinsing of the flow instrument between samples. The flow cytometers are considerably faster than the image analysis instruments in actual cell analysis rates and are for that reason more appropriate for the analysis of large samples. Therefore, the method of choice for automated detection of rare

cells at present is flow cytometry. All of the examples shown in this
paper were obtained using a flow cytometer with more general use than
analyzing blood cells, viz., a FACS light-activated cell sorter (Becton
Dickinson, Sunnyvale, Ca., U.S.A.). Flow cytometers for general applica-
tion are commercially available through several manufacturers: Becton
Dickinson FACS systems (Sunnyvale, Ca., U.S.A.), Bruker Spectrospin SA
(Wissembourg, France), Coulter Electronics (Hialeah, Fl., U.S.A.), Leitz
(Wetzlar, FRG), Ortho Diagnostic Systems (Westwood, Mass., U.S.A.),
Partec AG (Bottmingen, Switzerland) and Show Denko KK (Tokyo, Japan).

Table 1: Speed of commercially available devices for automated blood
cell analysis.

	number of samples per hour	number of cells analyzed per sample
Image analysis		
Hematrak 480 (Geometric Data)	60	100
Diff. 3 (Coulter)	35	100-500
ADC-500 (Abbott)	40	500
Flow cytometry		
Hemalog-D (Technicon)	90	10^4
ELT-8 (Ortho)	40	10^4

The larger the sample size the longer the duration of the measurements and the greater the contribution of artifacts from both the
machine and the sample. Some of the artifacts can be excluded from
further electronic processing and data storage by using more than one
parameter for classification of the cells. Figs. 3, 4 and 5 may serve to
illustrate this. Figures 4 and 5 show fluorescence histograms obtained
with mouse bone marrow cells which contained low (Fig. 4B) and very low
(Fig. 5B) concentrations of fluorescent cells. Fig. 3 shows a dot plot

of forward (FLS) versus perpendicular light scatter (PLS) intensities of
these bone marrow cells as well as a square box electronic selection
window around the "blast" cell compartment (refs. 18, 19, 54, 56). Without such electronic gating, the fluorescence histogram of untreated bone
marrow cells contains a tail at higher intensities (Fig. 4A, dotted
line) which is absent if only the fluorescence of the blast cells is
recorded (Fig. 4A, solid line). The presence of fluorescent subpopulations as shown in Fig. 4B (dotted line) can be clearly resolved and
enumerated as compared with untreated cells (Fig. 4B, solid line) if
electronic gating using FLS and PLS windows is employed. This would be
difficult, however, if the tail as shown in Fig. 4A would not have been
gated out of the date storage (cfr. Table 3). This demonstrates that the
stimultaneous measurement of several independent parameters is useful
and often required to gate out artifacts.

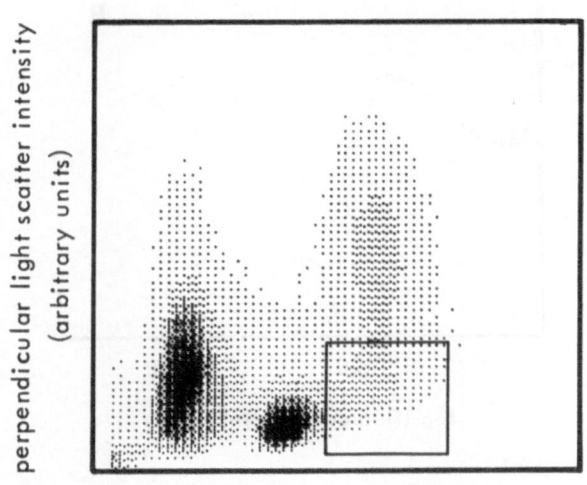

forward light scatter intensity
(arbitrary units)

FIGURE 3: Dot display of forward (FLS) versus perpendicular light
scatter (PLS) intensities of mouse bone marrow cells measured by a FACS
II. The square box indicates an electronic selection window for blast
cells (18, 19, 54, 56).

The limits of rare event detection by flow cytometry combining several parameters are illustrated by Fig. 5 and Table 3. With untreated cells from within the FLS-PLS blast window depicted in Fig. 3, the number of events with fluorescence signals above 150 (Fig. 5A, dots) is between 3.5 and 15 (Table 3) after analyzing 4×10^5 cells. This indicates that the background and artifact noise is between 1 and 4 per 10^5

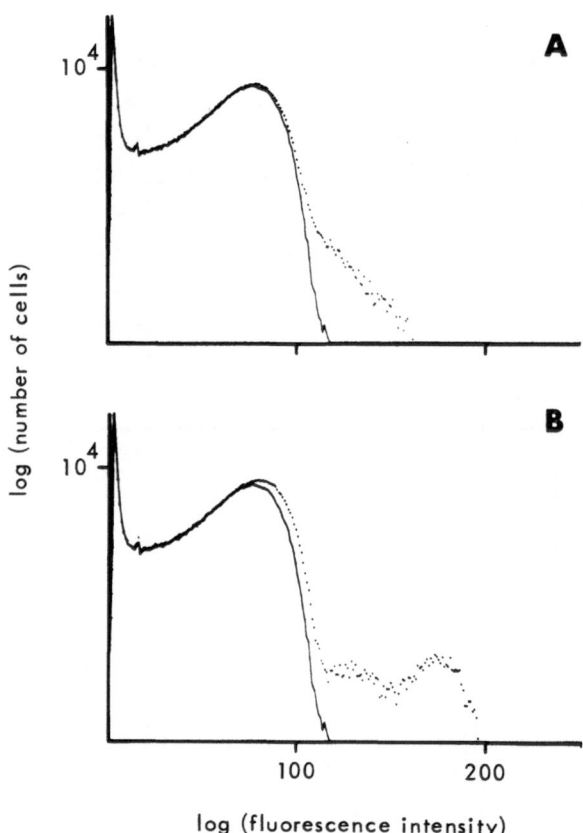

FIGURE 4: Frequency distributions of the fluorescence intensities of mouse bone marrow cells as measured by a FACS II. Both axes are plotted logarithmically. The number of cells per histogram equals 4×10^5.
A, dotted line: untreated cells without electronic window;
A and B, solid lines: untreated blast cells selected by the FLS-PLS window shown in Fig. 3; B, dotted line: sample containing fluorescent cells with FLS-PLS of blast cells.

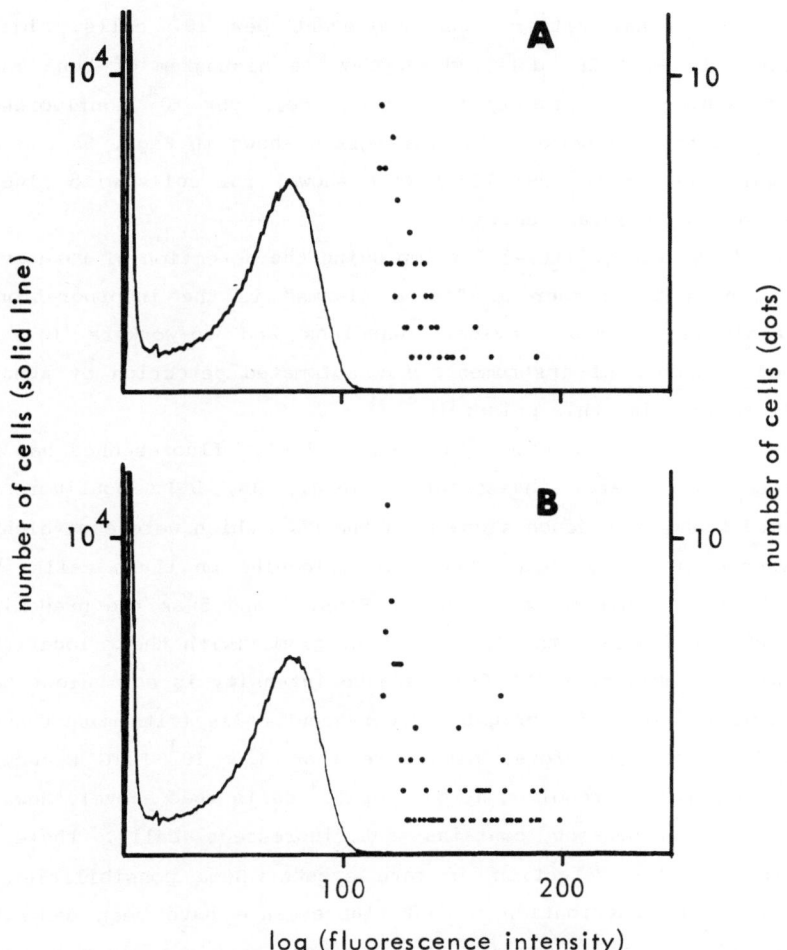

'IGURE 5: Frequency distributions of the fluorescence intensities of
louse bone marrow blast cells (FLS-PLS window of Fig. 3). The histograms
lave a different scaling along the ordinates on the left and the right
land sides. A: untreated cells. B: treated cells containing about one
'rightly fluorescent cell per 10^4 negative cells. 4 x 10^5 cells were
'ecorded per histogram.

ells. As can be seen in Table 2, this means that at least about 30
ositive events (per 4 x 10^5 cells) have to be counted in a labeled sus-
ension to find a significant difference. Therefore, the lower limit

for detection by flow cytometry of rare events which can be brightly labeled is somewhat better than one event per 10^4 cells. This is illustrated in Fig. 5B (dots) which shows a histogram of bone marrow cells containing one brightly fluorescent cell per 10^4 nonfluorescent ones. The difference between the histograms shown in Figs. 5A and B is also significant at the 99% level (not shown) for cells with fluorescence above 150 arbitrary units.

One of the possibilities for improving the detection of rare events by diminishing the number of "false alarms" is the incorporation of image analysis in flow devices. Wheeless and co-workers (33, 60) developed a number of instruments for automated detection of abnormal cervical cells using this principle.

The sensitivity of flow cytometers for FITC fluorescence has been quantitated by several investigators (e.g., 36, 53). Nonfluorescent cells were found to produce signals in the FACS which were equivalent to the presence of up to about 2000 FITC molecules on these cells. They contribute to the histograms shown in Figs. 4 and 5 as the predominant peak at 80 arbitrary units. In those histograms (with their logarithmic abscissa), a doubling of the fluorescence intensity is equivalent to an increase of 17 units. The brightly fluorescent cells (with more than 150 arbitrary units), therefore, bind more than 3×10^4 FITC molecules. These cells could be resolved at one per 10^4 cells (see above). However, if the cell suspension contains autofluorescent cells, these may interfere with the detection of rare events. Some possibilities for diminishing the contribution of autofluorescence have been described. Benson et al. (7) and Auben (2) have observed that autofluorescence is more intense in the green than in the red spectral area. This suggests that red fluorescent labels instead of FITC should be used if the measurements are distorted by autofluorescent cells. Hirschfield (28) has pointed out that preirradiation of the cells may bleach autofluorescence more than the fluorescence emission of dyes. Pinkel et al. (43) demonstrated this effect experimentally. On the other hand, Watt et al. (58) made use of autofluorescence to isolate neutrophils from mouse bone marrow.

INSTRUMENTATION

Flow cytometry

In flow cytometers, a random selection out of a suspension of single cells is analyzed. During the measurements, the cells are confined in a fluid jet which passes a focused light beam (Fig. 6). The concentration of cells in the suspension is chosen such that they pass the light beam ideally one by one. Photosensitive detectors which measure the light flashes from each passing cell are placed around the illuminated spot. The velocity of the jet is generally about 10 $m.s^{-1}$ and the light spot generally measures about 50 µm; therefore, the duration of each light flash is close to 5 µs. The electronics is set to process signals of this time duration so that much noise and artifacts are gated out. The processed signals are generally digitized and stored in a memory, ready for computer analysis. The storage of data in memory takes typically about 20 µs per cell. Most flow cytometers detect the presence of other cells during this 20 µs but do not analyse them. Cells which are coincident within the 5 µs measuring time are not processed separately; they produce signals which can mostly be recognized as being due to

Table 2: 95 and 99% confidence limits for "rare events" in large samples if between 10^4 and 10^7 cells are analyzed

Number of rare events counted	95% limits		99% limit	
0	0	- 3.7	0	- 5.3
10	4.8-	18	3.7-	21
20	12	- 31	10	- 35
30	20	- 43	18	- 47
40	29	- 54	26	- 59
50	37	- 66	34	- 71
60	46	- 77	42	- 83
70	55	- 88	50	- 94
80	63	-100	59	-110
90	72	-110	67	-120
100	81	-120	76	-130
200	180	-230	170	-240
300	270	-330	260	-340
400	370	-430	360	-440
500	470	-530	460	-540

Limits were iteratively approximated by computer (16, 44). For larger numbers of counted rare events, good approximations of the confidence limits are obtained by using: $x \pm c\sqrt{x(1-x/n)}$, where x is the number of counted rare events, n the total number of cells analyzed and c equals 1.96 for the 95% and 2.58 for the 99% confidence limits.

Table 3: Numbers of rare events according to the measurements shown in Figs. 4 and 5; 4 x 10^5 cells were analyzed per histogram. Confidence limits are calculated as given in Table 2.

	histogram area			
	130-200 arbitrary units		150-200 arbitrary units	
	number of events counted	95% conficence limits	number of events counted	95% confidence limits
all cells unlabelled (Fig. 4A, dotted line)	1063	999-1127	339	310-370
all cells labelled (not shown)	1134	1061-1192	389	359-425
blast cells* unlabelled (Fig. 5A).	39	28- 53	7	3.5- 15
blast cells* labelled (Fig. 5B)	73	58- 91	52	36- 73

*The blast cells were electronically selected for further analysis by their light scatter characteristics (Fig. 3).

aggregates. The rate of coincidences depends on the sample concentration. The probability follows Poisson statistics (57). Typically, the signals of about 10% of the cells are not analyzed if the sample rate is 3000 cells.s^{-1} and 30% is not processed at a rate of 10^4 cells.s^{-1}. Higher sample rates than 10^4 cells.s^{-1} are seldom used. Consequently, about 24 min are required to collect the data of 10^7 cells, which due to coincidences, implies running 1.4 x 10^7 cells through the device.

Most flow cytometers can be used to separate cells which are optically different. The fluid jet containing the cells breaks up into droplets after the passage of the light beam. These droplets can be electrically charged positively or negatively and so deflected by an electric field. The charging depends on the signals which are measured from the cell before the droplets break off. Optically different cells can thus be deflected within the droplets and collected in separate tubes, in culture wells, on microscope slides or otherwise. The rates of

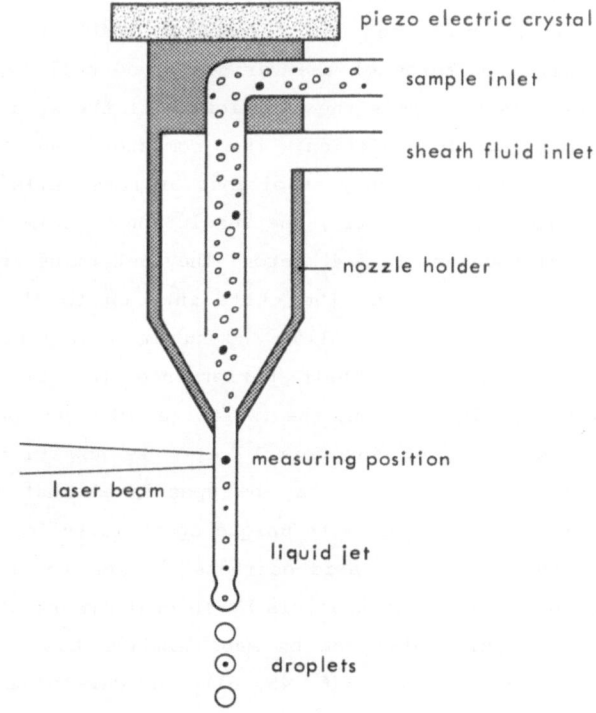

FIGURE 6:
Schematic representation
of nozzle and fluid jet
of a flow cytometer.

sorting are lower than the analysis rates. The frequency of droplet
formation is about $4 \times 10^4 .s^{-1}$. Typically, three droplets are deflected
per wanted cell. If only wanted cells must be deflected, the sorting has
to be inhibited if unwanted passengers are likely to be present within
one of these three droplets, i.e., within 75 μs. Consequently, a coin-
cidence rate of 10% is already reached at an analysis + sorting rate of
10^3 cells.s^{-1} (57).

Image analysis

Conventional microscope slides of blood and other samples can be
processed by automated computer-video-microscope combinations. The slide
is positioned in a light microscope with automated stage positioner and
self focusing (zoom) objective. In principle, an image of each field is
made on a video tube and the image is digitized and processed by a computer. The number of picture elements ("pixels") per field is finite and
the resolution depends on pixel density, magnification and staining. The

latter is quantitated by using the grey level per pixel. Each digitized image is processed by a computer which is programmed to recognize specific patterns of the various blood cell types. Generally, the computer also controls the positioning of the slide and the focusing of the objective. In addition, the computer can interactively facilitate reexamination of only suspicious or rare cells by the operator and the pathologist. Typically, the resolution of commercially available differential counters is 0.4 micron. They determine up to about 100 parameters per cell, subdivide the cells into up to 15 classes, classify up to about 10^3 cells per slide and automatically process between 20 and 60 slides per hour. Their performance in classifying rare cell types strongly depends on the software of the pattern recognition. The processing speed for normal cells is now in the order of 100 to 500 cells per minute. It may be speculated that the introduction of new staining techniques with unique specificity for certain rare cell types, together with the rapid decrease in computer process times, will speed up automated image analysis by several orders of magnitude. Technically, the analysis rates can be made similar to that of flow cytometers by using laser scanners (6, 45, 61). The development of new instruments and especially of the software designed to detect abnormal cell types is time comsuming if it has to be determined which of the possible hundred parameters are the most significant to discriminate the rare cell from the other cells and artifacts. However, using specific monoclonal antibodies and only one parameter (e.g., fluorescent or non-fluorescent), more generally applicable video microscope analyzers would rapidly become available. These would have a speed which is comparable to present day flow cytometers.

Automated image analyzers often need a learning set, slides containing a sufficient number of recognizable cells of the type which has to be detected automatically, so that the typical values of each measured parameter for the cell type can be determined. Therefore, if rare cells have to detected by the image analyzer, firstly, the rare cells have to be enriched at least once to such a degree that the preparation can serve as learning set. In general, this will require sorting by a flow cytometer.

In several aspects, automated image analyzers and flow cytometers can be regarded as complementary tools for the detection of rare cells

(17). Flow cytometers are capable of rapidly analyzing relatively large numbers of cells for a limited number of parameters. They can generally enrich for the rare cells and deposit them on slides so that they can be analyzed in more detail (i.e., more parameters) by the image analyzer.

SAMPLE PREPARATION AND STAINING

Blood and bone marrow cell suspensions contain many erythrocytes which are often not of importance for the enumeration of the rare cell types but which may use up significant processing time or data storage space in the automated analyzer. The erythrocytes can be removed prior to the analysis by effecting lysis or using relatively rapid procedures (62). Sometimes, the enumeration of rare events in the bone marrow has to be corrected for the blood contamination. Several procedures have been proposed for this. Holdrinet et al. (29) developed suitable methods using flow cytometry. In addition, de Witte et al. (62) and Latreille et al. (35) developed combinations of density gradient centrifugation, velocity sedimentation, elutriation and flow cytometry to analyze subpopulations of blast cells in the bone marrow in more detail.

Similar problems are caused by the presence of dead or dying cells in the suspensions. Dead cells often cause aggregation of cells in suspension which may give rise to both artifacts and clogging in flow cytometers. In addition, dead cells are often autofluorescent and they are easily labeled nonspecifically, thus contributing to sample noise. Dead cells can be recognized by dye exclusion tests or they can be removed by incubation of the cell suspension in low ionic medium. Aggregates due to dead cells can be disrupted by use of DNase. The dye exclusion determination can be performed simultaneously with other measurements: addition of a drop of propidium iodide solution (about 5 μg.ml^{-1}) to the cell suspension shortly before measurement will stain all dead cells brightly red fluorescent. One of the detectors may be used to probe for a red signal, the presence of which determines inhibition of further electronic processing of the cell.

A wide variety of staining and labeling procedures has been employed for analyzing rare hemopoietic cells. Some examples will be described below. In addition, an increasing number of lectins and especially antibodies is being tested for specifically labeling and analyzing early hemopoietic cells (8, 18, 19, 21, 22, 25, 40, 41, 51,

55, 57, 59). A staining procedure for analysis and isolation of poly-
ploid megakaryocytes has been described (39), combinations of stains for
complete blood differential counts have been developed (1, 32, 34, 46)
and a labeling procedure for analysis of fetal cells in maternal blood
(31) by flow cytometry has been described. New stains are continuously
being developed in this field for both image analysis and flow cytometry. The publications J. Histochem. Cytochem., Cytometry, and Analyt.
Quant. Cytol. cover the majority of the developments in staining and
apparatus; new antibodies are reported in a variety of immunology and
haematology journals. Some examples of new stains and antibodies will be
given below.

DATA ANALYSIS

The field of automated image analysis in completely dependent on
computerized data analysis. The development of pattern recognition
software for new cell types often requires the processing of up to 100
data per cell and up to 10^3 cells per specimen. Statistical analysis is
used to find the most significant parameters to distinguish the new cell
from all others and from artifacts. In addition, the optimal "false
positive" to "false negative" ratio has to be determined for the
specimen (13, 14). Extensive literature on these subjects is available
with respect to hematological specimens (e.g., 3, 4, 9, 11, 20).

Flow cytometers require less sophisticated data analysis. In principle, they can be operated without computers with only a pulse height
analyzer. On the other hand, comparison of histograms may require statistical analysis which is facilitated by using a computer. Statistics
similar to those used in the field of image analysis can be applied to
flow cytometry data (see, e.g., 63).

EXAMPLES

Quantitation of reticulocytes by flow cytometry

The incidence of reticulocytes in the peripheral blood can be taken
as a measure for the proliferative status of the hemopoietic system (10,
15, 27). Reticulocytes can be regarded as "rare cells"; their incidence
is normally below 1%. Tanke and co-workers (49, 50) have developed a
rapid procedure for quantitating human reticulocytes by flow cytometry.
In addition, the measurements provide qualitative information on the
maturation stage.

Peripheral blood (50 μl) is fixed in 25% formaldehyde and stained in suspension with 0.01% pyromin Y, a red fluorescent dye which is RNA specific. Subsequently, the sample is washed and the forward light scatter (FLS) and red fluorescence intensities of each cell are analyzed by a flow cytometer. The FLS measurement serves to distinguish thrombocytes from red cells and reticulocytes; the measurement of red fluorescence intensity discriminates between red cells, reticulocytes and leukocytes. The latter cells contain significantly more RNA than do reticulocytes and can be discriminated from those by their relatively strong red fluorescence intensity. The discrimination between red blood cells and reticulocytes on the basis of pyromin Y-RNA red fluorescence requires analysis of the histograms by computer. Fig. 7 shows fluorescence histograms of pyromin Y stained erythrocytes and reticulocytes of a patient with aplastic anemia before and after bone marrow transplantation. Eight days prior to transplantation, virtually no cells were observed with higher fluorescence intensities than erythrocytes. The take of the graft could be determined as early as between day 9 and 12 by the appearance

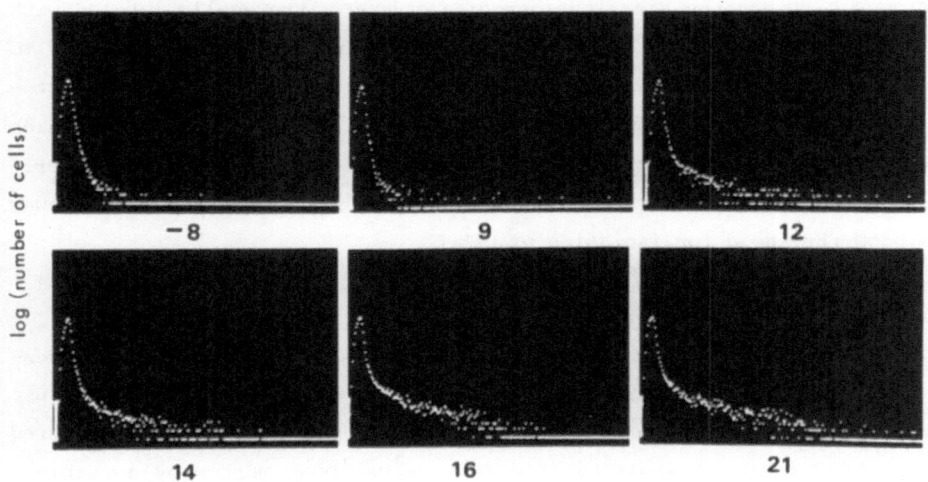

fluorescence intensity (arbitrary units)

FIGURE 7: Frequency distributions of pyromin Y stained red blood cells of a patient with aplastic anemia. Numbers indicate days before and after bone marrow transplantation (49, 50). Courtesy of H.J. Tanke, Leiden.

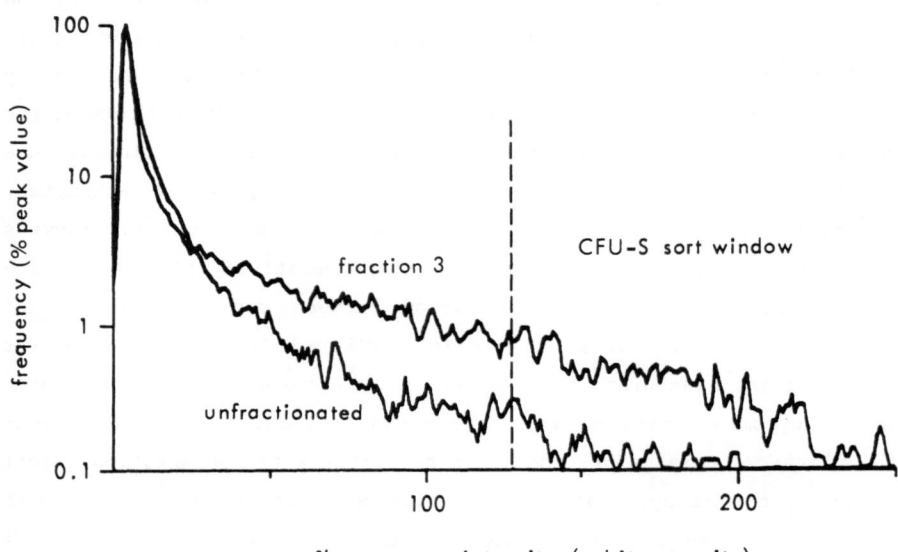

FIGURE 8: Frequency distributions of rat bone marrow cells labeled with a monoclonal anti-Thy-1.1 antibody and with rabbit-anti-mouse IgG-FITC (from ref. 12). The rats were pretreated with hydrocortisone. The histograms were recorded from unfractionated cells and from suspensions which were preenriched for Thy-1 positive cells by equilibrium density centrifugation (fraction 3). The dashed vertical line represents the lower window threshold for isolation of CFU-S.

Isolation of mouse pluripotent hemopoietic stem cells

The PHSC of the mouse cannot be isolated by methods such as described by Goldschneider et al. (21) and Castagnola et al. (12) because the mouse stem cells are Thy-1 negative (51). We recently discovered that PHSC could be isolated from adult mouse bone marrow by a combination of separation techniques. This combination was selected on the basis of earlier findings that mouse CFU-S are of relatively low density (18), medium forward light scatter (18, 54), low perpendicular light scatter (18, 54), wheat-germ-agglutinin positive (55) and H-2K positive (51). Therefore, bone marrow cells were firstly separated by equilibrium

of low numbers of cells with more fluorescence than the erythrocytes. The number of such cells, the reticulocytes, steadily increased between days 12 and 21. Although the computer analysis of these histograms requires interpretation of the transition from reticulocytes to erythrocytes, the histograms clearly demonstrate the potential of this method. Using arbitrary thresholds for discrimination between erythrocytes and reticulocytes, Tanke et al. found a significant increase in reticulocyte percentage from 0.23% to 0.58% at 5 hours after the donation of blood (50). These results show that flow cytometry of pyronin Y stained blood provides the possibility to quantitate reticulocytes and, particularly, changes in reticulocyte frequency at incidences of 1% and somewhat lower.

Analysis and purification of rat CFU-S

Goldschneider et al. (21) have described a procedure for isolating the pluripotent hemopoietic stem cells (PHSC) from rat bone marrow making use of Thy-1 labeling. Rats were given cortisone acetate for 3 days before their bone marrow was collected. The cortisone treatment reduced the percentage of Thy-1 positive cells from about 40 to about 10% of total nucleated cells (12, 21). Cells with different Thy-1 densities were sorted by a FACS after labeling with fluoresceinated anti-Thy-1 $F(ab)_2$ fragments. Simultaneous additional FLS sorting windows were used to sort CFU-S (colony forming units spleen). The 10% cells with the highest fluorescence intensity were 320-fold enriched for CFU-S in comparison with bone marrow of untreated rats. It was estimated that 80% of these cells were PHSC. The fluorescence histogram (Fig. 8) does not show a distinct subpopulation with high fluorescence intensity. Therefore, the difference in Thy-1 antigen content of PHSC and other cells is likely to be a gradual one and this label cannot easily be exploited to rapidly analyse and quantitate PHSC. On the other hand, Castagnola et al. (12) using the same method in combination with equilibrium density centrifugation confirmed the enrichment of CFU-S and additionally demonstrated that also the cell type providing radioprotection was similarly enriched for. Therefore, sorting of Thy-1 labeled bone marrow by a flow cytometer in combination with the CFU-S assay can be used to isolate and directly examine the PHSC of the rat.

density centrifugation. During this procedure, they were labeled with wheat germ lectin-FITC (WGA-FITC). The low density fraction was subsequently analyzed by the FACS and cells with medium forward light scatter (FLS), low perpendicular light scatter (PLS) and high WGA-FITC fluorescence were sorted. These sorted cells were between 60 and 100-fold enriched for CFU-S (56) and the labeling and sorting procedure did not affect the radioprotective capacity nor the seeding efficiency of the PHSC. Subsequently, the WGA-FITC was removed from the cells by incubation with N-acetyl-D-glycosamine (56). The cells were then labelled with a biotinylated monoclonal anti-H-2K antibody and with avidin-FITC. Fig. 9 shows a fluorescence histogram of the cells after this labeling step as determined by the FACS. Two subpopulations can be distinguished. After sorting, all CFU-S were found in the subpopulation with the high fluorescence intensity, i.e., high H-2K density. The average CFU-S enrichment in the sorted cells was 135-fold. The average (n = 15) incidence of spleen colony forming units was 6.5%. In the three

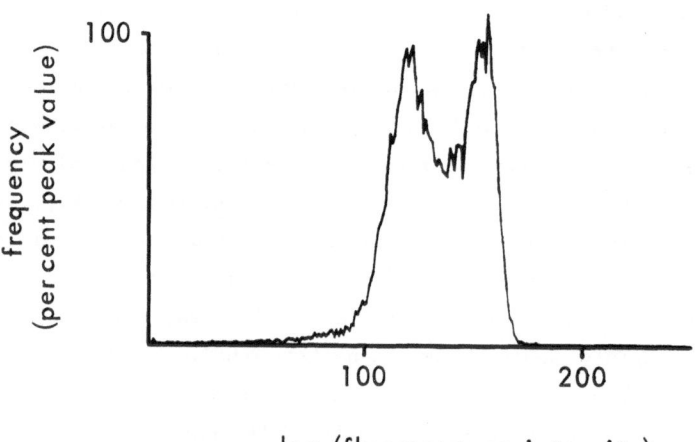

log (fluorescence intensity)

FIGURE 9: Frequency distribution of the fluorescence intensities of sorted mouse bone marrow cells after labeling with anti-H-2K-biotin and avidin-FITC. At this stage of the isolation procedure, the suspension is about 60-fold enriched for CFU-S.

experiments with the highest enrichment (180-220 fold), the incidence of CFU-S was 10 ± 1%. If it is assumed that the spleen seeding efficiency is 10%, this indicates that the cells in these three experiments are 100% pure PHSC. Radioprotection experiments indicated that the cell type preventing mortality by transplantation after lethal gamma irradiation was also enriched for by 130 to 220-fold. Therefore, this combination of flow cytometer techniques can be used to isolate and analyze the mouse PHSC. It may be performed in the future without sorting by analyzing bone marrow cells in a two-laser flow cytometer after labeling them with WGA and anti-HK-2 which are conjugated with different fluorochromes, e.g., FITC and phycoerythrin (42). On the other hand, the procedure now selects only 30 to 50% of all PHSC. Therefore, further study is required to determine unique markers for all of the PHSC. Nicola et al. (40, 41) have described several antigenic properties of fetal liver PHSC and committed progenitor cells. They achieved high enrichment factors employing pokeweed mitogen as a marker. Watt and co-workers (59) obtained a high enrichment for mouse progenitor cells employing combinations of monoclonal antibodies. To our knowledge, these monoclonals have not yet been tested for their specificity for CFU-S. However, such lines of experimentation are needed to provide unique PHSC markers. The apparatus is already sufficiently sensitive to quantitate rare cells such as PHSC with incidences of between 01 and 1% if those cells can be unequivocally labeled.

SUMMARY

Flow cytometry and image analysis can both be used for automated detection of rare hemopoietic cells. At present, flow cytometry can handle larger samples per unit of time and is therefore more suitable for rare event detection. It may be expected, however, that automated image analysis will soon become competitive in this respect.

The lower limit of detecting rare events is shown to be one abnormal cell per 10^4 to 10^5 normal cells if the abnormal one can be specifically labeled. About 3×10^4 FITC molecules bound per cell are sufficient to resolve specifically labeled cells above background signals from nonfluorescent cells.

38

ACKNOWLEDGEMENTS

This investigation is supported by a program grant from the Netherlands Foundation for Medical Research (FUNGO), which is subsidized by the Netherlands Organization for the Advancement of Pure Research (ZWO).

REFERENCES

1. Ansley, J., Ornstein, L. (1971). Enzyme histochemistry and differential white cell counts on the Technicon Hemalog D. Adv. Automated Anal. 1: 437.

2. Auben, J.E. (1979). Autofluorescence of viable cultured mammalian cells. J. Histochem. Cytochem. 27: 36.

3. Aus, H.M., Rüter, A., Ter Meulen, V., Gunzer, U., Nürnberger, T. (1977). Bone marrow segmentation by computer aided color cytophotometry. J. Histochem. Cytochem. 25: 662.

4. Bacus, J.W., Gose, E.E. (1972). Leucocyte pattern recognition. IEEE Trans. Sys. Man. Cyb, SMC-2: 513.

5. Bacus, J.W. (1973). The observer error in peripheral blood cell classificiation. Am. J. Clin. Pathol. 59: 223.

6. Bartels, P.H., Buchroeder, R.A., Hillman, D.W., Jonas, J.A., Kessler, D., Shoemaker, R.M., Shack, R.V., Towner, D., Vukobratovitsch, D. (1981). Ultrafast laser scanner microscope. Design and construction. Analyt. Quant. Cytol. 3: 55.

7. Benson, R.C., Meyer, R.A., Zaruba, M.E., McKhann, G.M. (1979). Cellular autofluorescence - Is it due to flavins? J. Histochem. Cytochem. 27: 44.

8. Beverley, P.C.L., Linch, D., Delia, D. (1980). Isolation of human haematopoietic progenitor cells using monoclonal antibodies. Nature 287: 332.

9. Bins, M., van Montfort, H., Timmers, T., Landeweerd, G.H., Gelsema, E.S., Helie, M.R. (1983). Classification of immature and mature cells of the neutrophil series using morphometrical parameters. Cytometry 3: 435.

10. Brecher, G. (1950). A time-saving device for the counting of reticulocytes. Am. J. Clin. Path. 20: 1079.

11. Brenner, J.F., Gelsema, E.S., Necheles, T.F., Neurath, P.W., Selles, W.D., Vastola, E. (1974). Automated classification of normal and abnormal leukocytes. J. Histochem. Cytochem. 22: 697.

12. Castagnola, C., Visser, J., Boersma, W., van Bekkum, D.W. (1981), Purification of rat pluripotent hemopoietic stem cells. Stem Cells 1: 250.

13. Castleman, K.R., White, B.S. (1980). Optimizing cervical cell classifiers. Analyt. Quant. Cytol. 2: 117.

14. Castleman, K.R., White, B.S. (1980). The tradeoff of cell classifier error rates. Cytometry 1: 156.

15. Cline, M.J., Berlin, N.I. (1963). The reticulocyte count as an indicator of the rate of erythropoiesis. Am. J. Clin. Pathol. 39: 121.

16. Documenta Geigy (1980). Scientific Tables. Diem, K., Lentner, C., eds., J.R. Geigy S.A., Basle, 7th Edition, p. 189, and Tables on pp. 107-108.

17. Driel-Kulker, A.M.J. van, Stöhr, M., Goerttler, K., Tanke, H.J. (1980). Analysis by image processing of cells sorted by two-parameter flow cytometry. In: Flow Cytometry IV, Laerum, O.D., Lindmo, T., Torud, E., eds., Universitetsforlaget, Bergen, pp. 453-457.

18. Engh, G.J. van den, Visser, J., Bol, S., Trask, B. (1980). Concentration of hemopoietic stem cells using a light-activated cell sorter. Blood Cells 6: 609.

19. Engh, G.J. van den, Bauman, J., Mulder, D., Visser, J. (1983). Measurement of antigen expression of hemopoietic stem cells and progenitor cells by fluorescence activated cell sorting. In: Haemopoietic Stem Cells. Sv.-Aa. Killmann, Cronkite, E.P., Muller-Bérat, C.N., eds., Munksgaard, Copenhagen, pp. 59-74.

20. Gelsema, E.S., Landeweerd, G.H. (1981). The use of ISPAHAN. Interactive system for statistical pattern recognition and analysis. Analyt. Quant. Cytol. 3: 195.

21. Goldschneider, I., Metcalf, D., Battlye, F., Mandel, T. (1980). Analysis of rat hemopoietic cells on the fluorescence activated cell sorter. I. Isolation of pluripotent hemopoietic stem cells and granulocyte- macrophage progenitor cells. J. exp. Med. 152: 419.

22. Greaves, M.F., Robinson, J., Sutherland, R., Newman, R.A. (1981). A library of monoclonal antibodies against human haemopoietic cells. Analysis of antigen expression during early haematopoietic differentiation and application to the differential diagnosis of leukemia. Br.J.Cancer 43: 564.

23. Green, J.E. (1979). A practical application of computer pattern recognition research. The Abbott ADC-500 differential classifier. J. Histochem. Cytochem. 27: 160.

24. Green, J.E. (1979). Rapid analysis of hematology image data. The ADC-500 preprocessor. J. Histochem. Cytochem. 27: 174.

25. Greenberg, P., Grossman, M., Charron, D., Levy, R. (1981). Characterization of antigenic determinants on human myeloid colony forming cells with monoclonal antibodies. Exp. Hematol. 9: 781.

26. Harms, H., Ganzer, U., Aus, H.M., Rüter, M., Hancke, M., Ter Meulen, V. (1979). Computer aided analysis of chromatin network and basophil color for differentiation of mononuclear peripheral blood cells. J. Histochem. Cytochem. 27: 204.

27. Heilmeyer, L., Westhäuser, R. (1932). Reifungsstadien an überlebende Retikulozyten in vitro und ihre Bedeutung für die Schätzung der täglichen Hämoglobin-produktion in vivo. Z. Klin. Med. 121: 361.

28. Hirschfield, T (1979). Fluorescence background discrimination by prebleaching. J. Histochem. Cytochem. 27: 96.

29. Holdrinet, R.S.G., van Egmond, J., Wessels, J.M.C., Haanen, C. (1980). A method for quantification of peripheral blood admixture in bone marrow aspirates; its relevance in cell kinetic research. In: Flow Cytometry IV. Laerum, O.D., Lindmö, T., Thorud, E., eds., Universitestsforlaget, Bergen, pp. 63-66.

30. Ingram, M., Preston, K., Jr. (1970). Automatic analysis of blood cells. Sci. Am. 223: 72.

31. Iverson, G.M., Bianchi, D.W., Cann, H.M., Herzenberg, L.A. (1981). Detection and isolation of fetal cells from maternal blood using the fluorescence activated cell sorter. Prenatal. Diagn. 1: 61.

32. Kaplow, L.S., Soman, S. (1980). Flow cytometric studies of human leukocyte enzymes: non-fluorescent methods and applications. In: Flow Cytometry IV. Laerum, O.D., Lindmo, T., Thornud, E., eds., Universitetsforlaget, Bergen, pp. 70-73.

33. Kay, D.B., Cambier, J.L., Wheeless, L.L. (1979). Imaging in flow. J. Histochem. Cytochem. 27: 329.

34. Lapen, D. (1982). A standardized differential stain for hematology. Cytometry 2: 309.

35. Latreille, J., Franco, J., Mellard, D., Meistrich, M., Fu, C.T., Barlogie, B. (1980). Centrifugal elutriation and flow cytometry of human bone marrow cells. Cell Tissue Kinet. 13: 684.

36. Loken, M.R., Herzenberg, L.A. (1975). Analysis of cell populations with a fluorescence-activated cell sorter. Ann. N.Y. Acad. Sci. 254: 163.

37. Mansberg, H.P., Saunders, A.M., Groner, W. (1974). The HEMALOG-D white cell differential system. J. Histochem. Cytochem. 22: 711.

38. Miller, M.N. (1976). Design and clinical results of HEMATRAK: An automated differential counter. IEEE Trans. Biom. Eng., BME-23: 400.

39. Nakeff, A., Valeriote, F., Gray, J.W., Grabske, R.J. (1979). Applications of flow cytometry and cell sorting to megakaryocytopoiesis. Blood 53: 732.

40. Nicola, N.A., Burgess, A.W., Staber, F.G., Johnson, G.R., Metcalf, D., Battye, F.L. (1980). Differential expression of lectin receptors during hemopoietic differentiation: enrichment for granulocyte- macrophage progenitor cells. J. Cell. Physiol. 103: 217.

41. Nicola, N.A., Metcalf, D., Von Melcher, H., Burgess, A.W. (1981). Isolation of murine fetal hemopoietic progenitor cells and selective fractionation of various erythroid precursors. Blood 58: 376.

42. Oi, V.T., Glazer, A.M., Stryer, L. (1982). Fluorescent phycobiliprotein conjugates for analysis of cells and molecules. J. Cell. Biol. 93: 981.

43. Pinkel, D., Dean, P., Lake, S., Peters, D., Mendelsohn, M., Gray, J., Van Dilla, M., Gledhill, B. (1979). Flow cytometry of mammalian sperm. Progress in DNA and morphology measurement. J. Histochem. Cytochem. 27: 353.

44. Rümke, Chr.L. (1976). De nauwkeurigheid van percentages; tabellen met betrouwbaarheidsintervallen. Ned. T. Geneesk. 120: 2052.

45. Shack, R., Baker, R., Buchroeder, R., Hillman, D., Shoemaker, R., Bartels, P.H. (1979). Ultrafast laser scanner microscope. J. Histochem. Cytochem. 27: 153.

46. Shapiro, H.M., Schildkraut, E.R., Curbello, R., Laird, C.W., Turner, R.B., Hirschfield, T. (1976). Combined blood cell counting and classification with fluorochrome stains and flow instrumentation. J. Histochem. Cytochem. 24: 396.

47. Smit, J.W., Gelsema, E.S., Huiges, W., Nawreth, R.F., Halie, M.R. (1979). A commercially available interactive pattern recognition system for the characterization of blood cells. Clin. Lab. Haematol. 1: 109.

48. Soman, S., Kaplow, L.S. (1980). Disaggregation of bone marrow spicules for studies by flow cytometry. In: Flow Cytometry IV, Laerum, O.D., Lindmo, T., Thorud, E., eds., Universitetsforlaget, Bergen, pp. 59-62.

49. Tanke, H.J., Nieuwenhuis, I.A.B., Koper, G.J.M., Slats, J.C.M., Ploem, J.S. (1980). Flow cytometry of human reticulocytes based on RNA fluorescence. Cytometry 1: 313.

50. Tanke, H.J., Rothbarth, P.H., Vossen, J.M.J.J., Koper, G., Ploem. J.S. (1983). Flow cytometry of reticulocytes applied to clinical hematology. Blood 61: 1091.

51. Trask, B., van den Engh, G. (1980). Antigen expression of CFU-S determined by light activated cell sorting. In: Baum, S.J., Ledney, G.D., van Bekkum, D.W., eds., Experimental Hematology Today, Karger, Basel, pp. 299.

52. Valet, G., Metzger, H., Kachel, V., Ruhenstroth-Bauer, G. (1972). Der Nachweis verschiedener Erythrozytenpopulationen bei der Ratte. Blut 24: 42.

53. Visser, J.W.M., Haaijman, J.J., Trask, B. (1978). Quantitative immunofluorescence in flow cytometry. In: Immunofluorescence and related staining techniques. Knapp, W., Holubar, K., Wick, G., eds., Elsevier/North Holland Biomedical Press, Amsterdam, pp. 147-160.

54. Visser, J.W.M., Van den Engh, G.J., Van Bekkum, D.W. (1980). Light scattering properties of murine hemopoietic cells. Blood Cells 6: 391.

55. Visser, J.W.M., Bol, S.J.L., Van den Engh, G. (1981). Characterization and enrichment of murine hemopoietic stem cells by fluorescence activated cell sorting. Exp. Hematol. 9: 644.

56. Visser, J.W.M., Bol, S.J.L. (1981). A two-step procedure for obtaining 80-fold enriched suspensions of murine pluripotent hemopoietic stem cells. Stem Cells 1: 240.

57. Visser, J.W.M., van den Engh, G.J. (1982). Immunofluorescence measurements by flow cytometry. In: Wick, G., Traill, K.N., Schauenstein, K., eds., Immunofluorescence Technology. Selected theoretical and clinical aspects. Elsevier Biomedical Press, Amsterdam, pp. 95-128.

58. Watt, S.M., Burgess, A.W., Metcalf, D., Battye, F.L. (1980). Isolation of mouse bone marrow neutrophils by light scatter and autofluorescence. J. Histochem. Cytochem. 28: 934.

59. Watt, S.M., Gilmore, D.J., Metcalf, D., Cobbold, S.P., Hoang, T.K., Waldmann, H. (1983). Segregation of mouse hemopoietic progenitor cells using the monoclonal antibody, YBM/42, J. Cell. Physiol. 115: 37.

60. Wheeless, L.L., Cambier, J.L., Cambier, M.A., Kay, D.B., Wightman, L.L., Patten, S.F. (1979). False alarms in a slit-scan flow system: causes and occurrence rates (implications and potential solutions). J. Histochem. Cytochem. 27: 596.

61. Wied, G.L., Bartels, P.H., Dytch, H.E., Pishotta, F.T., Bibbo, M. (1982). Rapid high-resolution cytometry. Analyt. Quant. Cytol. 4: 257.

62. Witte, T. de, Koekman, E., Plas, A., Blankenborg, G., Salden, M., Wessels, J., Haanen, C. (1982). Enrichment of myeloid clonogenic cells by isopicnic density equilibrium centrifugation in percoll gradients and counter flow centrifugation. Stem Cells 2: 308.

63. Young, I.T. (1977). Proof without prejudice: use of the Kolmogorov-Smirnov test for the analysis of histograms from flow systems and other sources. J. Histochem. Cytochem. 25: 935.

DETECTION OF MINIMAL RESIDUAL LEUKEMIA UTILIZING MONOCLONAL ANTIBODIES AND FLUORESCENCE ACTIVATED CELL SORTING (FACS)

ANTON HAGENBEEK AND ANTON C.M. MARTENS

INTRODUCTION

The major problem in the present treatment of human acute leukemia is the maintenance of a complete remission. So far, no information is available on the number of residual leukemic cells in the bone marrow after successful remission induction chemotherapy. Although the minimal efficacy of this initial treatment can be expressed as a 2 log leukemic cell kill (based on classical cytological methodology), the actual reduction in tumor load per individual patient remains unknown. Starting with 10^{12} leukemic cells prior to therapy, the number left in the phase of "complete remission" might thus vary between 0 and 10^{10} (Fig. 1).

As indicated in Fig. 1, two major approaches are presently being investigated for their efficacy to eradicate residual disease, i.e.

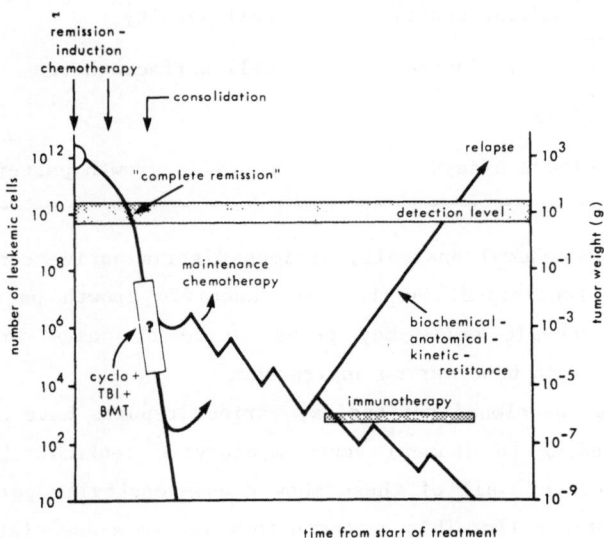

FIGURE 1. Acute leukemia: principles of treatment.

(maintenance) chemotherapy and high-dose chemotherapy (e.g. cyclophosphamide) in combination with total body irradiation (TBI) followed by
bone marrow transplantation (BMT). If these methods fail to eliminate
the clonogenic leukemic cells completely, leukemia relapse will occur.
Decreasing the detection level as regards residual leukemia is essential
for defining prognostic factors which lead to a more effective treatment
strategy per individual patient. The changes in tumor load could then be
quantified more accurately at various treatment stages and relapse could
be predicted earlier. Furthermore, the total duration of treatment could
be judged on a rational basis.

Several methods are presently being evaluated to detect "minimal
residual disease" (MRD; Table 1).

Table 1. Methods to detect residual leukemic cells

Technique	Leukemia-associated specific characteristic
1. Chromosome analysis	
a. cytometry	a. aneuploidy
b. premature chromosome condensation	b. proliferative-potential index
2. Concentration procedure	
a. monoclonal antibodies/FACS	a. specific antigens?
b. heterologous antibodies	b. malignant nucleolar antigens?
c. velocity sedimentation	c. cell size
d. density gradient centrifugation	d. cell density
e. free-flow cell electrophoresis	e. cell surface charge
f. combinations	
3. In vitro culture assays	specific growth pattern

Besides chromosomal analysis, various discriminative concentration
procedures are recognized. Furthermore, specific growth patterns of -
clonogenic - leukemic cells may prove to be of value in detecting
residual leukemia in bone marrow aspirates.

As regards monoclonal antibodies, various reports have appeared on
monoclonals binding to (human) acute myelocytic leukemia (AML) cells
(e.g., 1-4). However, all of these show cross-reactivity patterns with
normal hemopoietic cells. This suggests that leukemia-associated speci-

fic antigens do not exist. These antibodies rather detect differentia-
tion-antigens linked to the myeloid lineage. If there are differences in
the antigen density on the cell surface between normal- and leukemic
cells, leukemic cells might be specifically recognized by differences in
antibody-labeling intensity, to be detected by fluorescence activated
cell sorting (FACS). The present study describes the evaluation of a
monoclonal antibody (Rm124) directed against the BN rat acute myelocytic
leukemia (BNML) as regards the detection of small numbers of leukemic
cells in (a) artificial mixtures with - an overload of - normal marrow
cells; and (b) in bone marrow samples obtained at various times after
remission-induction chemotherapy.

MATERIALS AND METHODS
The rat leukemia model

The BN acute myelocytic leukemia (BNML), which was induced with
9,10-dimethyl 1,2-benzanthracene in a female Brown Norway rat, shows
striking similarities with human AML (5, 6). Some of its major characteristics are: a) a slow growth rate; b) a severe suppression of normal
hemopoiesis due to an absolute numerical decrease in the number of hemopoietic stem cells (CFU-S); c) the presence of clonogenic leukemic cells
(in vivo: LCFU-S; in vitro: clonogenic assays); d) response to chemotherapy as in human AML. An additional advantage of this model is that
normal stem cells (CFU-S) and leukemic clonogenic cells (LCFU-S) can be
selectively discriminated by modified spleen colony assays (7).

The Rm 124 monoclonal antibody

This monoclonal antibody (IgM) was produced and provided by Drs. H.
Kaizer and R.J. Johnson, Johns Hopkins University, Baltimore, Md.,
U.S.A.

Immunofluorescence labeling of cells

Bone marrow cell suspensions were prepared by flushing the femoral
shaft with Hanks Hepes buffered balanced saline solution (H.HBSS). The
cell suspension was centrifuged, resuspended in H.HBSS supplemented with
inactivated fetal calf serum (FCS, Flow Lab.; 5% v/v) and iodine azide
0.01% v/v), which is used throughout the whole labeling procedure. For
fluorescence labeling studies 10^6 cells were pelleted and labeled with

the MCA-Rm124 (50 µl) at various dilutions at 0°C for 45 minutes. After careful washing the cells were incubated with a Goat-anti-Mouse-IgM (Fc) coupled to Fluorescein Isothiocyanate (GAM/IgM(Fc)/FITC 1/30) for 30 min at 0°C. After washing the cells were resuspended and processed on the FACS II cell sorter.

Light activated cell sorter

After labeling the cells were analyzed on a modified FACS II (Beckton Dickinson, Sunnyvale, CA., U.S.A.) light activated cell sorter with the laser beam at 488 nm (0.4 W). FITC fluorescence was measured through a combination of a broad band multicavity interference filter (520-550 nm transmission, Pomfret, Stamford, Conn., U.S.A.) and a 520 nm cut off filter (Ditric) by an S-20 type photomultiplier. Perpendicular light scatter (PLS) intensity was measured by an S-11 type photomultiplier. PLS signals were linearly amplified. A logarithmic amplifier (Nozaki, T., Stanford, CA., U.S.A.) was used for the fluorescence signals.

RESULTS AND DISCUSSION

The fluorescence intensity profiles of normal rat bone marrow cells and BNML cells after labeling with the Rm124 monoclonal antibody (MCA) are shown in Fig. 2.

It is clear that the majority of leukemic cells are strongly positive. However, there is some overlap with a subpopulation of normal marrow cells. Upon sorting of the positive - normal - cells, they appear to be mainly mature granulocytes as judged by microscopical examination. Based on this cross-reactivity it is suggested that the Rm124 MCA detects a differentiation antigen. From studies to be reported elsewhere it is clear that the MCA does not bind to normal hemopoietic stem cells (8).

In subsequent experiments various artificial mixtures of normal- and leukemic marrow cells were incubated with Rm 124 and thereafter with Goat-anti-Mouse IgM Fluorescein Isothiocyanate (GAM-FITC). The fluorescence intensity profiles are shown in Fig. 3.

Up to a concentration of 1 leukemic cell per 10^4 normal marrow cells a small but distinct highly fluorescent subpopulation of cells is

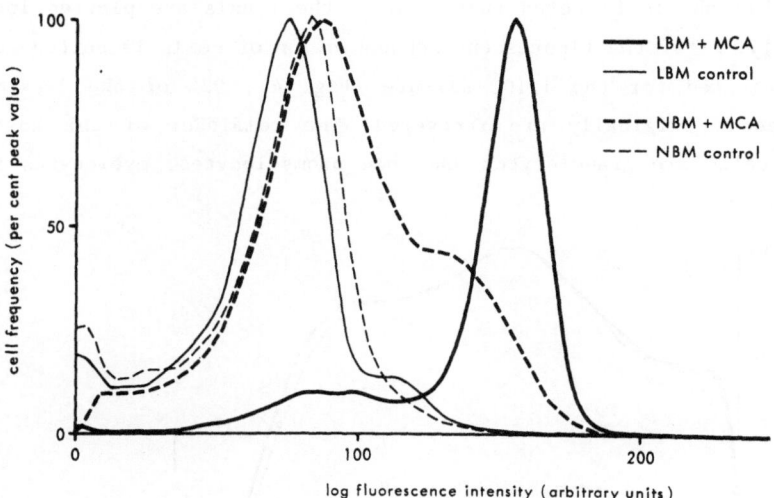

FIGURE 2. Fluorescence intensity profiles of normal rat bone marrow and BN leukemia bone marrow after labeling with the Rm 124 monoclonal antibody (MCA). LBM/NBM: leukemic/normal bone marrow cells.

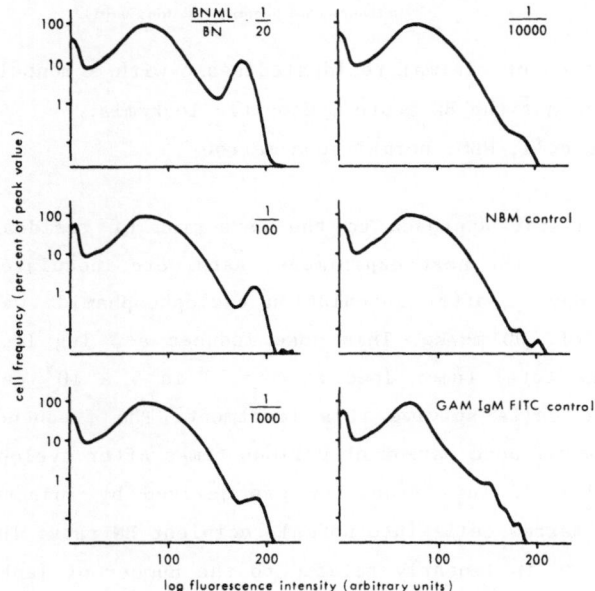

IGURE 3. Fluorescence intenstity profiles of various mixtures of normal BN) and leukemic (BNML) bone marrow cells after labeling with the CA-Rm124 (BN acute myelocytic leukemia). NBM: normal bone marrow cells.

observed. It should be noted that data on the Y-axis are plotted logarithmically. After the fluorescent subpopulation of cells is sorted out,
as is indicated for the 1/100 mixture (Fig. 4), 92% of the leukemic
cells present originally are recovered. The remainder of the sorted
positive cells are granulocytes and some promyelocytes, myelocytes and
metamyelocytes.

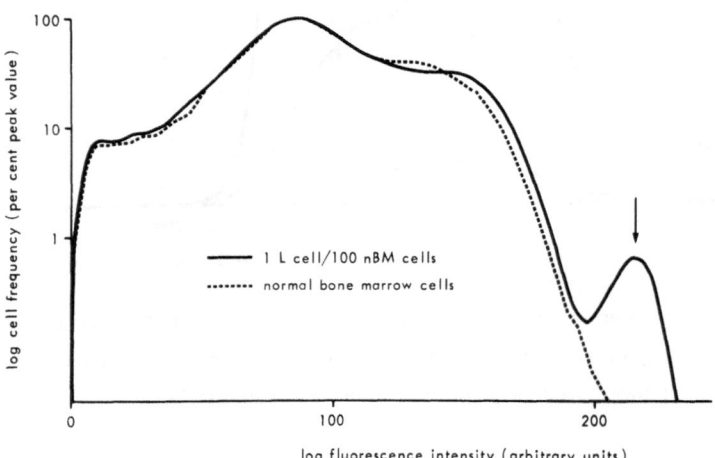

FIGURE 4. Detection of minimal residual disease with a monoclonal antibody (Rm 124) against the BN acute myelocytic leukemia.
L cell: leukemic cell; NBM: normal bone marrow.

A more realistic approach to the detection of residual leukemic
cells is offered in the next experiment. Rats were inoculated with 10^7
BNML cells. At day 13 after inoculation cyclophosphamide was injected
i.p. in a dose of 100 mg/kg. This dose induces a 5 log leukemic cell
kill (9). As the total tumor load at day 13 is 5×10^9 cells, about
5×10^4 leukemic cells survive this treatment. The frequency of BNML
cells in the femoral bone marrow at various times after cyclophosphamide
is given in Table 2. This frequency was derived by injecting graded
numbers of bone marrow cells into normal recipient BN rats. The survival
time of these rats is linearly related to the number of leukemic cells
present in the inoculum.

From Table 2, it appears that the frequency of leukemic cells among
normal cells decreases till around day 22, i.e., till 9 days after
cyclophosphamide treatment. This protracted decrease is due to the

Table 2. Detection of residual leukemic cells in the femoral bone marrow after remission-induction chemotherapy with cyclophosphamide

days after 10^7 BNML cells i.v.	days after cyclophosphamide	frequency of BNML cells*
17	4	1/1000
20	7	1/3500
22	9	1/16000
24	11	1/7800

Cyclophosphamide: 100 mg/kg i.p. at day 13.
*determined by survival bio-assays.

regrowth of normal marrow which is faster than that of the leukemic cell population.

The fluorescence intensity profiles of marrow suspensions incubated with the Rm 124 MCA at similar time intervals after chemotherapy are shown in Fig. 5.

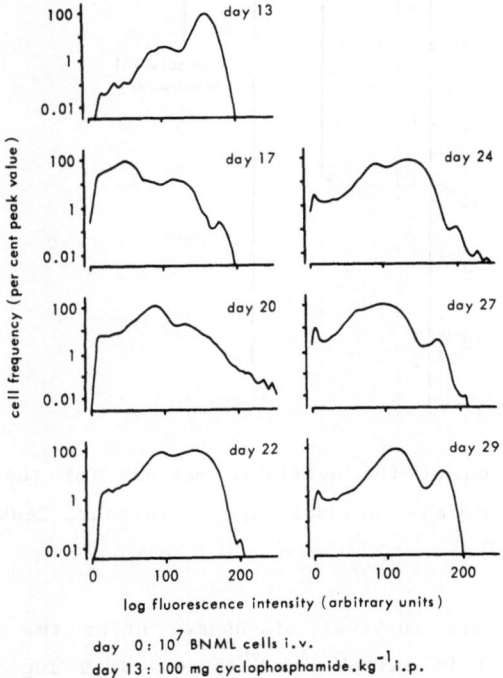

day 0: 10^7 BNML cells i.v.
day 13: 100 mg cyclophosphamide.kg^{-1} i.p.

IGURE 5. Detection of residual leukemia in the femoral bone marrow with he Rm 124 monoclonal antibody after high-dose cyclophosphamide treat-ent (BN acute myelocytic leukemia).

Apart from day 20, where apparently an overload of cell debris does not allow the detection of leukemic cells, a clear cut highly fluorescent cell population is observed at the other sampling times. After sorting, the cells are mainly leukemic. Thus, as low as 1 leukemic cell per 16,000 normal marrow cells (day 22, Table 2) can be detected with the monoclonal antibody approach.

Fig. 6 summarizes the presently available methods to detect minimal residual disease in the BN acute myelocytic leukemia.

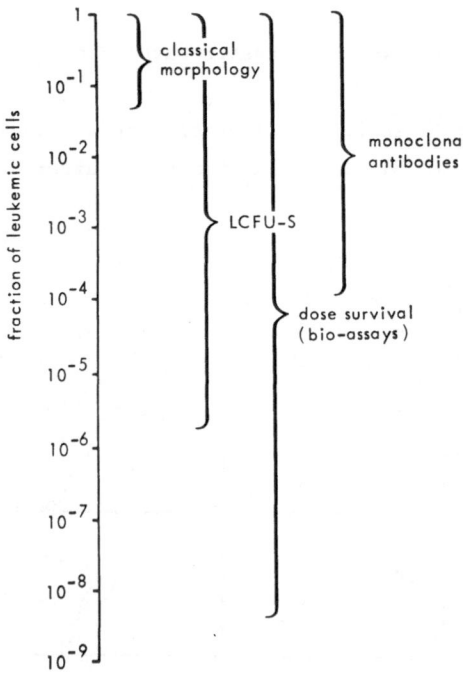

FIGURE 6. Limitation of the available methods for the detection and quantification of minimal residual disease in acute leukemia (BN acute myelocytic leukemia).

In general, dose survival bio-assays offer the most sensitive method of detection in animal model systems (8-9 log range). In the BNML, this is followed by clonogenic leukemic cell assays (LCFU-S; 5-6 logs) and detection with monoclonal antibodies (4 logs). The MCA approach adds 2.5 logs to the detection level feasible with conventional cytological means.

These animal model studies are meant to provide a base for clinical explorations. In this respect, it is recognized that the clinical conditions are more complex. First of all, the presently available monoclonal antibodies against AML show quite some cross-reactivity with normal marrow cells (1-4). Secondly, as only a relatively small fraction of the total marrow cellularity in man can be aspirated for diagnostic purposes and cell sorting technology is still rather "slow", the lower limit of detection of residual leukemia will be at the most in the order of 10^6 cells. This is illustrated in Fig. 7.

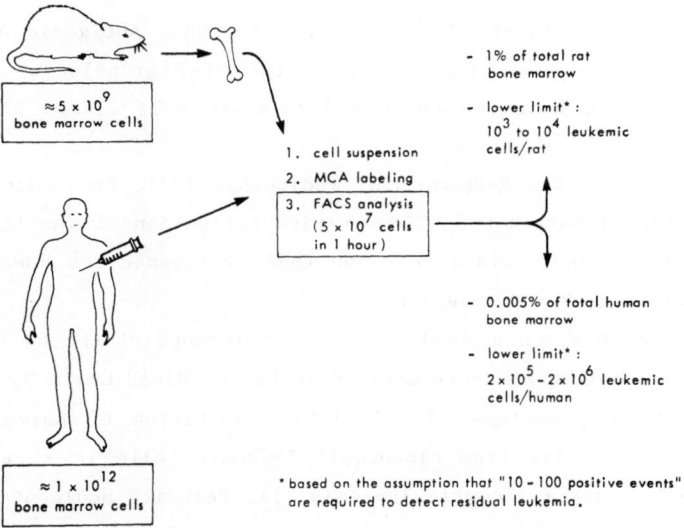

FIGURE 7. Lower limits of detection of minimal residual disease in acute leukemia: rat versus man.

With the clinical approach it will be necessary to combine various methods of concentrating and identifying residual leukemic cells. It is envisaged to combine density gradient centrifugation with (double) MCA labeling procedures and fluorescence activated cell sorting. Further analysis on the sorted cell fraction should include immunoperoxidase stains, karyotyping and/or electron microscopy.

ACKNOWLEDGEMENTS

These studies were supported by the Queen Wilhelmina Fund of the Dutch National Cancer League (grant: RBI 80-1).

REFERENCES

1. Linker-Israeli, M., Billing, R.J., Foon, K.A., Terasaki, P.I. 1981. Monoclonal antibodies reactive with acute myelogenous leukemia cells. J. of Immunol. 127, 2473.

2. Majaic, O., Liszka, K., Lutz, D., Knapp, W. 1981. Myeloid differentiation antigen defined by a monoclonal antibody. Blood 58, 1127.

3. Billing, R.J., Luaro, K., Shi, B.J., Terasaki, P. 1982. A new acute leukemia associated blast cell antigen detected by a monoclonal antibody. Blood 59, 1203.

4. Strauss, L.C., Stuart, R.K., Civin, C.I. 1983. Antigenic analysis of hematopoiesis. I. Expression of the MY-1 granulocyte surface antigen on human marrow cells and leukemic cell lines. Blood 61, 1222.

5. Hagenbeek, A., Van Bekkum, D.W. (editors). 1977. Proceedings of a International Workshop on "Comparative evaluation of the L5222 and the BNML rat leukaemia models and their relevance for human acute leukaemia". Leukemia Research 1, 75.

6. Van Bekkum, D.W., Hagenbeek, A. 1977. Relevance of the BN leukemia as a model for human acute myeloid leukemia. Blood Cells 3, 565.

7. Hagenbeek, A., Martens, A.C.M. 1981. Separation of normal hemopoietic stem cells from clonogenic leukemic cells in a rat model for human acute myelocytic leukemia. II. Velocity sedimentation in combination with density gradient separation. Exp. Hemat. 9, 573.

8. Martens, A.C.M., Hagenbeek, A. 1983. Characteristics of a monoclonal antibody (Rm124) against acute myelocytic leukemia cells. Exp. Hemat., in press.

9. Hagenbeek, A., Martens, A.C.M. 1982. High-dose cyclophosphamide treatment of acute myelocytic leukemia. Studies in the BNML rat model. Eur. J. Cancer Clin. Oncol. 18, 763.

DISCRIMINATION BETWEEN NORMAL HEMOPOIETIC STEM CELLS AND MYELOID
LEUKEMIA CELLS USING MONOCLONAL ANTIBODIES

BEVERLY LANGE, DARIO FERRERO, SILVANA PESSANO, HOWARD HUBBELL,
ANTONIO PALUMBO, SUN KAI LAI AND GIOVANNI ROVERA

1. INTRODUCTION

The maturation process of normal hemopoietic cells can be
recognized by in vitro clonogenic assays as a progression from
multipotent stem cells (1) to pluripotent colony-forming cells
(GFU-GEMM) (2) to colony-forming cells with a relatively
restricted commitment to erythroid (BFU-E, CFU-E) (3) or
granulocytic-monocytic differentiation (CFU-GM). Hybridoma
technology has provided a tool for analysis of the maturation of
hemopoietic cells using monoclonal antibodies. Our laboratory
and several other laboratories have generated an assortment of
monoclonal antibodies that react with antigens present on the
hemopoietic cells of different lineages expressed at discrete
stages of differentiation within the lineage (5-16).

Leukemic cells in AML have been compared to normal hemopoietic cells by morphology, growth in vitro, and by surface
phenotype. Lineage-related antigens as determined by monoclonal
antibodies are present on leukemic blasts, but often are expressed in an uncoordinated, unpredictable manner (5,7,9,11,
13,15).

There has been speculation that the clonogenic cells in
myeloid leukemias are analogous, in some respects, to normal
clonogenic cells in that they may be the cells responsible for
perpetuating the leukemia in vivo just as normal clonogenic
cells give rise to the whole array of hemopoietic cells in the
blood and marrow in vitro (17). The present study describes a
series of experiments using a panel of six cytotoxic monoclonal
antibodies known to react with lineage-related and differentiation-related antigens of myelomonocytic cells to determine the
antigenic phenotype of clonogenic cells in AML (2,11,14,15).

2. PROCEDURE

2.1 Monoclonal antibodies

The 6 monoclonal antibodies used in this study (Table 1) ha been previously described (9,11,14,15). Antibody 9-19 was a gift of Dr. Massimo Trucco.

Table 1. Panel of cytotoxic monoclonal antibodies.

Antibody	Immunogen	Isotype	Antigen
Anti-DR (9-19)	B-lymphocytes	IgG$_2$ a	gp28, gp3:
S3-13	AML	IgM	p29
S8-6	AML	IgM	gp61
S16-144	CML (K562)	IgM	ND
S4-7	AML (KG1)	IgM	gp150
R1B19	AML	IgM	gp145, gp

2.2 Cells

Normal peripheral blood and marrow cells were obtained fro adult volunteers. Leukemic cells were obtained from blood or marrow of children or adults with AML at the time of diagnosi or relapse when at least 70% of the cells were morphologicall blasts. Immunologic, morphologic (FAB) (18) and cytogenetic classification of leukemic cells was performed at Children's Hospital of Philadelphia, Hahnemann Hospital, or Ospedale S. Giovanni Battista, Torino.

Mononuclear cells were isolated on a Ficoll-Hypaque gradie (19) and for clonogenic assays most cases were depleted of co taminating T lymphocytes by gradient separation of E-rosettir cells (20). Aliquots of 10-20 x 10^6 cells were cryopreservec DMSO and stored at -70°C for repeated use.

2.3 Cytofluorimetry and cell sorting

Cells were treated with undiluted supernatant fluid of aso tes usually diluted 1:100, washed repeatedly, and then treate with fluorescein-isotiocianate-conjugated goat F(ab') anti-mo F(ab')$_2$ anti-serum and washed again repeatedly. Fluorescenc was measured in Ortho Cytofluorograph 50HH cells sorter as described (8,9,14).

Fluorescence-negative and positive-population were collected and analyzed for morphology and growth in vitro.

2.4 Growth of colonies in vitro

Growth of normal colonies has been described (1-4,14). Conditions for leukemic colony formation were established by growing mononuclear cells at various concentrations (1×10^4-2×10^5 cells/35mm^2 scored Petri dish) in fetal calf serum, horse serum, or human serum with either lymphocyte-conditioned medium (21) or GCT supernatant (GIBCO) for colony-stimulating activity (22). For most cases 0.9% methylcellulose, 30% Reheis fetal calf serum and .0% GCT supernatant allowed optimal growth. Cultures were incubated at 37°C in 5% CO_2 and colonies ($\geq$40 cells) and clusters 3-39 cells) were counted on days 7, 10, and 14. The morphology of colonies was determined by picking and spreading single colonies or by cytocentrifuge spreads of washed cells.

.5 Cytotoxicity

The ability of cytotoxic monoclonal antibodies to eliminate certain populations of cells was determined by treating cells first with antibody, at 4°C, then adding absorbed rabbit complement (Low Tox, Cedarline Laboratories) incubating at 37°C for 0-90 minutes, washing in PBS and plating as described above. Growth in complement without antibody was used for controls.

.0 RESULTS
.1 Antigenic phenotype of normal cells

Figure 1 is a schematic representation of the antigenic phenotype of morphologically recognizable myeloid and monocytic cells based on cytofluorometric studies of cells from normal donors. Antibodies S3-13 and DR react both with monocytes and the earliest recognizable granulocytic series.

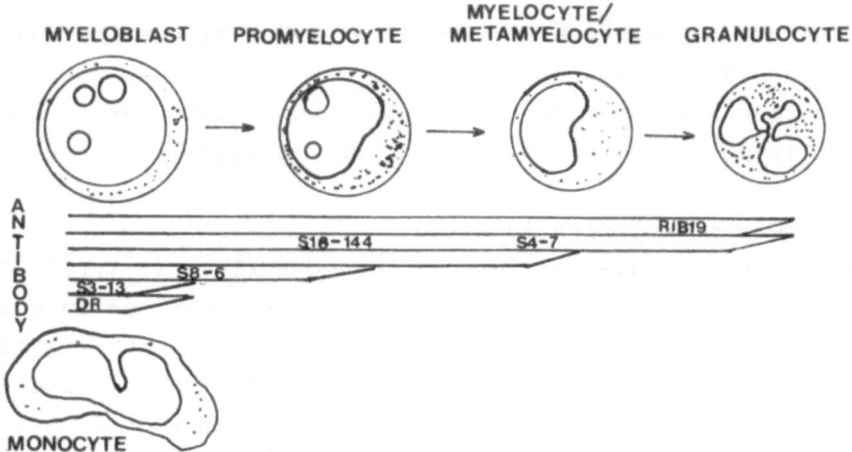

FIGURE 1. Antigenic phenotype of normal myeloid and monocytic cells as determined by indirect immunofluorescence and cell sorting with monoclonal antibodies.

3.2 Antigenic phenotype of normal clonogenic cells

Figure 2 is a schematic representation of the antigenic ph‹ notype of colony-forming cells as determined by growth of colonies in soft agar or methycellulose after treatment with antibody and complement or after sorting of fluorescence posi‹ tive and negative populations (14).

Antibodies S3-13, anti-DR, S8-6 and S16-144 react with all colony-forming cells that could be measured by available assa Antibodies S4-7 and RlBl9 react only with the more mature col forming cells committed to granulocytic or monocytic differen tion.

3.3 Antigenic phenotype of blasts in AML

Figure 3 shows the results of indirect immunofluorescent analysis of the surfaces of blasts from 50 adult or pediatric patients with AML. Figure 3 implies that not all blasts from given patient express all of the antigens and that the AML patients as a group show heterogeneous patterns of reactivity with the various antibodies. There is no correlation between the FAB classification and the immunologic phenotype as deter mined by this panel or the more extensive panel of 15 monocl‹

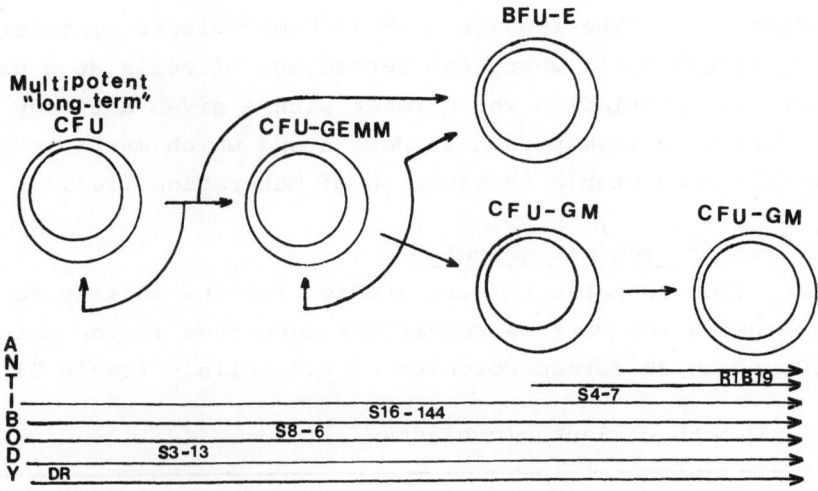

FIGURE 2. Antigenic phenotype of normal hemopoietic colony-forming cells as determined by complement-mediated cytotoxicity or cell sorting with monoclonal antibodies.

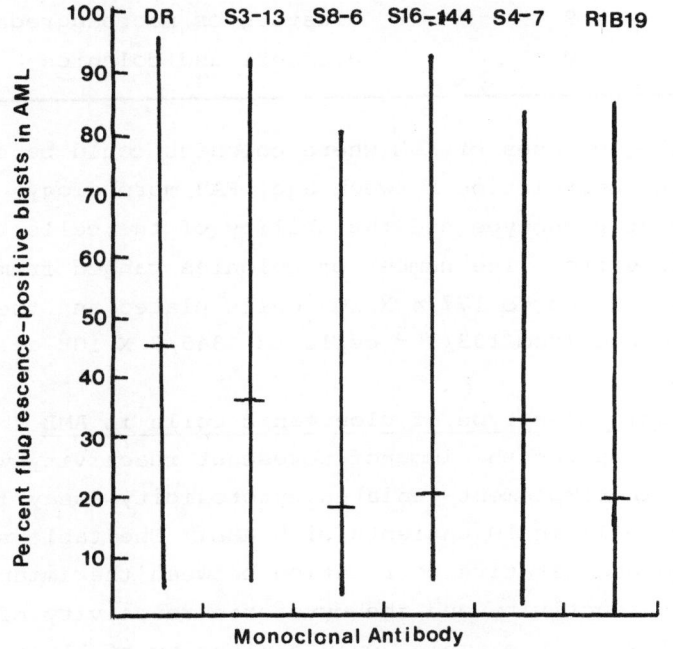

FIGURE 3. Reactivity of monoclonal antibodies with leukemic blasts. The vertical lines represent the range of percentages of blasts showing positive fluorescence for a given monoclonal antibody based on analysis of 3×10^5 cells per antibody from 50 patients with AML (9,15). The bar represents the median percentage showing positive fluorescence.

antibodies (15). The results with leukemic blasts contrast wi
those of normal cells where the percentage of cells at a given
level of differentiation which react with a given antibody sho
little variation from person to person and which manifest an
orderly and predictable progression of maturation (14).

3.4 Growth of leukemic colonies

Blasts from 28 patients were studied for the ability to gro
in vitro using the various conditions described in the methods
Only 10 of the 28 formed colonies of >40 cells. (Table 2).

Table 2. Growth of leukemic blasts.

Number of cases	Pattern of growth
5	no growth
4	increase in cell number
9	clusters or macroaggregates
10	clusters and colonies

Among the 10 cases of AML where colonies could be detected,
there was no correlation between age, FAB morphology, and immu
nofluorescent phenotype and the ability of the cells to form
colonies in vitro. The number of colonies ranged from
$8/10^5$ cells plated to $177/4 \times 10^4$ cells plated and the number
clusters ranged from $133/10^5$ cells to $4345/7 \times 10^4$ cells plate

3.5 Antigenic phenotype of clonogenic cells in AML

Table 3 compares the immunofluorescent reactivity with the
reactivity in complement-mediated cytotoxicity assay for the
clonogenic cells in 10 patients with AML. The table shows tha
there is no quantitative correlation between the immunofluorescent reactivity and the cytotoxic reactivity of colony-
forming cells. For example, only a minority of blasts (3% to
47%) show immunofluorescent reactivity with antibody S8-6;
however, virtually all of the clonogenic cells are eliminated

Table 3. Comparison of immunofluorescent and cytotoxic reactivity
of clonogenic leukemic cells with monoclonal antibodies.

Antibody	Immunofluorescence mean (range)	Cytotoxicity mean (range)
Anti-DR	50.2 (6-91)	97.9 (94-100)
S3-13	31.7 (3-90)	99.7 (97-100)
S8-6	16.4 (3-47)	99.1 (95-100)
S16-144	20.9 (1-51)	99.5 (98-100)
S4-7	25.9 (6-70)	59.7 (96-100)a
		(0-78) b
R1B19	29.2 (2-42)	70.0 (95-100)a
		(0-84) b

The mean and range percentage immunofluorescence is cytofluorometric analysis of 3 X 10^5 cells per antibody for the 10 patients
whose cells formed colonies in vitro. The mean and range percentage cytotoxicity represents percentage inhibition of colonies
compared to the complement control based on the mean of tripli-
cate cultures grown under conditions described in methods.
Cytotoxic inhibition for antibodies S4-7 and R1B19 is subdivided
to emphasize to patterns of reactivity: a) 4 of 10 cases where
virtually all clonogenic cells were eliminated by these antibodies and b) 6 of 10 cases where clonogenic cells were incom-
pletely eliminated by these 2 antibodies.

this antibody. These lack of correlation between immunofluorescence and cytotoxicity is seen in all cases with all
antibodies. These findings imply that the immunofluorescent
phenotype may not predict the phenotype of the clonogenic cells,
that is, those cells that are presumed to perpetuate the
disease.

For 4 of 10 patients the six antibodies eliminated all or
nearly all clonogenic cells. However, in 6 of 10 cases antibodies S4-7 and R1B19 that react with the more mature normal
clonogenic cells (Figure 2) did not eliminate all the clonogenic
leukemic cells ([Table 3] rows a. and b., respectively). Thus,
the cases in which all clonogenic cells are eliminated by all 6

antibodies have the phenotype of the more mature colony formir
cells as shown in Figure 2. The cases in which clonogenic cell
are not completely eliminated by antibodies S4-7 and R1B19 hav
the phenotype of the less mature colony-forming cells. Presuma
in the former cases the normal progression of maturation has ק
gressed to or beyond the level of the CFU-GM whereas in the
latter cases maturation may have been arrested anywhere from t
level of the multipotent stem cell to or beyond the late CFU-C

The ability of monoclonal antibodies to eliminate clonogeni
cells selectively in complement-mediated cytotoxicity was compared to the ability of antibodies to select clonogenic cells
using the fluorescence-activated cell sorter. Table 4 shows
that the majority of colony-forming cells are in the populatic
that is positive for the antigens detected by S3-13 or HLA-DR
antibodies while clonogenic cells are present in both the S4-7
antigen-negative and antigen-positive populations. Again, Tak
4 shows that while only a small fraction of the total leukemic
population may react with a particular antibody, almost all th
clonogenic cells react with the antibody. This is especially
apparent with antibody S3-13.

Table 4. Growth of leukemic colonies after fluorescence-activa
sorting of cells reacting with monoclonal antibodies

Case 7

		Number of colonies	
Antibody	% Fluorescence	Fluorescence positive population	Fluoresce negativ populatj
Anti-DR	85	246	18
S3-13	15	208	16
S4-7	70	55	68

4.0 DISCUSSION

Monoclonal antibodies which detect lineage-related and differentiation-related antigens on the surfaces of normal hemopoietic cells have allowed this laboratory and several other laboratories to characterize the surface phenotype of the leukemic blasts in AML. Our results have shown that the leukemic population as a whole does express antigens found on normal myelomonocytic precursors but expresses the antigens in an aberrant uncoordinated manner (9,11,15). These results are essentially in agreement with those of other laboratories (5,13).

Because those cells which are capable of repeated cycles of multiplication and division are those that are most likely the ones that are responsible for perpetuating the leukemia in vivo, (17), we studied the phenotype of the clonogenic cells in AML. Our studies were limited to analysis of those cases which formed colonies of >40 cells in methylcellulose. We found that the clonogenic cells were found in a small fraction of the population that expresses the antigens detected by these antibodies and that the phenotype of the total population as determined by indirect immunofluorescence did not quantitatively correlate with phenotype of the clonogenic cells as determined by cytotoxicity. In general, a relatively small percentage of the total leukemic population reacted with the antibodies using immunofluorescence while virtually all the cells reacted with 4 of 6 antibodies using cytotoxicity.

The composite phenotype of the clonogenic cells resembles that of the clonogenic cells in the normal peripheral blood and marrow (14). However, two distinct patterns of reactivity were found: 1) a pattern like that of the early hemopoietic precursors from the CFU-GEMM or early CFU-GM and 2) a pattern like that of clonogenic cells extending from the CFU-GEMM to the level or beyond the level of late CFU-GM. Using G6PD isozyme analysis, Fialkow has also found two distinct variants of AML (24). In the case of the more mature pattern it may be possible to eliminate all the clonogenic leukemic cells with antibodies such as S4-7 and R1B19 that react with the more mature normal clonogenic cells while preserving less mature normal-clonogenic cells at or before the level of the CFU-GEMM.

64

5.0 ACKNOWLEDGEMENT

Dr. Lange is a recipient of JCFC #564 from the American Can Society. Dr. Ferrero is supported in part by a Gigi Ghirotti Fellowship. The work is supported by grants from the National Cancer Institute CA-14489, CA-10815, CA-24273, CA-25875 and by The Eagles Fly for Leukemia. We thank Dr. Massimo Trucco for the gift of anti-HLA-DR antibody and Mrs. Elaine Burton for typing the manuscript.

6.0 REFERENCES

1. Nakahata T and Ogawa M. 1982. Hemopoietic colony forming cells in umbellical cord blood with extensive capability generate mono and multipotential hemopoietic progenitors. J. Clin. Invest. 70:1324-1327.
2. Ash RC, Detrick RA and Zanjani ED. 1981. Studies of human pluripotential hemopoietic stem cells (CFU-GM) in vitro. Blood. 58:309-315.
3. Iscove NN, Sieber F and Winterhalter KH. 1974. Erythroid colony formation in cultures of mouse and human bone marr analysis of the requirement for erythropoietin by gel filtration and affinity chromatography on agarose-concanavalin. A.J. Cell Physiol. 83:309-319.
4. Pike BL and Robinson WA. 1970. Human bone marrow colony growth in agar-gel. J. Cell Physiol. 76:77-88.
5. Griffin JD, Ritz J, Nadler LM and Scholssman SS. 1981. Ex pression of myeloid differentiation antigens in normal an malignant myeloid cells. J. Clin. Invest. 68:932-941.
6. Majdic O, Liszke K, Lutz D and Knapp W. 1981. Myeloid dif ferentiation antigen defined by a monoclonal antibody. Blood. 58:1127-1133.
7. Linker-Israeli M, Billing RJ, Foon KA and Terasaki PI. 19 Monoclonal antibodies reactive with acute myelogeneous leukemia cells. J. Immunol. 127:2473-2477.
8. Perussia B, Trinchieri G, Lebman D, Jankiewicz J, Lange B and Rovera G. 1982. Monoclonal antibodies that detect dif ferentiation surface antigens on human myelonocytic cells Blood. 59:382-392.
9. Pessano S, Bottero L, Faust J, Trucco M, Palumbo A, Pegoraro L, Lange B, Brezim C, Borst J, Terhorst C and Rovera G. Differentiation antigens of human hemopoietic cell: patterns of reactivity of two monoclonal antibodies Cancer Research, in press.
10. Ball ED and Fanger MW. 1983. The expression of myeloid sp cific antigens on myeloid leukemia cells: Correlations wi leukemia subclasses and implications for myeloid differen tiation. Blood. 61:456-463.

11. Pagliardi GL, Pessano S, Palumbo A, Levis A, Bottero L, Ferrero D, Lange B and Rovera G. 1982. Differentiation, maldifferentiation or arrested differentiation in human acute myelogenous leukemias. Symposia of 13th International Cancer Congress. E.A. Mirand (ed). A.R. Liss, New York, in press.

12. Mannon P, Janowicka-Wieczorek A, Turner AR, McGann L and Truc JM. 1982. Monoclonal antibodies against human granulocytes and myeloid differentiation antigens. Human Immunology, 5:309-323.

13. Van der Reijden HJ, van Rhenen DJ, Lansdorp PM, vant Veer M, Langehujsen MMAC, Engelfrezt CP and von dem Borne AEGK. 1983. A comparison of surface marker analysis and FAB classification in acute myeloid leukemia. Blood. 61:443-448.

14. Ferrero D, Pagliardi GL, Broxmeyer HE, Venuta S, Lange B, Pessano S and Rovera G. 1983. Two antigenically distinct subpopulations of myeloid progenitor cells (CFU-GM) are present in human peripheral blood and marrow. Proc. Natl. Acad. Sci. 80:4114-4118.

15. Pessano S, Ferrero D, Palumbo A, Bottero L, Hubbell H, Lange B and Rovera G. 1983, in press. Differentiation antigens of normal and leukemic myelomonocytic cells in normal and neoplastic hematopoiesis. UCLA symposium on molecular and cellular biology, vol. 9, Alan R. Liss, Inc. NY, NY.

16. Andrews RG, Torok-Strob B and Bernstein ID. 19 . Myeloid associated antigens on stem cells and their progeny identified by monoclonal antibodies. Blood. 62:129-133.

17. McCulloch EA and Till JE. 1981. Blasts cells in acute myelogenous leukemia. A model. Blood Cells. 7:63-77.

18. Bennett JM, Catovsky D, Daniel MT, Flandering G, Galton DAG, Gralnicle HR and Sultan C. 1976. Proposal for classification of the acute leukemias. Br. J. Hematology. 33:451-458.

19. Boyum A. 1968. Separation of leukocytes from Blood and bone Scan. J. Clin. Lab. Invest. 21 (Suppl. 97) 7-91.

20. Minden MD, Buick RN and McCulloch EA. 1979. Separation of blast cell and T-lymphocyte progenitors in the blood of patients with acute myeloblastic leukemia. Blood. 54:186.

21. Aye Mt, Niho Y, Till JE and McCulloch EA. 1974. Studies of leukemic cell populations in culture. Blood. 44:205-219.

22. DiPersio JF, Brennan JK, Lichtman MA, Abboud CN and Kirkpatrick FH. 1980. The fractionation, characterization and subcellular localization of colony stimulating activities released by the human monocyte cell line, GCT. Blood. 58: 717-727.

23. Broxmeyer HE. 1982. Relationship of cell-cycle expression of Ia like antigenic determinants on normal and leukemic human granulocytec-macrophage progentor cells to regulators in vitro by acidic isoferritins. J. Clin, Invest. 69:632-642.

24. Fialkow PJ, Singer JW, Adamson JW, Vaidyt K, Dow LW, Ochs J and Moohr JW. 1981. Acute non-lymphocytic leukemia: Heterogeneity of stem cell origin. Blood. 59:1068-1073.

DETECTION OF MINIMAL RESIDUAL DISEASE IN TdT POSITIVE T CELL MALIGNANCIES
BY DOUBLE IMMUNOFLUORESCENCE STAINING

J.J.M. VAN DONGEN , H. HOOIJKAAS , K. HÄHLEN , K. BENNE , W.M. BITTER ,
A.A. VAN DER LINDE-PREESMAN , I.L.M. TETTERO , M. VAN DE RIJN , J. HILGERS ,
G.E. VAN ZANEN AND A. HAGEMEIJER .

1. INTRODUCTION

Identification of small numbers of residual malignant cells is one of
the major goals in cancer research. Detection of minimal disease enables
better staging of the malignant process and provides information about
residual disease. As a consequence individual adjustment of the therapy
as well as avoidance of under- or overtreatment of the patient is possible.

In the Netherlands 82% of childhood leukemias are acute lymphoblastic
leukemias (ALL) (1). With immunological techniques five different immunological subtypes of ALL have been distinguished: null-ALL: 10.5%, common
ALL (cALL): 55%, pre-B ALL: 11%, B-ALL: 1.5%, T-ALL: 22% (2).

For the detection of small numbers of leukemic cells, large numbers
(10^5-10^6) of cells have to be screened at the single cell level, and specific
markers are needed. However, the markers that are frequently associated
with ALL such as terminal deoxynucleotidyltransferase (TdT), cALL antigen
and T6 antigen, are normal differentiation-linked structures. It has been
demonstrated that leukemic cells from null-ALL (HLA-DR$^+$/cALL$^-$/TdT$^+$), cALL
(HLA-DR$^+$/cALL$^+$/TdT$^+$) and even pre-B-ALL (HLA-DR$^+$/cALL$^+$/cytoplasmic IgM$^+$/TdT$^+$)
have their normal counterparts in normal and regenerating bone marrow (BM)
(3,4). In contrast, cells with the T-ALL phenotype (T cell marker$^+$/TdT$^+$)
have been found in the thymus only and not in normal or regenerating BM
and peripheral blood (PB) (3,5-8). This T cell marker$^+$/TdT$^+$ phenotype occurs
in T-ALL as well as in some T cell non-Hodgkin lymphomas (T-NHL), especially
lymphoblastic lymphomas (9).

We employed double immunofluorescence staining for the detection of T
cell markers and TdT at the single cell level, using two different fluorochromes (5,10). To determine the sensitivity of this combined immunofluorescence (IF) assay for the detection of minimal residual disease in TdT
positive T cell malignancies, we performed dilution experiments using T-NHL
cells as well as thymocytes. Both were positive for TdT and the common
thymocyte antigen T6, which normally is exclusively found on thymocytes
(11) and on Langerhans cells in the skin (12), and not in normal BM and
PB (11). In parallel, using the T6 antigen as the specific marker, we
determined the detection limit of the fluorescence activated cell sorter
(FACS), since it was suggested that low percentages of specifically labeled
cells can be detected by FACS analysis (13,14).

Finally, the immunological data of two patients with T cell malignancies are presented, illustrating the potential value of the combined IF assay in the detection of minimal (residual) disease.

2. MATERIALS AND METHODS

2.1. *Origin of cell samples*. To obtain control values for the TdT determination and for the combined IF assay (T cell marker/TdT), cell samples were used from children treated for non-T-ALL or non-T-NHL: 52 BM samples from 23 patients, and 51 PB samples from 23 patients. In addition, 60 cerebrospinal fluid (CSF) samples from 27 ALL or NHL patients were used. The thymus sample was derived from a 3-yr-old girl undergoing cardiac surgery and a thymocyte suspension was made as described elsewhere (15). From patient 1 BM, PB, pleural effusion (PE) and CSF samples were analyzed, whil from patient 2 BM, PB and CSF samples were studied (see case reports).

2.2. *Cell sampling*. Cells from BM, PE and CSF were obtained by needle aspiration and PB cells by venapuncture. For immunological studies the BM, PB and PE samples were heparinized and, in principle, 1 ml BM, 10 ml PB and 5-10 ml CSF were used.

2.3. *Morphological analysis*. The morphological diagnosis was made on BM and PB smears and on PE and CSF cytocentrifuge preparations after staining with May-Grünwald-Giemsa and was confirmed by additional histochemical stainings including a.o. acid phosphatase (16).

2.4. *Immunological characterisation*. Mononuclear cells from BM and PB were isolated by Ficoll Paque (Pharmacia, Uppsala, Sweden) density centrifugation (17) and the cells in the PE and CSF were centrifuged and washed. All washings were performed in phosphate buffered saline (PBS) with 1% bovine serum albumin (BSA), pH 7.8. Any remaining red blood cells were removed by NH_4Cl lysis (18). To detect surface membrane markers, the cell suspensions were incubated with optimally titrated relevant monoclonal antibodies and conventional antisera (see Table 2; references 19-31). If necessary, this was followed by incubation with an appropriate second step antiserum, either labeled with fluorescein isothiocyanate (FITC) or tetramethylrhodamine isothiocyanate (TRITC). Finally, the cells were mounted on slides in glycerol/PBS (9:1) with 1 mg/ml phenylenediamine to prevent fadi of the fluorescence (32). E rosette tests were performed with 2-aminoethylisothiouranium bromide (AET)-treated sheep erythrocytes (21). For TdT determinations cells were cytocentrifuged on slides and subjected to indirect immunofluorescence staining with rabbit-anti-TdT antiserum and FITC-conjugated goat-anti-rabbit-Ig antiserum (19). Determination of cytoplasmic immunoglobulin μ heavy chain (cIgM) was also performed on cytocentrifuge preparations (33).

2.5. *Combined IF assay*. For double immunofluorescence staining the cells were successively incubated with 66IIIE5, Leu-1 or WT1 and TRITC-conjugate goat-anti-mouse-Ig antiserum. Subsequently, two cytocentrifuge preparation of these labeled cells were subjected to indirect immunofluorescence staining with rabbit-anti-TdT anti-serum and FITC-conjugated goat-anti-rabbit-Ig antiserum.

2.6. *Fluorescence microscopy*. Fluorescence staining was evaluated using Zeiss and Leitz microscopes with Osram HBO mercury lamps and filter combinations for the selective visualization of FITC and TRITC. The microscopes were equipped with phase contrast facilities. For microphotography we exclusively used an Orthoplan Leitz microscope with a Ploemopak fluorescer epi-illuminator and a Leitz Vario-Orthomat Camera. In routine determinatic at least 200 cells were evaluated in the suspension preparations and 1000 cells for the assessment of TdT or cIgM. In double labeling experiments routinely at least 20,000 cells from 2 cytospins (each cytospin with at least 10,000 cells) were evaluated for cells positive for both TdT and the T cell marker used.

2.7. *FACS analysis.* For FACS analysis we used a FACS II (Becton Dickinson, Sunnyvale, CA) equipped with a Spectrophysics argon-ion laser type 164-05 (Spectrophysics, Mountainview, CA) at 547 nm using a 70 μm nozzle. FITC fluorescence was measured above 520 nm by using a combination of K510, K515 (Schott Optical Glass Inc., Duryea, PA) and LP520 (Ditric Optics Inc., Malboro, MA) filters. Routinely 20,000 cells were examined.

2.8. *Dilution experiments.* For dilution experiments either infant thymocytes or T6 antigen positive T-NHL cells (patient 1) were diluted with a suspension of mononuclear PB cells of a single healthy adult donor. The T6 antigen was used as a specific marker. However, it must be remarked that it is not possible to use this antigen for the detection of low numbers of tumor cells in all cases of T-ALL and T-NHL, since only 40% of these malignancies are positive for the T6 antigen (34). The following dilutions were made: 1 in 3, 1 in 10, 1 in 30, 1 in 100, 1 in 300, 1 in 1000, 1 in 3000, 1 in 10,000, 1 in 30,000, 1 in 100,000 and 1 in 300,000. One part of the diluted cell suspensions and the appropriate controls were incubated with the monoclonal antibody 66IIIE5 (anti-T6 antibody) and a FITC-conjugated second step antiserum. Samples from each suspension were simultaneously analyzed with the fluorescence microscope and the FACS. Another part of each diluted cell suspension was incubated with 66IIIE5 followed by a TRITC-conjugated second step antiserum. Afterwards the latter suspensions were centrifuged on slides and subsequently subjected to indirect immunofluorescence staining with rabbit-anti-TdT antiserum and a FITC-conjugated second step antiserum. The cytospin preparations were evaluated for cells positive for both 66IIIE5 and TdT. At least 1000 cells were evaluated in both the suspension preparations and the cytospin preparations. If less than 1% of the cells were positive for both markers, at least 20,000 cells were examined as described above.

The PBS/BSA 1% solution, the monoclonal antibodies and the antisera used in these dilution experiments were filtered through 0.22 μm filters to remove particles that might disturb the FACS analysis.

3. RESULTS

3.1. *Incidence of cells positive for both a T cell marker and TdT in BM and PB.* To evaluate the validity of the use of the different T cell markers in the combined IF assay for detection of minimal residual disease we determined the incidence of TdT, WT1/TdT, T6/TdT and Leu-1/TdT positive cells in BM and PB samples of patients treated for non-T-ALL or non-T-NHL, which at the time of sampling were in clinical and hematological remission. The percentage of TdT positive cells ranged from 0.5 to 10% in BM (52 samples/23 patients) and from 0 to 0.2% in PB (51 samples/23 patients). T6 positive cells were never detected in 20 BM and PB samples from 20 patients. Cells positive for both Leu-1 and TdT were never observed in 10 BM and PB samples from these patients. However, in 6 out of 6 BM samples from 6 patients up to 5% of all TdT positive cells evaluated were also positive for WT1 (Table 1). Screening of 5 PB samples from 5 patients did not reveal a single cell positive for both WT1 and TdT. In all cases at least 20,000 nucleated cells per sample were analyzed.

TABLE 1

Cells positive both for WT1 and TdT in the BM of patients in remission of non-T-ALL or non-T-NHL

Patient	% TdT$^+$ (per mononuclear cells)	% WT1$^+$ (per TdT$^+$ cells)	% WT1$^+$/TdT$^+$ (per mononuclear cel
A	5	1.6 (8/500)	0.08
B	4	1.6 (8/500)	0.06
C	1	1.3 (3/220)	0.01
D	2.5	4.7 (8/169)	0.12
E	5.4	1.7 (8/460)	0.09
F	7.7	2.3 (11/500)	0.17

3.2. Incidence of TdT positive cells in the CSF of ALL and NHL patients during follow-up. In 5 out of 60 CSF samples from 22 ALL and 5 NHL patient in follow-up high percentages of TdT positive cells, ranging from 30 to 95 were detected. This correlated with the cytomorphological diagnosis of central nervous system (CNS) relapse. In 3 samples less than 0.2% TdT positive cells were detected. In the patients concerned no CSF relapse occurred within 3 to 4 months after diagnosis. In the other 52 samples, containing 10 to 2,000 nucleated cells, no TdT positive cells were observe

3.3. Sensitivity of the assay systems employed. To determine the sensitivi of the double IF assay and the FACS analysis, thymocytes and T6 positive NHL cells were diluted with a mononuclear PB cell suspension from a health donor. The results of two such experiments are given in Figure 1A (thymo-cytes) and Figure 1B (T-NHL cells). Analysis of cytocentrifuge preparation using the fluorescence microscope enabled the detection of small numbers o combined T6/TdT positive cells down to 1 in 10,000 cells. All TdT positive cells were also T6 positive as is demonstrated in Figure 2 (1 in 3 dilutio of T-NHL cells). The detection limit of the fluorescence microscope in evaluating suspension preparations, however, is not as good as the one in evaluating cytocentrifuge preparations due to the smaller number of cel that can be screened. Moreover, in our hands the lowest detection limit of the FACS appeared to be 2 positive cells among 100 cells (Figure 1). Although there was a great difference in fluorescence intensity between th T6 negative and the T6 positive cells (Figure 3), the FACS detected false positive cells as frequent as 1%, even in dilutions down to 1 in 300,000.

4. CASE REPORTS

4.1. Patient 1. A 13-yr-old boy presented with complaints due to mediastin: and hilar enlargement and right-sided pleural effusion. Examination of the pleural fluid revealed pathological lymphoblasts which, according to immuno logical marker analysis, were identified as T lymphoblasts. They formed E rosettes and were positive for TdT, WT1, 66IG10 (anti-transferrine recepto: antibody), 66IIIE5 (anti-T6 antibody), Leu-1, Leu-2, Leu-3 and VIL-A1 (weal expression) (Table 2). PB, BM and CSF were morphologically normal. Thus, a clinical diagnosis of T-NHL, stage II, was made. However, combined IF assay (WT1/TdT, 66IIIE5/TdT, Leu-1/TdT) revealed that the lymphoma cells were al: present in the BM (0.5%) and PB (3%) (Figure 4), while in the CSF 2% TdT positive cells were detected, indicating a more widespread dissemination than suspected on morphological criteria only. The response to chemotherap;

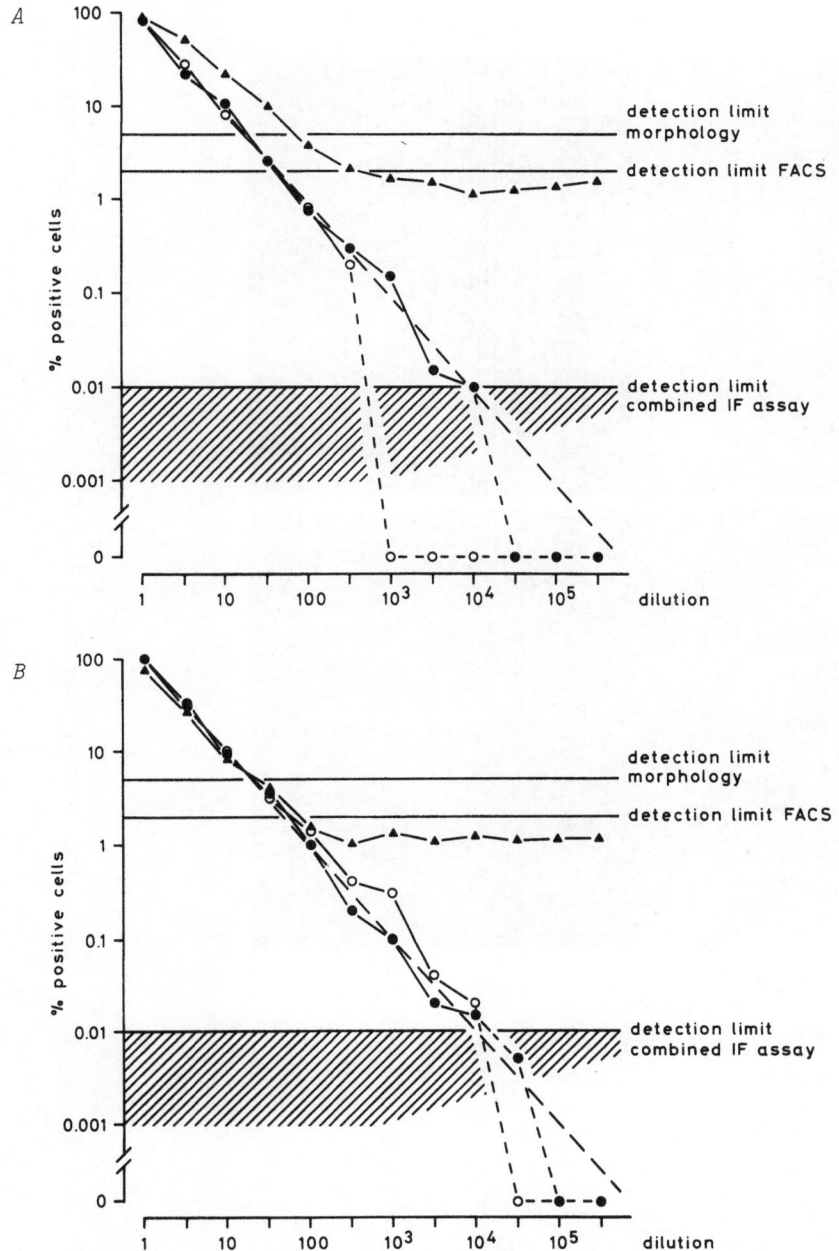

Figure 1. Sensitivity of FACS analysis and the combined IF assay as deter-mined by dilution of thymocytes (A) and T-NHL cells (B) with a mononuclear PB cell suspension. The T6 antigen was used as a marker for detection of the thymocytes and T-NHL cells.
    ▲—▲\: FACS; ○—○ \: suspension preparations; ●—● : cytocen-trifuge preparations, using the combined IF assay (T6/TdT).

72

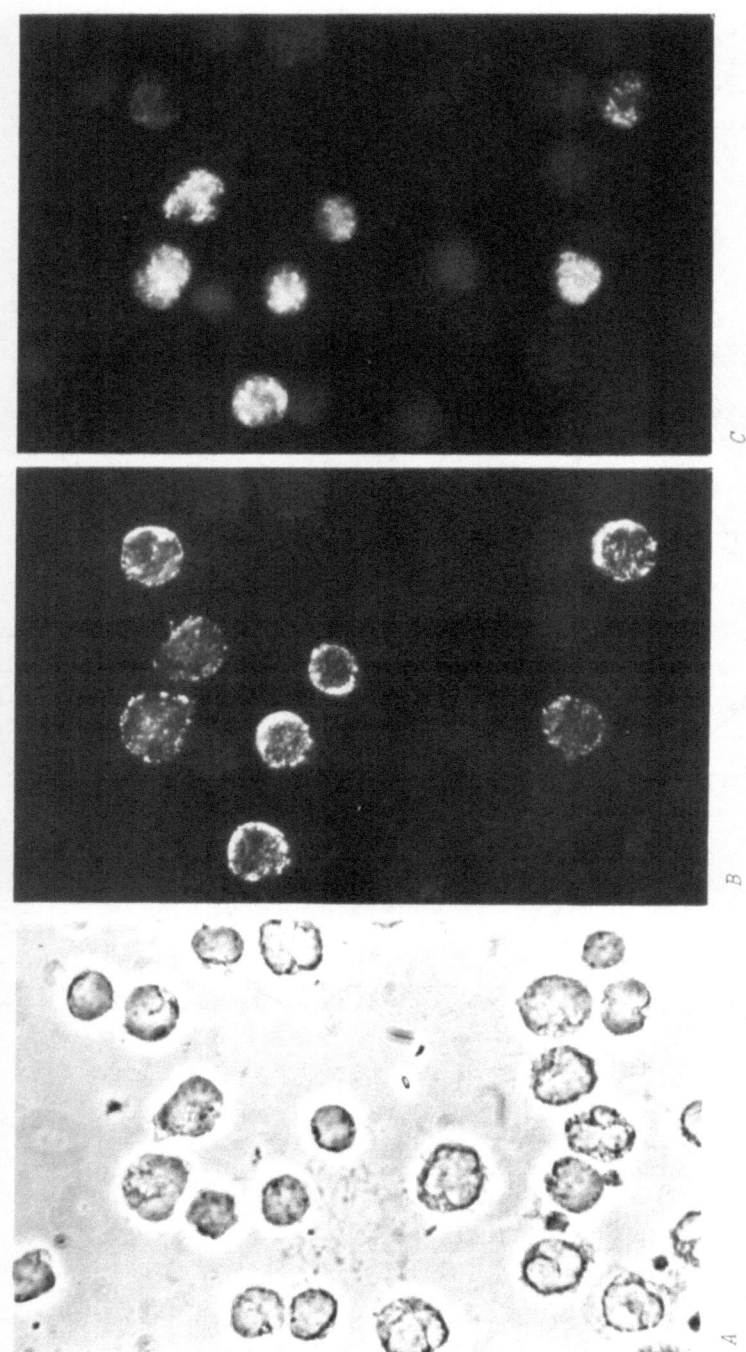

Figure 2. Micrographs of T-NHL cells diluted with a mononuclear PB cell suspension (dilution 1 in 3).
A: phase contrast morphology; B: 66IIIE5 (T6) positive cells (TRITC-labeled); C: TdT positive cells
(FITC-labeled). The combined IF assay demonstrates that all TdT postive cells are also positive for
T6.

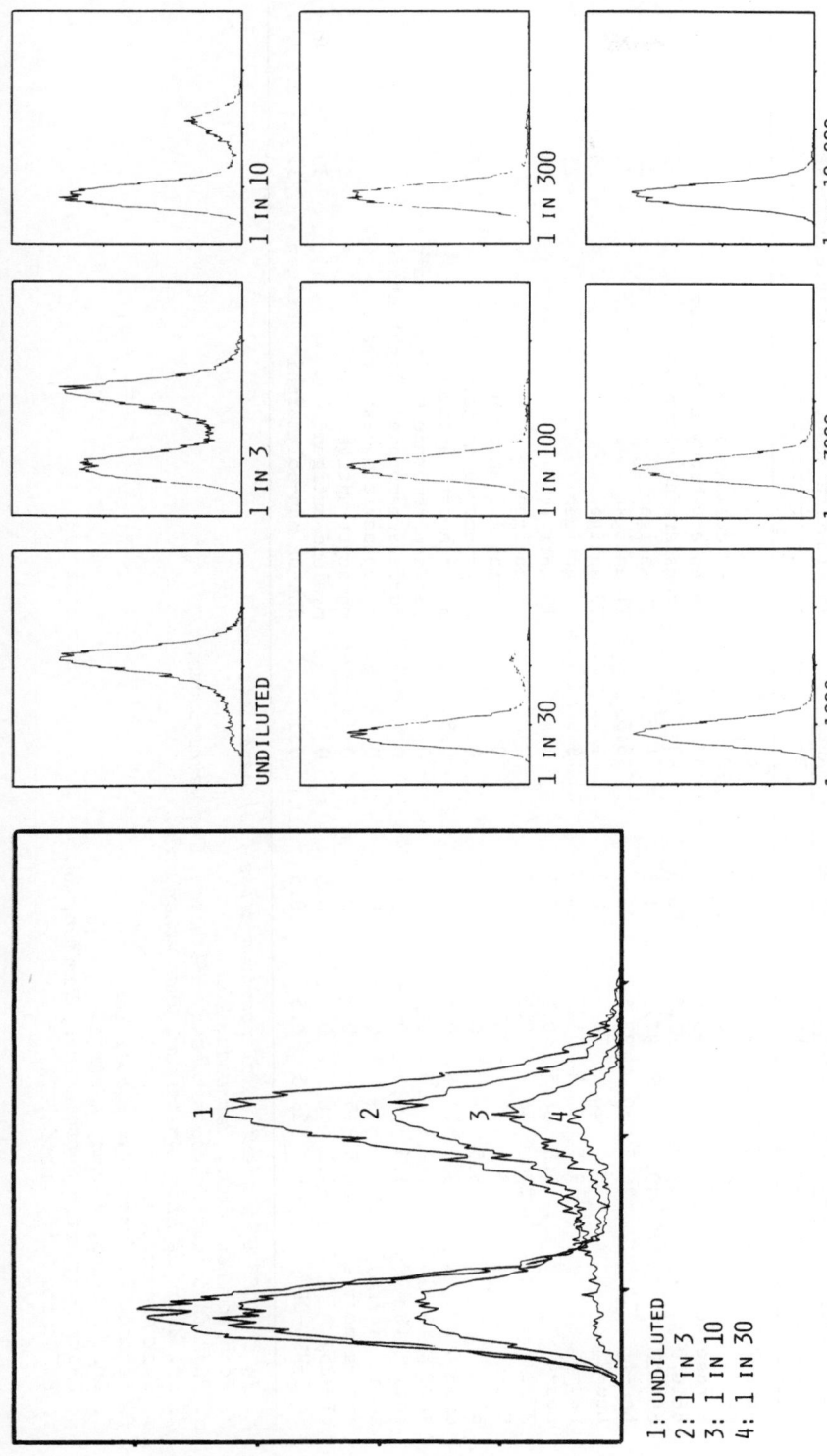

1: UNDILUTED
2: 1 IN 3
3: 1 IN 10
4: 1 IN 30

Figure 3. Fluorescence histograms from FACS analysis of thymocytes diluted with a mononuclear PB cell suspension, using the T6 antigen as a specific marker.

TABLE 2

Immunological characterization of patient 1 (T-NHL) and patient 2 (T-ALL) at diagnosis

Antibodies/ rosette	Patient 1 (T-NHL)[a]			Patient 2 (T-ALL)		Information about the antibodies/rosette used: Antigen recognized	Reference
	% positive cells						
	BM	PB	PE	BM	PB		
anti-TdT[b]	2.5	3.1	96.5	97.5	98	TdT	19
WT1[c]	16	43.5	98	98	100	pan-T cell antigen	20
E rosette	14	70	95	22.5	37	sheep erythrocyte receptor	21
66IG10[d]	11.5	4	92.5	86.5	99	transferrine receptor	22
66IIIE5[d]	0.5	3	97.5	1.5[e]	1.5[e]	T6 antigen	23
Leu-1[f]	26.5	50.5	98.5	97	96.5	T1 antigen	24
Leu-2[f]	23	26	78	0.5	1	T8 antigen	25
Leu-3[f]	9.5	37.5	41	14.5	16	T4 antigen	25
Leu-4[f]	19.5	36.5	0.5	0.5	1.5	T3 antigen	26
WT32[c]	21	46	0.5	0.5	0	T3 antigen	
VIL-A1[g]	3	2	74[e]	0.5	0	common ALL antigen	27
B1[h]	8.5	11	0	0.5	0.5	B lymphocyte antigen	28
Leu-10[f]	19.5	11.5	0.5	0.5	0.5	B lymphocyte antigen	
anti κ (Smκ)[i]	1	0.5	0	0	0	surface membrane κ light chain	
anti λ (Smλ)[i]	1.5	0.5	0	0	0	surface membrane λ light chain	
anti μ (cIgM)[b]	1	1	0	0	0	cytoplasmic μ heavy chain	
anti-monocyte	18.5	15	0	0	0	monocyte antigen	29
VIM-D5[g]	34.5	0	0	0.5	0	myeloid antigen	30
anti-HLA-DR[f]	41	23.5	0.5	0.5	0.5	HLA-DR non-polymorphic antigen	31

a. In the CSF of patient 1 TdT positive cells (2%) were detected.
b. Bethesda Res. Lab., Bethesda, MD.
c. Rijksinstituut Volksgezondheid, Bilthoven, The Netherlands.
d. Dr. M. van de Rijn, Amsterdam, The Netherlands.
e. Weak expression.
f. Becton Dickinson, Sunnyvale, CA.
g. Dr. W. Knapp, Vienna, Austria.
h. Ortho Diagnostic Systems Inc., Raritan, NJ.
i. Kallestad Lab., Austin, TX.

was successful and 4 months after diagnosis the patient is in complete
remission according to morphological criteria as well as combined IF assay
analyses, using WT1, 66IIIE5 and Leu-1 as T cell markers.
4.2. Patient 2. An 8-yr-old girl was diagnosed as having a T cell leukemia
with mediastinal enlargement and high white blood cell (WBC) count. The
lymphoblasts in BM and PB formed E rosettes and were positive for TdT, WT1,
66IG10 and Leu-1 (Table 2). After 6 weeks of induction treatment a remission
according to morphological criteria was achieved. Repeated morphological
BM examinations up to 4 months after diagnosis were consistent with
remission. However, immunological monitoring with the combined IF assay
revealed that cells with the T-ALL phenotype were still present in all BM
and PB samples tested (Table 3 and Figure 5). In the two CSF samples
tested no TdT positive cells were detected.

TABLE 3

Monitoring of patient 2 (T-ALL) up to 4.5 months after diagnosis.

	Apr.27 Diagnosis	May 26	June 7	June 29	Aug.25	Sept.1	Sept.15
Morphological characterization:							
BM cellularity x 10^9/l	1000	22	40	90	42	NT^a	NT
% lymphoblasts	96	7	4	1	1		
% lymphocytes	2	10	36	6	6		
acid phosphatase of blasts	+	+	NT	NT	NT		
PB WBC x 10^9/l	212	2.4	1.0	4.2	0.6	1.2	1.0
% lymphoblasts	93	3	0	0	0	0	0
% lymphocytes	4	41	62	11	20	43	29
Interpretation	T-ALL	PR^b	CR^c	CR	CR	CR	CR
Immunological characterization:							
BM % TdT	97.5	NT	1.2	NT	5.6	NT	NT
% WT1/TdT^d	97.5		0.2		4.9		
% Leu-1/TdT	97		0.2		4.4		
% T-ALL cells	97.5		0.2		4.4		
PB % TdT	98	NT	0.2	NT	2.6	0.22	1.75
% WT1/TdT	98		0.04		2.4	0.22	1.72
% Leu-1/TdT	96.5		0.04		2.4	0.21	1.70
% T-ALL cells	98		0.04		2.4	0.21	1.70
Interpretation	T-ALL		NR^e		NR	NR	NR

a. *NT = not tested;* b. *PR = partial remission;* c. *CR = complete remission;*
d. *% cells positive both for Leu-1 and TdT;* e. *NR = no remission*

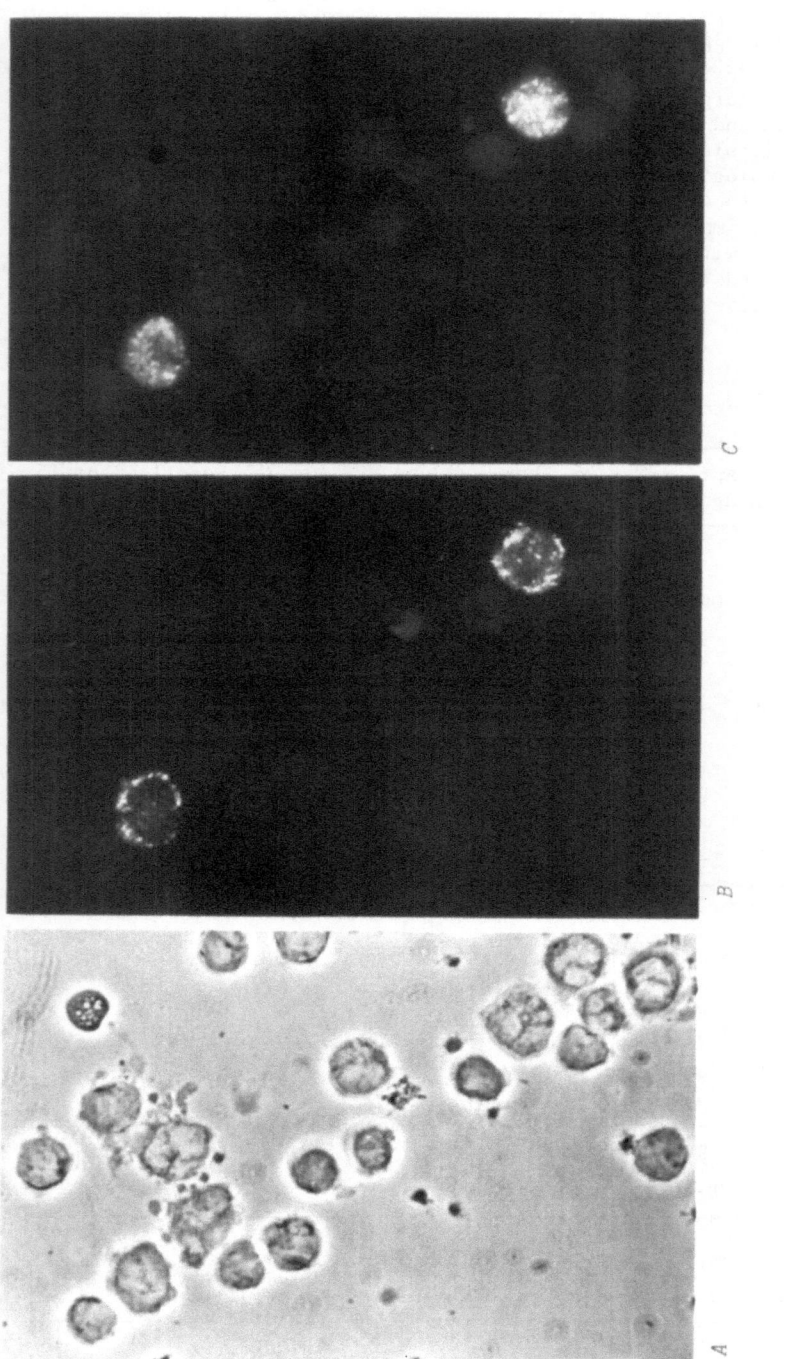

Figure 4. Micrographs of PB cells from patient 1 at diagnosis.
A: phase contrast morphology; B: 66IIIE5 (T6) positive cells
(FITC-labeled); C: TdT positive cells (TRITC-labeled); C: TdT positive cells
(FITC-labeled). The combined IF assay demonstrates that all TdT positive cells in the PB are also
positive for T6.

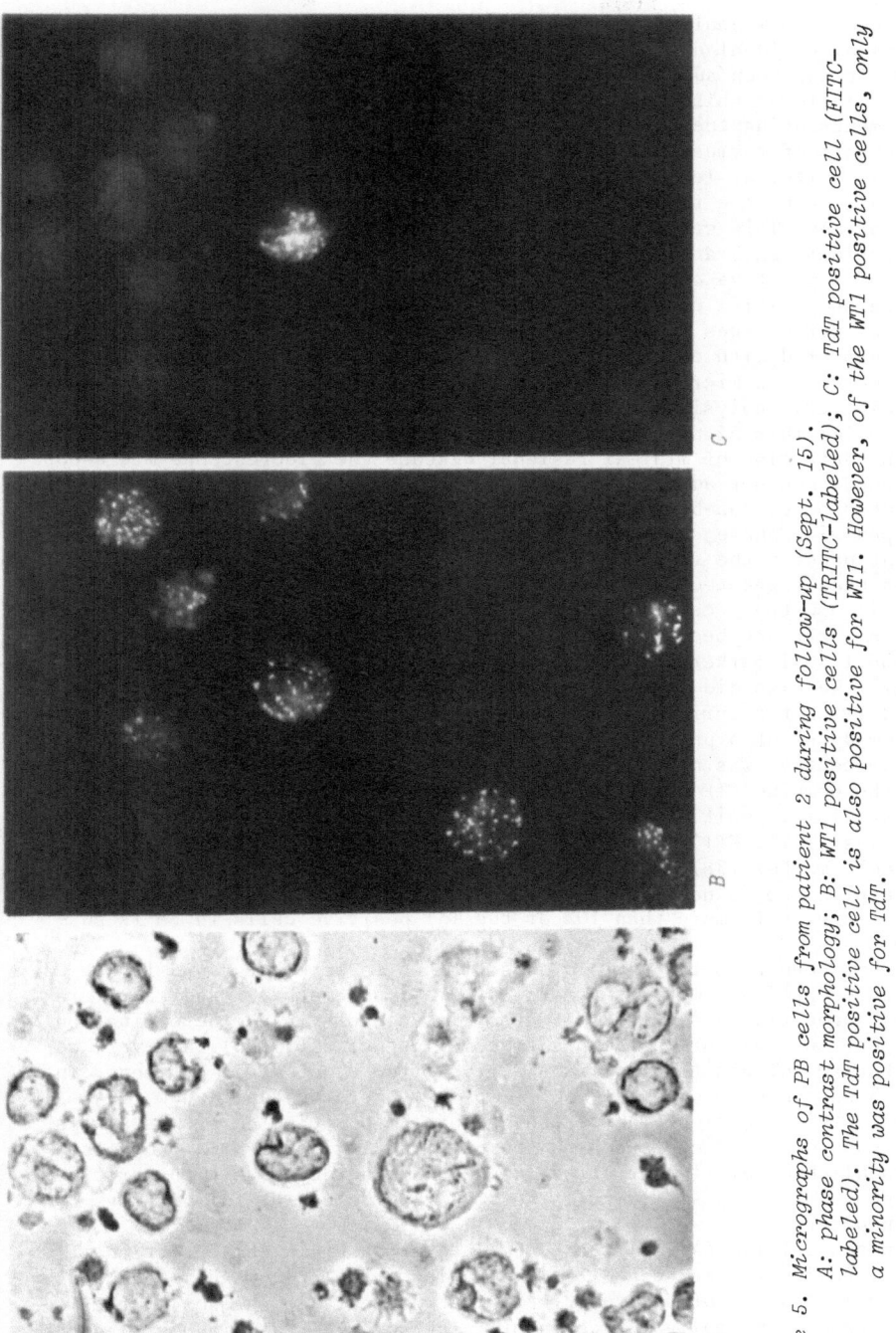

Figure 5. *Micrographs of PB cells from patient 2 during follow-up (Sept. 15). A: phase contrast morphology; B: WT1 positive cells (TRITC-labeled); C: TdT positive cell (FITC-labeled). The TdT positive cell is also positive for WT1. However, of the WT1 positive cells, only a minority was positive for TdT.*

5. DISCUSSION

Morphological analysis of BM smears has set the limit for the detection of minimal residual disease in leukemia patients at 5% of the nucleated cells. It has been suggested that the use of the combined IF assay or the FACS could lower this detection limit (5,10,13,14). Indeed, in dilution experiments using the T6 antigen as a specific marker we were able to detec low numbers of thymus cells and T-NHL cells. Very small numbers of T6 positive cells, at least down to 1 in 10,000 were detectable in the combine IF assay, using the fluorescence microscope to examine cytocentrifuge preparations. This sensitivity can be further enhanced by screening more preparations. FACS analysis of the same suspensions revealed a detection limit of 2 positive cells in 100 only, and in more diluted suspensions even false positive cells were scored. This indicates, in our opinion, that low percentages of positive cells detected by FACS analysis have to be interpreted with caution. Thus examination of the relevant markers with the fluorescence microscope is 500 times more sensitive than conventional morphological analysis and 200 times more sensitive than FACS analysis (Figure 1). This significant lower sensitivity of the FACS implies that for the detection of minimal residual disease the fluorescence microscope is needed. Another advantage of the use of the fluorescence microscope is that morphology can be correlated with immunological markers, if it is equipped with phase contrast facilities (3,35). For these reasons we doubt that at present the fluorescence microscope can be replaced by the FACS as has been suggested by some investigators (36).

Until now the T cell marker$^+$/TdT$^+$ phenotype, detectable by the combined IF assay, has not been found in extra-thymic locations (3,6-8). Even WT1, a broad T cell marker, has not been detected on TdT positive cells in the BM (37). We also did not find Leu-1$^+$/TdT$^+$ or T6 antigen$^+$/TdT$^+$ cells in BM and PB, but surprisingly, we did detect WT1$^+$/TdT$^+$ cells in regenerating BM from 6 out of 6 patients treated for non-T cell malignancies. However, this percentage was never higher than 5% of the TdT positive cells. Therefore the combined IF assay is indeed useful for the detection of minimal disease of TdT positive T cell malignancies, except perhaps for pre-T cell leukemias (TdT$^+$, WT1$^+$, E rosette$^-$, Leu-1$^-$, T6$^-$), which express only WT1 as T cell marker (38). In these cases the combined IF assay might still be useful since we never detected WT1$^+$/TdT$^+$ cells in PB and detection of WT1 positivity in more than 10% of the TdT positive cells in BM is suspicious.

It has been reported that TdT positive cells were not found in the CSF from three patients without hematologic malignancies (39) and therefore it was suggested that the TdT IF assay is valuable in the determination of meningeal involvement in TdT positive malignancies (39,40). However, we did observe TdT positive cells in the CSF from 3 out of 55 patients. In these 3 patients no clinical CNS relapse has occurred until now, 3-4 months after detection. The percentage of TdT positive cells was always lower than 0.2%, which resembles the critical limit for PB as suggested by Froehlich et al. (41). Further studies are needed to set the critical percentage of TdT positive cells for CNS involvement of TdT positive malignancies.

A potential limitation of the combined IF assay in the detection of minimal residual disease and the prediction of relapse might be caused by phenotypic changes of the tumor cells. At present, comparison of the phenotypes of the malignant cells of T-ALL and T-NHL at diagnosis and at relapse, however, suggests that the observed changes mostly concern minor alterations in the cell surface phenotype within the T cell differentiation lineage (10,34,41,42). Thus to avoid misdetection, a well chosen panel of T cell markers is needed.

Relapses in extra-medullary sites such as CNS or testis are frequently found in T-ALL. Therefore the combined IF assay (T cell marker/TdT) or at least the detection of TdT positive cells only must be used for the examination of the nucleated cells in the CSF (40), and, if possible, also in the evaluation of testis biopsies. Since the cells of most T-ALL and T-NHL relapses have a short doubling time, it is important to lower the detection level of the screening technique. However, the prediction of relapse is not only dependent on the sensitivity of the assay, but also on the frequency of the immunologic monitoring during follow-up. The high sensitivity of the combined IF assay in combination with a frequent control of the patient can partly overcome this problem.

As an illustration of the potential value of the combined IF assay we studied two patients with a TdT positive T cell malignancy.
Patient 1 presented with a T-NHL, classified according to clinical and morphological criteria as stage II. Using a.o. the combined IF assay, the lymphoma cells were not only detected in the PE, but also in BM, PB and CSF, revealing a more extensive dissemination of the lymphoma cells. Therefore, a stage IV classification should be more appropriate. In some NHL protocols local therapy alone is applied for stage I or II, but the percentage of patients with disease free survival is disappointingly low (44). Our findings explain why local treatment is insufficient in the majority of these patients and underline the tendency of NHL to be more widespread than suspected according to the usual morphological criteria. Thus the use of the combined IF assay leads to a better detection and consequently to better staging of TdT positive T-NHL.
Patient 2, who presented with a T-ALL, is in continuous complete remission according to clinical and morphological criteria. During 4.5 months of follow-up low percentages of leukemic T cells were persistently detected in the BM and PB using the combined IF assay with WT1 and Leu-1 as T cell markers. According to these immunological data this T-ALL patient actually never attained hematological remission. So far, however, the follow-up period is too short to evaluate the significance of this finding. If this patient indeed relapses within the next half year of maintenance treatment these immunological positive findings retrospectively may imply predictive value. Such findings can then be taken as an early indication to deliver more intensive or alternative treatment.

Summarizing we conclude that the described dilution experiments demonstrate that a routinely performed combined IF assay can detect small numbers of TdT positive T-ALL and T-NHL cells, down to 1 in 10,000 cells. Furthermore, the two case reports demonstrate that this technique can be used not only for the detection of minimal residual disease in TdT positive T cell malignancies, but also for the staging of TdT positive T-NHL at diagnosis, both having therapeutical consequences. The value of the combined IF assay for the prediction of relapse has still to be evaluated.

ACKNOWLEDGMENTS

We gratefully acknowledge Prof.Dr. R. Benner for his continuous support, Prof.Dr. W. Hijmans and Mrs. H.R.E. Schuit for their advice in immunofluorescence techniques, Mrs. I. Dekker for technical assistance, Dr. T. van Os for excellent photographic assistence, Dr. M. Poot for the help with FACS analyses and Mrs. C. Meijerink-Clerkx for typing the manuscript.

This work was supported by the Fund 'Geven voor Leven' of the Netherlands Cancer Foundation (Koningin Wilhelmina Fonds).

REFERENCES

1. Van Steensel-Moll HA, Valkenburg HA, van Zanen GE. 1983. Br J Cancer 47, 471.
2. Van der Reijden HJ, van Wering ER, van de Rijn JM, Melief CJM, van 't Veer MB, Behrendt H, von dem Borne AEGKr. 1983. Scand J Haematol 30, 356.
3. Janossy G, Bollum FJ, Bradstock KF, Ashley J. 1980. Blood 56, 430.
4. Greaves M, Delia D, Janossy G, Rapson N, Chessels J, Woods M, Prentice G. 1980. Leuk Res. 4, 15.
5. Bradstock KF, Janossy G, Hoffbrand AV, Ganeshaguru K, Llewellin P, Prentice HG, Bollum FJ. 1981. Br J Haematol 47, 121.
6. Bradstock KF, Janossy G, Pizzolo G, Hoffbrand AV, McMichael A, Pilch JR, Milstein C, Beverley P, Bollum FJ. 1980. J Nat Cancer Inst 65, 33
7. Janossy G, Tidman N, Papageorgiou ES, Kung PC, Goldstein G. 1981. J. Immunol. 126, 1608.
8. Greaves MF, Rao J, Hariri G, Verbi W, Catovsky D, Kung P, Goldstein G. 1981. Leuk Res 5, 281.
9. Kung PC, Long JC, McCaffrey RP, Ratliff RL, Harrison TA, Baltimore D. 1978. Am J Med 64, 788.
10. Bradstock KF, Janossy G, Tidman N, Papageorgiou ES, Prentice HG, Willoughby M, Hoffbrand AV. 1981. Leuk Res 5, 301.
11. Reinherz EL, Kung PC, Goldstein G, Levey RH, Schlossman SF. 1980. Proc Natl Acad Sci USA 77, 1588.
12. Fithian E, Kung P, Goldstein G, Rubenfeld M, Fenoglio C, Edelson R. 1981. Proc Natl Acad Sci USA 78, 2541.
13. De Bruin HG, Astaldi A, Leupers T, van de Griend RJ, Dooren LJ, Schellekens PThA, Tanke HG, Roos M, Vossen JM. 1981. J Immunol 127, 2
14. Ault KA. 1979. New Engl J Med 300, 1401.
15. Benner R, van Oudenaren A, Koch G. 1981. Immunological Methods, Vol. I. Lefkovits and B. Pernis, eds. (Academic press New York), p. 247.
16. Flandrin G, David MT. 1981. Methods in Hematology, Vol. 2, The Leukem Cell. D. Catovsky ed. (Churchill Livingstone, London), p. 29.
17. Böyum A. 1968. Scand J Clin Lab Invest 21, 77.
18. Roos D, Loos JA. 1970. Biochim Biophys Acta 222, 565.
19. Goldschneider I, Gregoire KE, Barton RW, Bollum FJ. 1977. Proc Natl Acad Sci 74, 734.
20. Tax WJM, Willems HW, Kibbelaar MDA, de Groot J, Capel PJA, de Waal RMW, Reekers P, Koene RAP. 1982. Protides of the Biological Fluids, Vol. 29, H. Peeters, ed. (Pergamon Press, Oxford), p. 701.
21. Moore AL, Zusman J. 1978. J Immunol Meth 23, 275.
22. Van de Rijn M, Geurts van Kessel AHM, Kroezen V, van Agthoven AJ, Terhorst C, Verstijnen K, Hilgers J. 1983. Cytogenet Cell Genet, in press.
23. Lerch PG, van de Rijn M, Schrier P, Terhorst C. 1983. Hum Immunol 6, 13.
24. Engleman EG, Warnke R, Fox RI, Dilley J, Benike CJ, Levy R. 1981. Proc Natl Acad Sci USA 58, 1791.
25. Engleman EG, Benike CJ, Glickman E, Evans RL. 1981. J Exp Med 153, 19
26. Ledbetter JA, Evans RL, Lipinski M, Cunningham-Rundles C, Good RA, Herzenberg LA. 1981. J Exp Med 153, 310.
27. Knapp W, Majdic O, Bettelheim P, Liszka K. 1982. Leuk Res 6, 137.
28. Stashenko P, Nadler LM, Hardy R, Schlossman SF. 1980. J Immunol 125,
29. Ugolini V, Nunez G, Smith GR, Stastny P, Capra JD. 1980. Proc Natl Acad Sci USA 77, 6764.
30. Majdic O, Liszka K, Lutz D, Knapp W. 1981. Blood 58, 1127.

31. Lampson LA, Levy R. 1980. J. Immunol. 125, 293.
32. Johnson GD, de C. Nogueira Araujo GM. 1981. J Immunol Meth 43, 349.
33. Raff MC, Megson M, Owen JJT, Cooper MD. 1976. Nature 259, 224.
34. Roper M, Crist WM, Metzgar R, Ragab AH, Smith S, Starling K, Pullen J, Leventhal B, Bartolucci AA, Cooper MD. 1983. Blood 61, 830.
35. Schuit HRE, Hijmans W. 1980. Clin Exp Immunol 41, 567.
36. Barr IG, Toh BH. 1983. J Clin Immunol 3, 184.
37. Tax W, Tidman N, Janossy G, Trejdosiewicz L, Willems R, Leeuwenberg J, de Witte T, Capel P, Koene R. Clin Exp Immunol in press.
38. Vodinelich L, Tax W, Bai Y, Pegram S, Capel P, Greaves MF. 1983. Blood in press.
39. Bradstock KF, Papageorgiou ES, Janossy G. 1981. Cancer 47, 2478.
40. Bradstock KF, Papageorgiou ES, Janossy G, Hoffbrand AV, Willoughby ML, Roberts PD, Bollum FJ. 1980. Lancet ii, 1144.
41. Froehlich TW, Buchanan GR, Cornet JAM, Sartain PA, Smith RG. 1981. Blood 58, 214.
42. Borella L, Casper JT, Lauer SJ. 1979. Blood 54, 64.
43. Bernard A, Raynal B, Lemerle J, Boumsell L. 1982. Blood 59, 809.
44. Chen MG, Prosnitz LR, Gonzalez-Serva A, Fisher DB. 1979. Cancer 43, 1245.

DETECTION OF EARLY RELAPSE AND MINIMAL RESIDUAL DISEASE IN CHILDREN WITH
ACUTE LYMPHOBLASTIC LEUKEMIA BY ENUMERATION OF TERMINAL DEOXYNUCLEOTIDYL
TRANSFERASE-POSITIVE CELLS IN PERIPHERAL BLOOD

GEORGE R. BUCHANAN AND R. GRAHAM SMITH

.. INTRODUCTION

Nearly 95% of children with acute lymphoblastic leukemia (ALL) enter
complete remission following 4 weeks of two- or three-drug induction
chemotherapy. However, recent advances in chemotherapy design, CNS
prophylaxis, and stratification according to risk factors have not prevented
leukemic relapse in nearly one-half of these patients (1,2).

One of the greatest stumbling blocks in the management of ALL is the
inability to detect minimal residual disease and accurately predict which
patients are destined to relapse (1). At the time of achieving complete
remission, affected patients are estimated to have leukemic burdens of 10^9
cells (3), but these malignant cells cannot be detected by standard
morphologic techniques in peripheral blood or bone marrow. Thus it is
uncertain whether a given patient in a chemotherapy-induced remission
has a cell burden of 10^9, 10^6, 10^3 or 0 - i.e., is in fact cured. The
possible detection of minimal residual disease in ALL has been a
subject of great interest. Discovery of a sensitive and specific
marker of minimal disease would be extremely useful at many stages of
the illness - (1) immediately after achievement of complete remission
in order to detect those patients destined to develop early relapse),
) during the prolonged course of maintenance therapy, and, in
particular, (3) at the time of elective cessation of chemotherapy.
Following 2-3 years of maintenance therapy, 20 to 25% of patients
develop a relapse (1), and a successful test which predicts imminent
relapse by detecting residual leukemic cells might allow
intensification of therapy with curative intent.
Several tests have recently been proposed as markers of minimal
residual disease in ALL. Leukemia-associated membrane antigens such as the

common ALL antigen initially seemed like promising candidates, but the presence of such antigens on populations of normal marrow cells (4) has ma the use of these membrane markers less attractive. In one study marrow fro ALL patients destined to relapse reacted in vitro with autologous peripher blood lymphocytes, whereas patients remaining in remission exhibited no su autoreactivity (5). Other investigators have examined marrow chromosomes b direct karyotyping or by analyzing DNA content by flow cytometry in ALL patients with aneuploid cell populations (6). Additional proposed markers minimal residual disease in leukemia have included serum ferritin measure- ments (7,8) and plasma fibrinopeptide A levels (9). Certain enzymes prese in ALL cells have also been studied as possible markers of persistent disease activity (10). For example, Glader has identified increased levels of adenosine deaminase in the marrow cells of children with T-cell ALL in remission who later develop a relapse (11). In our laboratory and in others, much attention has focused on terminal deoxynucleotidyl transfera (TdT) (12,13,14), and the purpose of this report is to describe results of our continued preliminary studies of TdT positive cells in peripheral bloo as a possible marker of minimal residual disease and predictor of early relapse in ALL.

2. TERMINAL DEOXYNUCLEOTIDYL TRANSFERASE

Terminal deoxynucleotidyl transferase (TdT) is an enzyme with the properties of a DNA polymerase which is present in normal thymocytes, in a small population of bone marrow mononuclear cells (15), and, as shown in c laboratory, in a minute number of circulating peripheral blood lymphocytes (12). In 1973 McCaffrey and Baltimore demonstrated that TdT was present ir the malignant cells of children with ALL (16), and subsequent studies fron their laboratory and others showed that the cells from the vast majority (over 90%) of patients with T cell and non-T cell ALL contain large quantities of the enzyme, as measured by direct assay or indirect immunofluoresence techniques (17). The presence of the enzyme in disease states is not specific for ALL however (15). The malignant cells in patier with lymphoblastic lymphoma, a closely related childhood T-cell malignanc) also contain the enzyme (15). Moreover, thirty percent of patients with chronic granulocytic leukemia in blast transformation have circulating Td1 positive leukocytes, which in most cases morphologically resemble lymphoblasts, and approximately 5 to 10% of patients with acute myelogenou leukemia exhibit cells containing the enzyme (17). Finally, TdT positive cells are observed in large numbers (up to 20%) in the mononuclear cell fraction from bone marrow in normal children and in patients with diverse malignancies (including solid tumors) who are recovering from chemotherapy-induced aplasia (17). These cells probably represent an expansion of the TdT-positive cell population present in normal marrow (18).

Since the development of techniques to accurately measure TdT-positive cells in peripheral blood and marrow, investigators have used these assays for two purposes: (1) as a diagnostic test for ALL, and (2) as a possible marker of minimal residual disease in patients with ALL in hematologic remission (15). The cell lineage of a significant percentage of leukemias in both children and adults is poorly defined by standard morphological techniques, and the presence of TdT positivity provides strong evidence for a lymphoid origin (15). The presence of the enzyme in the great majority of lymphoblasts in patients with ALL has generated much interest in the measurement of TdT positive cells during remission to determine whether minimal disease is present (13,15).

DETECTION OF MINIMAL RESIDUAL DISEASE BY MEASURING TdT-POSITIVE CELLS:
Since TdT positivity is a sensitive albeit somewhat non-specific marker of leukemic lymphoblasts, the numbers of TdT-positive cells or the TdT enzyme activity within a cell population have been measured in ALL patients during remission in order to determine whether elevations persist during remission in some patients and then increase prior to relapse as defined by standard morphologic techniques (12,13,18).

Most studies thus far have focused on serial measurements of TdT in bone marrow. The marrow in patients with ALL contains large numbers of TdT positive cells at diagnosis and also at the time of marrow relapse (13,18). Several studies have shown that during remission TdT-positive cells in marrow are usually within the normal range - i.e., less than 2% of the total (19-21). Miller et al studied TdT in 23 marrow samples from 15 patients with ALL in remission and were unable to detect the enzyme in 13 patients. One subject with 4% positive cells developed a marrow relapse 5 weeks later, and another patient remained in remission despite having persistently elevated (2-4%) TdT-positive cells over a 6 month period (20). Of 19 patients with ALL in remission studied by Muelich et al (19) only 2 had greater than 2% TdT-positive cells in their bone marrow. In addition, 38 c 49 ALL patients studied by Stass et al (21) had fewer than 1% TdT-positive cells in their marrow during remission. Of 11 patients with elevated values, only 2 subsequently developed a marrow relapse, and both of them ha less than 1% TdT-positive marrow cells 3 months earlier. Lauer and co-workers (14) studied 52 patients with ALL using a new technique (countercurrent centrifugal elutriation) to concentrate the bone marrow lymphoid cells and found similar numbers (7-10%) of TdT-positive cells in normal subjects and ALL patients in remission who did not subsequently relapse. However, 11 additional patients who later relapsed had 25-80% TdT-positive lymphoid cells at a time when relapse could not be confirmed (morphologic grounds alone (14).

There are several problems with reliance on serial study of TdT-positive cells in marrow specimens for detection of minimal disease. Firstly, the high "background" of 1% or more TdT positive cells in many normal marrow specimens precludes such an analysis from being particularly sensitive (17,18). TdT may be present in up to 30% of marrow cells during recovery from chemotherapy-induced myelosuppression (15), so this test would be of little value in patients with high risk ALL receiving inten-sive intermittent chemotherapy treatments. Secondly, an accurate test for minimal residual disease should allow for frequent serial sampling without great discomfort and expense to the patient (12). Most ALL treatment protocols require surveillance bone marrows only every 2-4 months, interva not sufficiently frequent for the desired close monitoring of disease activity.

For these reasons, several years ago our laboratory began to examine peripheral blood of normal subjects and patients with ALL in remission in order to determine whether these measurements might accurately predict relapse. Since the TdT enzyme assay is insensitive when small numbers of enzyme-containing cells are present (12,15,18), we developed a method for counting TdT-positive cells by the standard indirect immunofluorescence technique using anti-sera against purified bovine TdT (12). Normal subjec were found to have small numbers (3 to 4 per 10,000 mononuclear cells) of TdT-positive cells circulating in their peripheral blood. Values for TdT-positive cells were similar in normal children (0.036 ± 0.014%) and adults (0.030 ± 0.015%). Children without ALL who were receiving cyclic chemotherapy for solid tumors had a similar value (0.040 ± 0.031%) but a wider degree of fluctuation. TdT-positive cells were also examined in 15 patients with ALL or lymphoblastic lymphoma in remission. Three of these patients subsequently developed a marrow relapse during the period of study, and each of them demonstrated elevated (over 0.11%) and/or progressively increasing numbers of TdT-positive cells 3-8 weeks prior to marrow relapse. These increased numbers of TdT-positive cells were present without abnormal physical findings, altered routine hematologic parameters, presence of blasts on peripheral blood smear, or other clinical or laboratory evidence of relapse (12). Forty-six determinations of TdT in peripheral blood were made in the 8 patients with ALL who continued in remission, and none of them exhibited elevated numbers of TdT-positive cells. Three additional patients in marrow remission but with extramedullary relapse were studied. One of them sporadically had slightly increased numbers of TdT-positive cells during treatment of a refractory meningeal relapse, but no progressive increase was present. An additional patient in this initial study had serial TdT peripheral blood measurements during induction of remission (12). Abnormally increased numbers of TdT-positive cells in peripheral blood persisted despite rapid disappearance of morphologically identifiable blasts. Four weeks later the patient's aspirated bone marrow contained large numbers of blasts, suggesting that failure of TdT positive cells to rapidly decline into the normal range might indicate a persistent leukemic cell burden and predict induction failure (12).

The only other published study evaluating the utility of serial blood sampling for TdT-positive mononuclear cells during remission of ALL is that of Hutton and co-workers (13). Using the less sensitive quantitative enzyme assay, they observed that 64% of patients had elevated (3 standard deviations above the mean value during remission) TdT activity at the time of relapse. They concluded, however, that wide fluctuations in enzyme activity during remission precluded the use of this assay for predicting relapse (13).

CONTINUED STUDIES OF PERIPHERAL BLOOD TdT-POSITIVE CELLS IN ALL

During the past 2 years our laboratory has continued to examine the utility of assessing TdT-positive mononuclear cells in peripheral blood of patients with ALL in remission. Twenty-three children, whose cells were shown at diagnosis to contain TdT, were selected for study (Table 1). Thes children were in intermediate and high risk groups, and their parents consented to serial blood sampling for assay of TdT-positive cells. Eight c the children were in their initial complete remission, whereas 15 had previously developed one or more relapses, placing them into a particularly high-risk category (2). The patients were treated with a variety of chemotherapy regimens and all were followed closely with physical examinations and routine CBCs every 1 to 4 weeks. In some instances periodic surveillance bone marrow examinations were performed, but in 9 of the children marrow examinations were not required by protocol and hence n performed unless relapse was suspected.

TdT-positive cells in peripheral blood were analyzed according to previously described methods (12). Briefly, a 2 cc sample of peripheral blood was fractionated on a Ficoll-Hypaque gradient, and the mononucler cells were cytocentrifuged onto glass slides, air dried, and fixed. The cells were reacted with a specific rabbit antibody against bovine TdT and then counterstained with an immunofluorescent-labeled goat antibody agains rabbit immunoglobulin. The percentage of fluorescent cells was enumerated scanning several fields; a minimum of 10,000 cells were counted, and typically 30,000 to 100,000 cells were scanned in each assay.

During and after the 2-year period of study, 14 of the 23 patients continued in complete marrow remission. All of these patients (# 1 to 14 i Table 1) were studied on at least 5 separate occasions, and 5 patients wer studied on 10 or more separate occasions at intervals of 2 to 8 weeks. The median value for TdT-positive peripheral blood cells in these 14 patients was 0.024%. No TdT-positive cells were evident in 74 of the specimens, and only 1 of the 128 measurements was greater than 0.11%, a value shown in ou previous study to be the upper limit of normal (12). This single elevated value occurred in patient 12, a child with T-cell ALL who remains in complete marrow remission 14 months later and who has subsequently had several peripheral blood TdT measurements in the normal range. Each of th 14 patients remains in marrow remission 18 to 48 months since initiation this study. Chemotherapy has been electively discontinued in 10 of them; children still receive chemotherapy, one of whom has since developed extramedullary relapse (see below).

TABLE 1: DESCRIPTION OF STUDY POPULATION: 23 PATIENTS WITH ACUTE LYMPHOBLASTIC LEUKEMIA

Patient No.	Age at diagnosis (yr),sex		Site (number) of prior relapses	No. of separate measurements	TdT Assays % positive cells (Range)
Patients remaining in marrow remission during study:					
1	3	M	CNS	9	.016 - .022*
2	4	M	Testes	5	0 - .080
3	2	F		7	0 - .021
4	4	F	CNS	5	0 - .005
5	2	F		5	.013 - .034
6	1	M		9	0 - .073
7	4	F	BM	9	0 - .038
8	6	M		5	0 - .025
9	4	M		12	0 - .016
10	10	F		13	0 - .041
11	7	M		13	0 - .066
12	9	M		6	0 - .250
13	8	M	BM	10	0 -
14	3	M	BM,Testes	19	0 - .021
Patients developing marrow relapse during study:					
15	7	F	BM	6	0 - 1.8
16	13	M	BM	12	0 - 25.8
17	9	F	BM (2)	7	0 - 1.00
18	2	M	BM (2)	13	0 - 6.52
19	8	M	BM	2	.003 - .240
20	14	M	BM,CNS	3	0 - 1.47
21	2	M	BM,Testes	10	.004 - 62.4
22	1 4/12	M	BM	3	0
23	2	M	BM (2)	10	.014 - 44.0

Abbreviations: CNS = central nervous system; BM = bone marrow
A value of 0 means that no positive cells were seen in at least 10^4 cells examined; i.e., < 0.01% TdT-positive cells were present.

TABLE 2:   PATIENTS WITH INCREASED AND/OR RISING NUMBERS OF TdT-POSITIVE
           CELLS PRIOR TO MARROW RELAPSE*

Patient No.	Days prior to marrow relapse*	% TdT positive cells in peripheral blood	% Blasts in peripheral blood***
15	63	0	0
	21**	1.8	0
	0	-	42
16	52	0	0
	45	0	0
	38	0	0
	31**	4.2	0
	7	-	0
	0	25.8	9
17	80	.003	0
	28**	1.0	0
	0	-	11
18	70	0	0
	35**	0.28	0
	14	6.52	0
	7	-	0
	0	-	48
19	28**	0.24	0
	0	9	0
20	36	0	0
	26**	1.47	0
	20	0.17	0
	0	-	93
21	21**	0.52	0
	7	-	0
	0	62.4	1

* Relapse confirmed by presence of M_3 marrow on Day 0
**Elevated % of TdT-positive cells first observed
***As recorded on 100 to 250 cell differential WBC counts

Nine additional patients (#15 to 23) developed a bone marrow rel
during the period of study. Unfortunately, peripheral blood TdT spec
could not be obtained from each of them at regular intervals prior to
relapse. However, it can be seen in Table 2 that 7 of the 9 patients
elevated (>0.11%) numbers of TdT positive cells identifiable in perip
blood 21 to 35 days prior to any clinical or laboratory evidence of m
relapse. Several of the patients (e.g., # 16) had had multiple norma
measurements prior to the initial elevation preceding the relapse. Bo

marrow aspirates were not performed in these 7 patients at the time of the
first TdT elevation, since the assays were often performed retrospectively
after the relapse had been diagnosed. When relapse was confirmed by the
presence of an M_3 marrow (>25% lymphoblasts), the percentage of
TdT-positive cells in peripheral blood was always greater than the
accompanying percentage of morphologically identifiable blasts in the blood.
This observation is illustrated in Table 2 (patients #16 and 21), was
characteristic of several additional patients under study who were not among
the 23 children who had serial sampling performed (Table 3), and confirms
our earlier finding (12). The reasons for this difference are twofold.
First, mononuclear cells are concentrated prior to staining for TdT. This
enhances the detection of infrequent leukemic cells. Second, TdT positive
cells may be deceptively small, and when infrequent may be overlooked in
differential counts (12).

TABLE 3: THE PERCENTAGE OF TdT-POSITIVE CELLS AND THE PERCENTAGE OF BLASTS
IDENTIFIABLE BY MORPHOLOGY IN PERIPHERAL BLOOD AT TIME OF RELAPSE

Patient No.	% TdT positive cells in peripheral blood at time of relapse	% Blasts in peripheral blood* at time of relapse
25	3.73	0
	0.74	0
26	19.3	0
27	18.0	0
	4.76	0
	6.96	2

* As recorded on 100 to 250 cell differential WBC count.

Two patients (#22 and 23 in Table 1) developed a marrow relapse during
the study but did not exhibit increased TdT-positive peripheral blood
leukocytes when tested 28 and 63 days prior to confirmation of the relapse
(Table 4). In neither patient, however, was frequent sampling performed.

TABLE 4: PATIENTS WITHOUT INCREASED AND/OR RISING NUMBERS OF TdT-POSITIVE
CELLS PRIOR TO MARROW RELAPSE*

Patient No.	Days prior to marrow relapse*	% TdT positive cells in peripheral blood	% Blasts in peripheral blood**
22	76	0	0
	28	0	0
	0	-	0
23	104	.067	0
	63	.014	0
	28	-	0
	15	-	0
	0	31.0	2.5

* Relapse confirmed by presence of M_3 marrow on Day 0.
** As recorded on 100-250 cell differential WBC count.

Our initial study showed no progressive increase in TdT-positive
peripheral blood cells during extramedullary relapse (12). This finding
confirmed in 2 of our patients (#10 and 20) who, at the time of isolate
meningeal relapse, had no identifiable TdT-positive cells in their
peripheral blood. Although this finding suggests that there might be no
traffic of leukemic cells in the peripheral blood "en route" to the mar
from the central nervous system, the presence of extremely small number
these cells cannot be excluded.

5. DISCUSSION

The ideal test for detection of residual leukemia in ALL would be
capable of identifying one malignant cell among 10^3 to 10^6 normal cells
None of the proposed techniques for assessing minimal residual disease,
including the one described here, has this degree of sensitivity. Howe
assessment of bone marrow morphology usually allows only 10 to 20 cells
among 100 normal cells to be reliably identified as leukemic blasts. In
addition, bone marrow surveillance is expensive, time consuming, and
traumatic to the child. A test using peripheral blood would accordingly
many advantages, even if it lacked extreme sensitivity.

The search for a leukemia-specific marker has eluded investigators
far. The studies described here suggest that a non-specific test can t

utilized for detecting minimal disease and possibly predicting marrow relapse. Futher carefully designed prospective studies are necessary. Particular focus will need to be placed upon serial sampling of peripheral blood at rigorously defined intervals of 2-4 weeks in order to accurately assess the time pattern of TdT positivity and elevations prior to relapse. When elevated TdT-positive peripheral blood cells are first observed in selected study patients, the results must be promptly correlated with a Wright Giemsa-stained buffy coat preparation from peripheral blood and, in particular, with the morphology of the bone marrow aspirate. It is possible that a more detailed study of the peripheral blood and bone marrow by standard morphology may be just as senstive as enumeration of TdT-positive peripheral blood cells. If peripheral blood TdT positive cells are elevated and rising only when the marrow is clearly diagnostic of relapse i.e., M_3, the test proposed here may still have value in prompting the performance of a bone marrow examination when one would otherwise not be done. On the other hand, if the marrow does not confirm the presence of relapse, the finding of elevated peripheral blood TdT-positive mononuclear cells might truly be a marker of minimal residual disease and then allow for intensification of chemotherapy with potential cure still a goal. All of these considerations do assume that early identification of relapse is beneficial to the patient by allowing more intensive treatment, an hypothesis which is yet unproven (22).

6. CONCLUSION

The results of our continued studies confirm the preliminary observations that TdT-positive cells appear in peripheral blood prior to the appearance of blasts identifiable by morphology in children with ALL who develop marrow relapse. These measurements may be useful in predicting imminent relapse. It is uncertain at this time whether measurement of TdT-positive cells in peripheral blood represents a sensitive test for minimal residual disease, however. Perhaps a dual marker assay, using TdT as well as another enzyme present in leukemia cells or an associated chromosomal marker, might permit the necessary sensitivity . Additional studies in our laboratory will be aimed at further characterizing the sequential patterns of TdT-positive peripheral blood cell numbers during initial induction therapy, prior to marrow relapse, and in the presence of extramedullary leukemia.

REFERENCES

1. Simone JV. 1980. The treatment of acute lymphoblastic leukaemia.
    Br J Haematol 45:1-4.
2. Mauer AM. 1980. Therapy of acute lymphoblastic leukemia in
    childhood. Blood 56:1-10.
3. Arlin ZA, Fried J. Clarkson BD. 1978. Therapeutic role of cell
    kinetics in acute leukaemia. Clin Haematol 7:339-362.
4. Greaves M, Delia D, Janossy G, Rapson N, Chessells J, Woods M,
    Prentice G. 1980. Acute lymphoblastic leukaemia associated antigen.
    IV Expression on non-leukaemic 'lymphoid' cells. Leukemia Res
    1:15-32.
5. Kumar S, Carr TF, Hann IM, Jones PHM, Evans DIK. 1978. Immunological
    detection of residual leukaemic disease in the bone marrow of
    children with acute lymphoblastic leukaemia. Br Med J 1:544-546.
6. Walle A, Andreeff M, Clarkson BD. 1982. Monitoring of submicroscopic
    levels of aneuploid leukemia cells following induction therapy. Proc
    Amer Society of Clinical Oncology, p. 189.
7. Koller ME, Romslo I, Finne PH, Haneberg B. 1979. Serial
    determinations of serum ferritin in children with acute
    lymphoblastic leukemia. Acta Paediatr Scand 68:93-96.
8. Siimes MA, Wang WC, Dallman PR. 1977. Elevated serum ferritin in
    children with malignancies. Scand J Haematol 19:153-158.
9. Myers TJ, Rickles FR, Barb C, Cronlund M. 1981. Fibrinopeptide A in
    acute leukemia: relationship of activation of blood coagulation to
    disease activity. Blood 57:518-525.
10. Van Der Weyden MB, Ellims PH, Gan TE. 1983. Enzymatic markers in
    lymphoproliferative disorders. Am J Hematol 14:301-311.
11. Glader BE. 1983. Personal communication.
12. Froehlich TW, Buchanan GR, Cornet JAM, Sartain PA, Smith RG. 1981.
    Terminal deoxynucleotidyl transferase-containing cells in peripheral
    blood: implications for the surveillance of patients with
    lymphoblastic leukemia or lymphoma. Blood 58:214-220. Hutton JJ,
13. Coleman MS, Moffitt S, Greenwood MF, Holland P, Lampkin B, Kisker T,
    Krill C, Kastelic JE, Valdez L, Bollum FJ. 1982. Prognostic
    significance of terminal transferase activity in childhood acute
    lymphoblastic leukemia: a prospective analysis of 164 patients.
    Blood 60:1267-1276.
14. Lauer S, Lyman S, Kirchner P, Gottschall J, Camitta B, Casper J.
    Terminal transferase surveillance of remission bone marrows in
    childhood acute lymphoblastic leukemia: improved sensitivity with
    countercurrent centrifugal elutriation. Submitted for publication.
15. Bollum FJ. 1979. Terminal deoxynucleotidyl transferase as
    hematopoietic cell marker. Blood 54:1203-1215.
16. McCaffrey R, Smoler DF, Baltimore D. 1973. Terminal deoxynucleotidyl
    transferase in a case of childhood acute lymphoblastic leukemia.
    Proc Nat Acad Sci USA 70:521-525, 1973.
17. Kalwinsky DK, Weatherred WH, Dahl GV, Borman WP, Melvin SL, Coleman
    MS, Bollum FJ. 1981. Clinical utility of initial terminal
    deoxynucleotidyl transferase determinations in childhood acute
    leukemias. Cancer Res 41:2877-2881.
18. Bradstock KF, Janossy G, Hoffbrand AV, Ganeshaguru K, Llewellin P,

Prentice HG, Bollum FJ. 1981. Immunofluorescent and biochemical studies of terminal deoxynucleotidyl transferase in treated acute leukaemia. Br J Haematol 47:121-131.

19. Muehleck SD, McKenna RW, Gale PF, Brunning RD. 1983. Terminal deoxynucleotidyl transferase (TdT)-positive cells in bone marrow in the absence of hematologic malignancy. Am J Clin Path 79:277-283.

20. Miller WM, Stass SA, Schumacher HR, Bollum FJ. 1981. Terminal-deoxynucleotidyl-transferase immunofluorescence on bone marrow smears: serial studies on 28 patients. Am J Hematol 10:1-7.

21. Stass SA, McGraw TP, Folds JD, Odle B, Bollum FJ. 1981. Terminal transferase in acute lymphoblastic leukemia in remission. Am J Clin Path 75:838-840.

22. Komp DM, Fischer DB, Sabio H, McIntosh S. 1983. Frequency of bone marrow aspirates to monitor acute lymphoblastic leukemia in childhood. J Pediatr 102:395-397.

PRINCIPLES OF THERAPY OF MALIGNANCY EXTRAPOLATED FROM A RAT
MODEL OF LEUKEMIA TO MAN

P.J. BURKE

INTRODUCTION

Stimulation of tumor regrowth by the effect of the initial
drug in a sequence promotes sensitivity of the perturbed residual
tumor to cell cycle specific drugs. This persistent and predictable growth enhancement has led to the empiric design of trials in
man. Such schema assume that the proliferative rate of leukemia
is low, and the initial drug(s) is given to reduce tumor mass and
induce greater proliferation of the residual tumor. A repeat dose
of an antimetabolite given at the predictable time of greatest
sensitivity produces good antitumor effects. Our timed sequential
therapy includes cytosine arabinoside (ara-C), $2gm/m^2$ given by
continuous 72 h infusion begun on day 1 and repeated on day 10,
the predicted time of maximal tumor growth (Fig. 1). The high
dose rate of ara-C is based on pharmacologic considerations and
evidence from our laboratory models of a dose response of tumor
reduction and enhanced survival. These trials in man have resulted in a significant kill of leukemic cells and a high percentage of long, chemotherapy-free remissions (1,2).

During these human treatments we conducted similar studies
in a rat model of acute leukemia, collecting evidence that
following initial therapy the growth and thereby drug sensitivity
of the previously quiescent tumor relates directly to an effect
of the initial drug on the host. This host response, the elabora-
tion of substances that regulate normal bone marrow growth, but
similarly effect the growth of hematopoietic malignancy is proportional to the degree of bone marrow aplasia.

Because of the curative results of a second cycle of timed
sequential therapy in the leukemic rat with minimal residual

disease we extended our human trials to include 1 intensive
course of sequential drugs following induction of remission.
The duration of remission achieved in those 20 patients is sign
ficantly greater than that after one course.

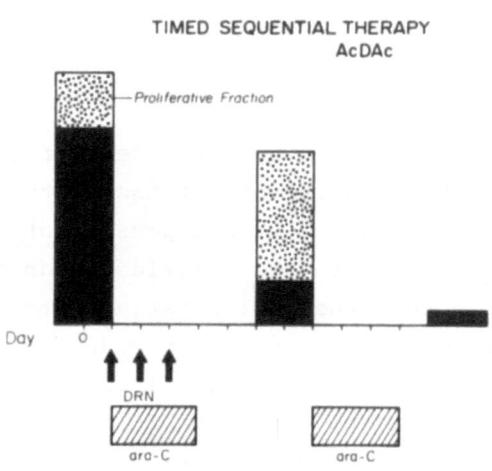

FIGURE 1. The therapeutic model of timed sequential chemothera
in man (AC-D-AC$_{10}$): 2 gm/m^2 of ara-C is given by continuous in
sion over 72 h, and 45 mg/m^2 DNR is given IV push on days 1,2
3. The ara-C infusion is repeated beginning on day 10. Closed
circles (o) represent cells in cycle, open circles (o) cells in
G_0. Arrows represent recruitment of cells from $G_0 \to G_1$. The dot
line represents the combined effect of the 1st drug on HSA. No
drugs are given in remission.

This report summarises these studies which demonstrate the
salutary effect of drugs given in high dose to reduce tumor mas
and recruit tumor cells to further high dose drug sensitivity.
The sequence trials and the dose-response curves support the
postulate that adequate initial tumor kill must be achieved to
produce an increase in the proliferative index of residual
leukemic cells. Maximal prolongation of life is achieved with
sequence at that time, confirming the temporal correlation of
tumor growth and response.

Methods and Results

Timed Sequential Therapy in Humans with AML-Remission Induction

One of the most effective drugs for the treatment of human AML, ara-C is toxic exclusively to cells which are actively synthesizing DNA. However, it is rapidly metabolized and therefore unavailable to leukemic cells in cycle but not synthesizing DNA or dormant at the time of administration. Consequently, the effectiveness ara-C can be increased by interrupted infusions in a timed sequence to take advantage of the increase in growth fraction resulting from perturbation by the initial drug.

In adults with AML we applied an empirically derived therapy (AC-D-AC$_{10}$) and withheld further drug in remission in order to study the effect of the initial induction therapy. The results relative to remission induction (60%) and the duration of unmaintained remission (UCR) are shown in Figure 2.

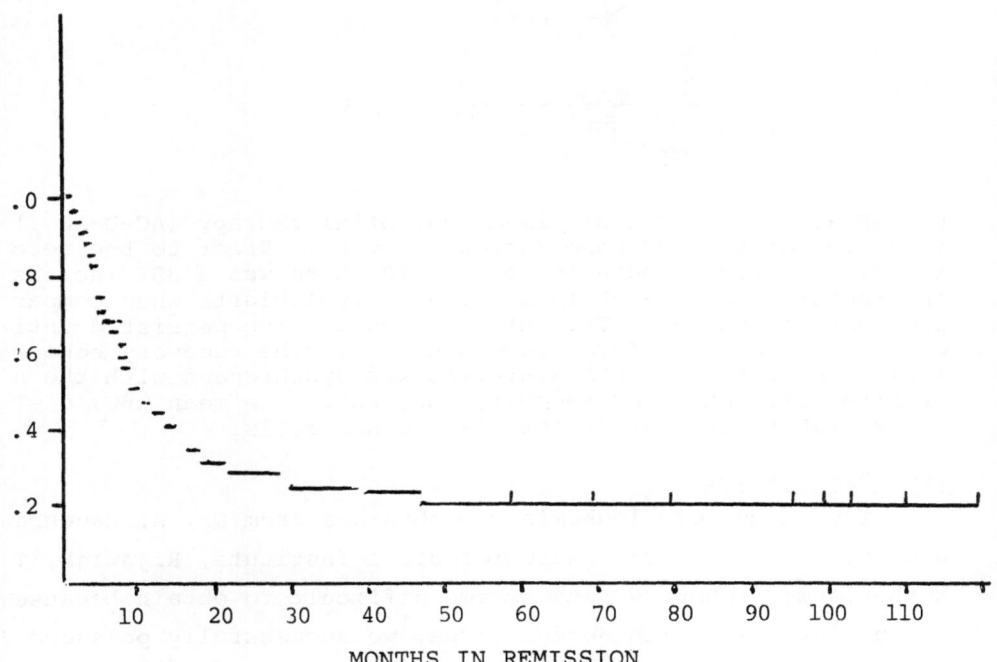

FIGURE 2. Probability of remaining in first complete remission without chemotherapy after a single cycle of AC-D-AC$_{10}$ (34 patients).

The effect of drug on bone marrow aplasia and recovery, and
the magnitude of induced humoral stimulatory activity (HSA)
and its kinetics are depicted in Figure 3.

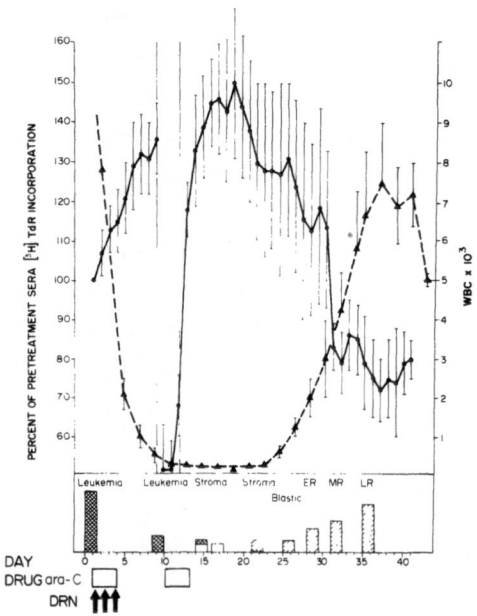

FIGURE 3. The effect of timed sequential therapy (AC-D-AC$_{10}$)
induction of HSA and bone marrow recovery. Prior to the seco
infusion of ara-C beginning on day 10 there was a 35% increas
incorporation of ^{3}H-TdR into cultured myeloblasts when compar
pretreatment values. This stimulation in vivo persisted unti
early proliferative forms were present in the recovery bone m
(ER). Inhibition of DNA synthesis was synchronous with the n
proliferative phase of recovery (MR, LR). = mean WBC, o =
CPM ^{3}H-TdR incorporation into target AML cells.

The LBN-ML Model

The BN myeloid leukemia was obtained from Dr. A. Hagenbe
and Dr. DW van Bekkum, Radiobiological Institute, Rijswijk, T
Netherlands. When BN rats became difficult to obtain because
colony infection with Sendai virus, we successfully passaged
tumor in available F$_1$ hybrid Lewis by BN (3). Growth charact
tics and morphology appear unaltered after 100 passages. Our
data, and those obtained by A. Hagenbeek, et al, clearly demc
strate that this tumor has characteristics desirable in an ar

model of AML. Following intravenous (IV) inoculation, there is wide dissemination and growth of cells in the spleen, liver, and bone marrow, which have cytologic and histochemical characteristics of progranulocytic leukemia (4). As in the human, these cells fail to form normal colonies in agar, and suppress colony formation by normal bone marrow CFU-c and hematopoiesis in vivo (5). Analysis of cell kinetics parameters with an [3H] TdR pulse-labeling technique and autoradiography reveal that characteristics developing during the natural cause of the disease are quite comparable to those observed in human AML (6). In the LBN rat, there is a dose-response survival curve with 100% mortality in a close time-span. Five days prior to death, the normal femoral bone marrow elements are completely replaced by a monotony of cells with the morphology of progranulocytes, and easily accessible for sequential kinetic determinations. Death occurs with a rapidly rising cell count associated with disseminated intravascular coagulation and leukostasis.

Sequential Therapy in the Rat

Using a rodent model with late stage disease (LSD) as a bioassay, we have been able to conduct large numbers of trials not possible in man to develop principles of therapy (7). These demonstrated that the dose of the initial drug in sequence truly correlates with an increased tumor growth and bestows sensitivity to cytotoxic drugs. Demonstration of this enhancement of drug effect in sequence requires that the dose of initial drug be great enough to reduce the tumor mass, and stimulate HSA and growth of residual tumor. No synergistic effect on increased life span (ILS) was achieved at the initial dose of ara-C (50 mg/kg Q8h x 6), which did not cause an increase in the LI on day 6, whereas doubling that dose resulted in an increased LI and ILS. Enhanced survival was achieved in all groups treated in sequences up to day 8, the maximal in group 0,6. When compared using the Wilcoxan Rank Sum test, the survival of those treated on day 0,6 was significantly longer than in those treated by longer sequences (P<0.001) by shorter sequences (P<0.005). The extent to which survival is increased by sequential therapy corresponded to the increase HSA and the LI of the residual tumor at the time of beginning

102

the second course of treatment. The most marked effect of
prolonged survival occurred in the 0,6 group, in which the sec
drug was administered at the time of peak HSA and tumor LI
(Figure 4).

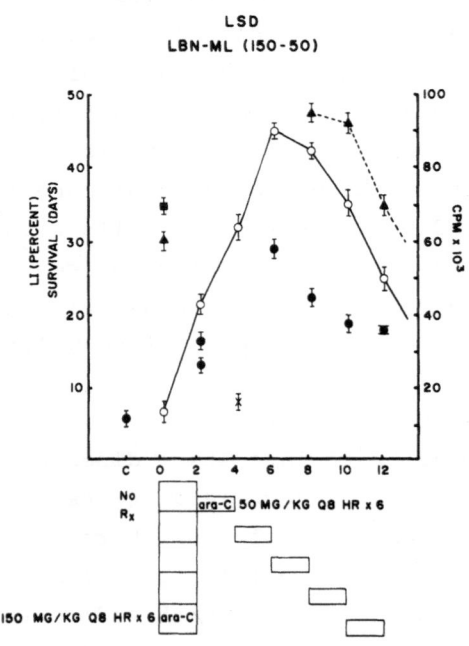

FIGURE 4. The effect of sequential courses of ara-C examinec
a function of the interval between courses relative to the pr
liferation of leukemia and HSA induced by the initial drug.
Animals were treated on day 17 of tumor with an initial dose
ara-C, 100 mg/kg Q8h x 6, followed by a dose of ara-C, 50 mg/
Q8h x 6, in sequence. The effect of the initial dose on tumc
LI (----), and HSA (o---) are depicted. Vertical bars re
sent ± 1 SEM (C) is survival of control animals. The surviva
those treated with ara-C in sequence are represented by (o).

Chemotherapy of Minimal Residual Disease (MRD) in the LBN-ML Model

We have shown the efficacy of timed sequential therapy of this rat model with LSD, but no matter the dose and schedule, no cures were achieved. To test the hypothesis in MRD, further studies were done in animals induced into remission, but destined to relapse and die.

For these experiments, complete remission was routinely induced with 100 mg/kg of cyclophosphamide (CY) given IP 3-7d prior to death of controls. Chemotherapy in remission was begun 14d after CY when bone marrow and peripheral blood recovery were complete and no leukemia could be seen in smears of spleen or bone marrow. Since control rats given no chemotherapy in remission live 22-28d beyond 14d, the amount of residual tumor at the time chemotherapy in remission was begun was calculated to be between 10^5 and 10^6 leukemic cells. The MTD of ara-C given as 2-day course of Q8h injections 14d after CY (consolidation) was determined to be 200 mg/kg/dose (total dose 1,200 mg/kg).

This dose of ara-C given as consolidation or in early relapse (30d after CY) produced 20d prolongation of median survival. More toxicity was seen in early relapse than in early remission, but no significant numbers of cures resulted from this dose and schedule of ara-C given at either time. A second consolidation course of ara-C given 14d after the first increased toxicity had only additive therapeutic effect. The same total dose (1,200 mg/kg) of ara-C given in a variety of lower single dose intermittent or continuous schedules (maintenance) also produced no significant numbers of cures and was quite toxic. Median survival was not prolonged with tolerable toxicity longer than the duration of any of the continuous therapy schedules examined, and no significant numbers of cures were obtained with any "maintenance" therapy (8) Table 1).

Table 1. Toxicity and therapeutic effect of chemotherapy for MRD

Therapy	Cure rate	Toxic deaths	Median survival
No therapy in remission	0/29 (9%)	0/29 (0%)	--
ara-C 1200 mg/kg			
as consolidation	1/23 (4%)	7/23 (30%)	18
as maintenance	1/42 (2%)	22/42 (52%)	17
as reinduction	0/10 (0%)	3/10 (30%)	17

Whereas few or no cures resulted from administration of 1,200 mg/kg of ara-C "consolidation," "maintenance," or "rein duction" chemotherapy, significant numbers of cures resulted this dose of ara-C was given in early remission in timed sequ An initial 2-day infusion of 150 mg/kg Q8h x 6 was followed 2 6, 8 or 10d later by 50 mg/kg Q8h x 6, since this dose distri tion was proven to be less toxic with similar therapeutic ben to equal, divided doses in sequential therapy of LSD. Toxici was found to be inversely proportional to the time interval o sequence, with the greatest toxicity occurring with the short interval sequential therapy (0,2) in which ara-C was given cc ously for 4d. On the other hand the therapeutic effect appea to be maximal with 4, 6 and 8d interval sequential therapy bu diminished at 10d (Figure 5).

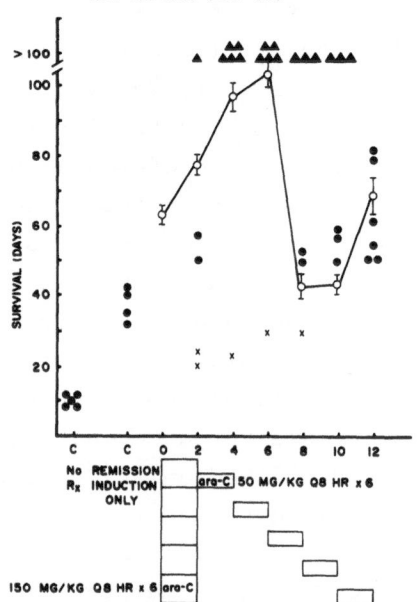

FIGURE 5. The effect of sequential courses of ara-C (1200 m relative to HSA induced by the initial drug. Rats in remiss received an initial dose of ara-C, 100 mg/kg Q8h x 6, follow a dose of ara-C, 50 mg/kg, Q8h x 6 in sequence. The effect initial dose on HSA (o). Survival of untreated controls (o) remission duration after CY (C), after ara-C (o) and cures (are depicted.

Additional studies confirmed these results obtained with 200 mg/kg of ara-C, but only with sequential therapy in remission Table 2).

able 2. Toxicity and therapeutic effect of various chemotherapy or residual leukemia after CY-induced CR of LBN-ML. Combined esults from several experiments of timed sequence in remission.

herapy		Cure rate	Toxic deaths	Median survival of remainder
50/50*	d0/2	5/18 (28%)	13/18 (72%)	--
	d0/4	9/17 (53%)	7/17 (41%)	47
	d0/6	8/16 (50%)	5/16 (31%)	11
	d0/8	9/17 (53%)	0/17 (0%)	19
	d0/10	3/17 (18%)**	4/17 (24%)	34
otal		34/85 (40%)	29/85 (34%)	20

150 mg/kg Q8h x 6 followed by 50 mg/kg Q8h x 6 beginning 2,4,6,8 or 10d later as indicated

*P < 0.0001 compared to results of other therapies MRD, x^2

rinciples of Therapy, Transferred from Rat to Man

In our clinical trials long chemotherapy-free remissions ere obtained in patients with AML when using 1 cycle of high ose infusions of ara-C in a timed sequence designed to exploit predictable and measurable increase in leukemia cell pro- iferation occurring during treatment (2). However, the ajority of patients relapsed after this therapy, indicating that iable noncycling or resistant residual leukemia cells were resent after initial treatment. Since direct study of the inetics, tissue distribution, and drug sensitivity of residual ut undetectable leukemia in complete remission is not possible, e extrapolated the observed effect of various treatment chedules in the LBN rat model with MRD to man. The gratifying esults of sequence in those rodent trials prompted the use of second course of timed sequential therapy in patients with 1L in remission.

Patients Given a Second Cycle of Timed-Sequential Chemotherapy in Early First Remission

Twenty-six (58%) of 45 evaluable previously untreated patients achieved CR with a single cycle of AC-D-AC. The patients were similar to the patients in the historical contro groups and other unselected series of patients with respect to age (median 50 years), presenting manifestations (frequency of infection, preleukemia prodrome, elevated WBC or low platelet count, presence of extramedullary disease, etc.) and all othe: known or suspected risk factors including distribution of FAB phenotype. The percentage of patients responding to therapy and the percentage achieving CR after the first cycle of AC-D also were not different from the historical controls.

Twenty of the 26 patients who achieved CR after a first cycle of AC-D-AC in this trial received a second cycle of AC-D-AC in early first remission (by day 70). These 20 patie were not different by any clinical parameter examined from th historical control group of 34 patients who did not receive a second cycle of AC-D-AC unless relapse occurred. The second cycle of AC-D-AC was well tolerated despite a median of 36 da until first WBC count greater than 1000/UL and a similar peri of severe thrombocytopenia. One patient became refractory to platelet transfusions and died of an intracerebral hemorrhage day 26.

Ten (50%) of these 20 patients remain in CR from 40 to 161 weeks from hospital discharge with a median follow up of 125 weeks. The median duration of CR for this group of patients has not been reached but will be at least 1 1/2 year Comparing these data to the historical controls it can be cal lated that the probability of remaining in first CR after 2 c of AC-D-AC as initial therapy is significantly (p < .001, log greater than the probability of remaining in first CR after only a single cycle of this therapy (Figure 6).

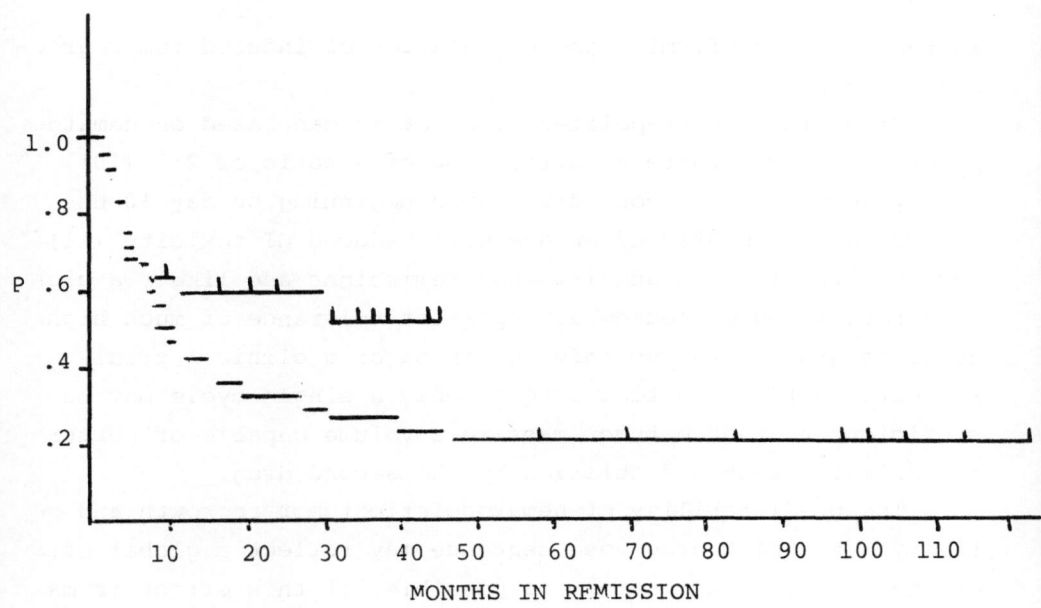

FIGURE 6. Probability or remaining in first CR without further chemotherapy after 2 cycles of AC-D-AC_{10} as initial therapy (20 patients, bold lines) compared to probability of remaining in first CR without chemotherapy in remission after only a single cylce of AC-D-AC_{10} (34 patients, narrow lines), p < .001, longrank.

DISCUSSION

In these studies in man and rat with leukemia we have perturbed a kinetically heterogeneous tissue and measured the induced
changes, taking advantage of the more homogenous enforced growth
to increase the cytotoxicity of cycle active drugs given at the
optimum time and to produce greatest tumor cell kill. With an
aim to elucidating controls of cell growth and drug sensitivity,
we have used the LBN rat with progranulocytic leukemia, an ideal
model, since cure can be achieved, but only with meticulous manipulation of the timing of dose. We can relate this relative resistance to quiescent residual tumor which can be recruited to drug
sensitivity only by accurately timed sequential treatment (9).

These studies demonstrate the salutary effect of drugs given
in high dose to reduce tumor mass and recruit tumor cells to further drug sensitivity. The sequence studies support the postulate
that prolongation of life can be achieved with the sequence given

at that time, confirming the correlation of induced tumor grov
and response.

With timing extrapolated from rat to man based on hematopoietic regrowth patterns after drug of a ratio of 2:3 (10),
the cycle with the second drug given beginning on day 10 has
allowed a therapeutic advantage with reduced GI toxicity (11)
and resulted in long unmaintained remissions and likely a higl
cure rate in human leukemia. Apparent tolerance of much high
doses of ara-C given by infusion in ongoing clinical trials
suggests that the initial drug in only a single cycle may be
sufficient to reduce tumor mass to a volume capable of perturl
to maximal growth and ablation by the second drug.

The predictability of hematopoietic tumor regrowth and s
tivity after high drug dose sequence may reflect a global eff
of induced stimulation. It is possible, if this effect is ma
mal, that the heterogenicity of growth kinetics of malignancy
relate to local environmental factors and tumor density might
overcome. If so, and with effective drugs, an increased cure
should be achieved.

REFERENCES

1. Burke PJ, Karp JE, Braine HG, Vaughan WP. Timed sequential therapy of human leukemia based upon the response of leukemic cells to humoral growth factors. Cancer Res. 1977; 37:2138-46.
2. Vaughan WP, Karp JE, Burke PJ. Long chemotherapy remissions after single-cycle timed sequential chemotherapy for acute myelocytic leukemia. Cancer 1980; 45:859-65.
3. Vaughan WP, Burke PJ, Jung JW. BN rat myeloid leukemia transferred to the (LEW x BN) F_1 rat. J. Natl. Cancer Inst. 1978; 61:927-9.
4. Hagenbeek, A. Introduction of the BN myelocytic leukemia. Leukemia Res. 1977; 1:85.
5. Van Bekkum DW, Van Oosterom P, Dicke KA. In vitro colony formation of transplatable rat leukemias in comparison with human acute myeloic leukemia. Cancer Res. 1976; 36:941-6.
6. Hagenbeek A, Martins AC, van Bekkum DW, et al. Proliferation kinetics of the BNML leukemia in vivo. Leukemia Res. 1977; 1:99.
7. Burke PJ, Vaughan WP, Karp JE. A rationale for sequential high-dose chemotherapy of leukemia timed to coincide with induced tumor proliferation. Blood 1980; 55:960-68.
8. Vaughan WP, Burke PJ. Development of a cell kinetic approach to curative therapy of acute myelocytic leukemia in remission using the cell cycle-specific drug 1-β-D-arabinofuranosylcytosine in a rat model. Cancer Res. 1983; 43:2005-9.
9. Burke PJ, Vaughan WP, Karp JE, et al. Recruitment of quiescent tumor by humoral stimulatory activity: requirements for successful chemotherapy. Blood Cells 1982; 8:519-33.
10. Burke PJ, Karp JE, Vaughan WP. Chemotherapy of leukemia in mouse, rat and man relating to humoral stimulation, tumor growth, and clinical response. J. Natl. Cancer Inst. 1981; 67:529-38.
11. Burke PJ, Vaughan WP, Karp JE, et al: The correlation of maximal drug dose, tumor recruitment, and sequence: schedule-dependent toxicity of cytosine arabinoside. Med. Ped. Onc. Supl. 1982; 1:201-8.

EVALUATION AND CHEMOTHERAPY OF RESIDUAL DISEASE IN ACUTE
LEUKEMIA

R. ZITTOUN, J.P. MARIE

During the last fifteen years major progress   has
been accomplished in the induction treatment of acute leuke-
nia in adults, with about 70 % complete remission (CR), achieved in acute myelogenous leukemia (AML) and in acute lymphoblastic leukemia (ALL), except in old and poor prognostic
patients - secondary leukemias, blast crisis -. However in
most center the number of long term survivors is still lower
than 5 % (30). In our department, only 2 % of the 806 patients
referred during the 11 last years are alive in their first
CR for more than 4 years. The risk of relapse after a prolonged CR is low : we have observed two such AML patients who
relapsed after 5 and 8 years of CR, but this occurs unfre-
quently - 2.8 % of cases in a large multicentric study (30)-.
Extensive histologic examinations have shown a high frequency of occult foci of leukemic cells in various tissues when
such surveys were made shortly after the establishment of CR
(20), whereas similar studies in ALL patients in continuous
CR for three or more years revealed only few positive testicular biopsies (17). One can hypothesize consequently that
the leukemic cell burden in most patients in short term CR
is relatively high, not far under the 10^{10} cells corresponding to the limit between overt disease and CR. Cytogenetic
studies have shown that most relapses - even after bone
marrow allogenic transplant - originate from the initial
clone, taking into account clonal evolution and/or subclones
expansion. Evaluation and treatment of the residual disease,
once a CR is obtained, is therefore actually the major task

in the treatment of acute leukemia.

1.- EVALUATION OF THE RESIDUAL DISEASE

1.1.- Monitoring of complete remission

Besides morphological examinations, many methods have been proposed for monitoring of CR. Table 1 shows the comparative results of morphological examination of bone marrow (BM) smears, agar BM culture, search for a decrease of the ^{3}H-thymidine LI (27) and use of immunologic markers in AML (3). One can see that combinations of kinetic and immunologic methods can help to predict relapse ; however, whatever the method employed, relapses were also observed without any previous abnormality during the very last weeks. We observed recently normal BM agar culture in patients with already recurrent blastic infiltration. It can be concluded that several types of residual disease exist according to the level of plateau - if such plateau can be extrapolate from multiple myeloma to leukemia -, to the kinetics of the expanding clone which will engender the full relapse, and to the interactions with normal tissues.

Table 1.- Results of various methods for monitoring complete remission in AML.

Method	Time to relapse (mths)	Normal	Abnormal (%)
BM morphology[1] (Auer rods and/or small increase of blasts)	1 - 4	23	7 (23 %)
In vitro abnormal growth[1] (agar culture)	1 - 6	12	11 (48 %)
3H-thymidine LI $<$ 20 %[2]	3	9	8 (47 %)
Immunologic markers[3]	1 - 6	5	21 (80 %)

1.- Personnal data
2.- P. Stryckmans et al. See reference 27
3.- Baker et al. See reference 3

In ALL the definition of CR should be question-
ed, and efforts must be made to differentiate during CR the
residual leukemic lymphoblasts (1.9 $\pm$ 1.2 % in 21 of our
patients) from the normal myeloblasts. The use of the markers for cALL antigen is hampered by the presence of positive
cells in normal regenerating BM, by occurence of relapses
without previous increase of cALL + cells, and of phenotypic
shift with loss of cALL antigen (8). In 19 of our patients,
the remission duration was no different whether the level of
cALL + cells at the beginning of CR was low or undetectable,
or higher than 2 %. The main clinical interest of anti-cALL
or TdT antibody is to rule out false CR (with BM infiltration by cells resembling mature lymphocytes but presenting
the typical leukemic phenotype), and to help identifying
leukemic cells in CSF and testis. Immunologic markers are
more useful in T-ALL since the phenotype of this leukemia
(HUTLA +, TdT+) is not found in normal BM : double labeling
has been proposed to detect as few as 0.5 % leukemic cells.
However, again phenotypic heterogeneity and changes may occur corresponding to subclone selection (5).

1.2.- Prognostic factors for duration of complete remission.
These are far less numerous than for remission
induction. Age, initial blood count, and Auer rods in AML,
are more predictive for the induction of remission than for
its duration (34). Besides some interesting initial biological parameters such as LDH or fibrin level, which need
confirmation, the major prognostic factors for duration of
remission, resulting from recent multivariate analysis, relate to kinetic parameters and sensitivity to induction treatment : labeling index, in vitro agar colony growth, halving
rate of leukemic cells in the blood and number of courses
to CR (14). It can be assumed consequently that the leukemic cell burden at the begining of the CR depends on the
proliferative capacity of the leukemic cells and the rate of
cell kill by induction treatment. Later on, other factors
will interfere such as hostfactors, sanctuaries, and develop-

ment of resistant subclones.

Immunologic factors, after excessive vogue, and contradictory conclusions of numerous trials on immunotherapy, suffer now from excessive discredit. The role of graft versus host disease in reducing the risk of relapse after allogenic BM transplant, the new therapeutic possibilities raised by specific monoclonal antibodies show clearly that immunologic status remain important, at least in patients with minimal residual disease.

CNS and testicular sanctuaries have been extensively reviewed in ALL. Asymptomatic CNS involvement is not unfrequent in AML, especially in young people and in monocytic subtypes, but remission duration was not substantially longer in patients who received CNS prophylaxis with radiotherapy and intrathecal chemotherapy than in other series (7

Spleen tissue may represent a favorable microenvironment for leukemic residual disease (9) but splenectomy performed early in remission of childhood AML did not significantly influence the duration of CR (6).

The overgrowth of resistant clones seems in fact the major problem in acute leukemia and the major cause of relapse after remission induction. Besides experimental models, the only ways to study alternate treatments able to eradicate these clones are :
a) the study of response rate to new drugs and combinations in relapsing and refractory patients,
b) randomized comparison of continuous versus alternate consolidation during remission

2.- SELECTION OF ALTERNATE TREATMENTS IN ACUTE LEUKEMIA
2.1- Subclones resistant to the first line drugs.

Skipper and Schabel have developped models of kinetics of the residual disease following a first treatment of L1210 or P388 leukemias by Cytosine-arabinoside (Ara-C). Optimal schedule of Ara-C failed to cure mice with large body burden of leukemic cells, with death due to the overgrowth of an Ara-C resistant subpopulation originating from one stable mutant cell in 10^6 L1210 sensitive cells (24).

It was assumed therefore that an Ara-C resistant cohort is usually present in the Ara-C sensitive human acute leukemia at diagnosis ; this could explain in human leukemia the progressively shorter duration of CR with repeated courses of induction treatment and the final failure of response to chemotherapy.

In AML the rate of development of resistant subpopulations varies from patient to patient, with 10 - 20 % already resistant to the first induction treatments. Second and more CR are actually easily obtained using conventional drug combinations, with however a higher rate of CR when reinduction treatment includes drug which was not utilized previously (22). One can hypothesize that therapeutic synergism between Ara-C and anthracycline drugs may postpone the development of resistance, each drug being active on the subpopulation of cells resistant to the other. However the proportion of resistant cells increases at each successive relapse.

We have tested the in vitro cell kill of Ara-C and anthracycline drugs (Daunomycin or Adriamycin) on AML clonogenic cells growing with a PHA-leucocyte conditionned medium (18). The study was performed repeatedly on 2 or 3 separate occasions at 1 - 17 months interval (median : 5 mths) in 13 AML patients. The second and third studies were performed after failure of a conventional anthracycline - Ara-C induction regimen, or at time of relapse after a first CR was achieved by such treatment. The results are shown in figure 1. The development of in vitro resistance to Ara-C was observed in 5/12 cases, to anthracycline drugs in 6/12 cases, and to both drugs in 4/13 cases. Of interest were 2 patients with clonogenic cells initially resistant to Ara-C, and secondarily of intermediate sensitivity after treatment by high doses Ara-C plus AMSA. Another patient with a high in vitro cell kill by daunomycin became intermediately in vitro resistant after 2 months, then recovered its full in vitro sensitivity. The rapid emergence of resistant clones in our observations may be biased by the selection of patients

116

refractory to the first induction treatment or studied during early relapse. However it gives some consistency to the postulate of Schabel et al, according which treatment should be changed at time of nadir of the leukemic cell burden by introducing, early after achievement of CR,

drugs which are cytotoxic for both residual Ara-C sensitive cells and also for Ara-C resistants cells (24). Such early change should be preferred to increasing the number of drugs in the first combination treatment protocol, which cannot prevent from development of resistance (25).

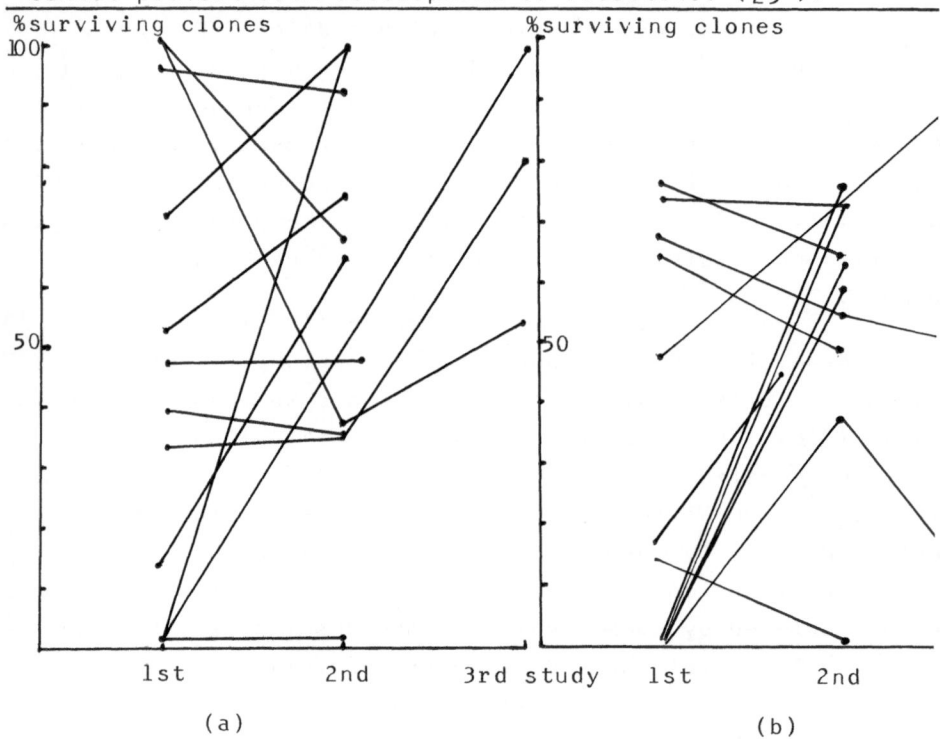

(a)   (b)

FIGURE 1.- % Surviving clones in 2 or 2 consecutive studies in AML patients. Cells were cultured in methyl cellulose with a PHA-LCM conditionned medium. Cells were exposed a) continuously to Ara-C 10^{-6} b) 10 minutes to Adriamycin 10^{-5} M or Daunomycin 10^{-6}M

2.2.- Selection of drugs for Ara-C resistant cells.

Cells resistant to Ara-C have a collateral sensitivity for drugs inhibiting the de novo pyrimidine synthesis,
since they lack deoxycytidine and are totally dependent on
the de novo synthesis for replication. Such collateral sensitivity of Ara-C resistant cells have been shown in experimental leukemia for PALA, pyrazofurin and 3-deazauridine (24).
Some drugs such as thymidine or hydroxyurea can modulate the
activity of Ara-C by decreasing the dCTP pool and increasing
the intra-cellular concentration of Ara-CTP (26). Other
drugs are also synergistic without any proven collateral sensitivity. A list of drugs with collateral sensitivity, modulation activity and/or therapeutic synergism with Ara-C is
presented in table 2.

Table 2.- ARA-C modulation, collateral sensitivity and
         synergism.

	Modulation	Collateral Sensitivity	Synergism
Thymidine	+		
Hydroxyurea	+		
M 26	+		
ethotrexate	+		
ALA	+	+	
Deazauridine	+	+	
FU	+	+	
yrazofurin	+	+	
ihydro-5-Azacytidine		+	
iOH Anthracenedione			+
M 26			+
hioguanine			+
. Asparaginase			+

Few clinical trials have been conducted, using
drugs for which Ara-C resistant cells had a collateral sensitivity in experimental models.
The first extensive trial with 3-deazauridine, a structural

analog of uridine which inhibits CTP - synthetase resulted
in no complete or partial remission in 36 adult acute leukemia, mainly AML, who had received extensive prior therapy
including Ara-C (33). Thymidine, after conversion into dTTP,
inhibits CDP-reductase and decreases the intra-cellular dCTP
pool. In a recent study, Van Echo et al observed, after simultaneous administration of thymidine and Ara-C 47 % responses (5 CR + 2 PR) in 21 relapsed patients having received
prior Ara-C therapy (28). After sequential administration
of thymidine-Ara-C or hydroxyurea - Ara-C, we   have
observed 34 % responses in 32 patients without documented
clinical resistance to Ara-C, but no response in 7 patients
refractory to previous Ara-C treatment. This difference is
not yet significant, but modulation of Ara-C with infra-
cytotoxic doses of thymidine does not seem to overcome markedly resistance to Ara-C. Such failure could be explained
if impaired activity of deoxycytidine(dC)-kinase is the major
mechanism of Ara-C. In that case, selective eradication of
Ara-C resistant leukemic cells could be obtained by administration of both cytotoxic concentrations of thymidine and dC
dC could protect the normal cells from the lethal effect of
thymidine, but not the leukemic cells devoided of dC-kinase
(4).
          Another method recently utilized to overcome re-
sistance   to Ara-C is to use high doses of this drug, which
could result, through passive diffusion, in high intra-
cellular concentrations. Infusions of $3g/m^2$ of Ara-C as single drug every 12 hours during 6 days resulted in 50 % CR
in 27 patients totalized from 3 different centers, with most
of these patients refractory to conventional doses of Ara-C
(13, 10, 31). Toxicity of such dose schedule is marked but
seems acceptable, and the first results are receiving confirmation   from several centers.

2.3.- Non cross-resistant interchalating agents.

          The search for non-cross resistant interchalating
agents can be made also on the basis of the in vitro clonogenic studies. 4 different anthracyclin drugs (daunomycin,

adriamycin, rubidazone, and aclacinomycin A), have been tested in our laboratory in 19 AML patients : complete in vitro
cross-sensitivity or cross-resistance was found in 10 cases ;
in 7 other cases, adriamycin activity differed from the 3
other drugs ; in 2 cases only   non - cross resistance between the 3 other anthracycline drugs was observed. Conclusions
can be hardly drawn since the in vitro results correlated
poorly with the clinical response, and adriamycin needs ten
fold greater in vitro concentrations to achieve the same level
of inhibition than the 3 other drugs.

In a recent clinical trial, Aclacinomycin was found
ctive in AML patients who appeared refractory to adriamycin
reviously administered (19).

Another drug of interest which has been extensi-
ely studied is AMSA. This drug is an acridine derivative,
ctive in acute leukemia and malignant lymphoma, with a res-
onse rate of 20 - 25 % in patients previously treated with
onventional therapy. In a recent trial, 28 % AML patients
chieved a CR, and no significant difference was observed
hether patients were refractory or not to anthracycline
rugs (15).

.4.- Other non-cross resistant drugs and drug combinations :
Resistance to vincristine and prednisone raises
he questions still unsolved of replacement of vincristine
y vindesine, and usual by high doses of prednisone. Inter-
ediate doses of methotrexate and high doses of VP 16-213
e also currently under study respectively in ALL and AML.

Various drug combinations are actually tried in
fractory acute leukemia. One of the most promising seems
he association of AMSA and high dose Ara-C. Using this asso-
ation (AMSA : 90 - 115 mg/m^2/d 1 to 5, Ara-C 3g/m^2 q 12 hrs
ys 1 and 2), we observed 8 CR out of 16 AML patients and
CR in 4 ALL, with the same rate of CR in case of resistance
conventional treatments. Using 6 days of Ara-C (3g/m^2 q
hrs) followed by 3 days of AMSA (75 - 100 mg/m^2/d), Hines
al observed 10 CR in 15 refractory AML (12). The hemato-
gic, buccal and hepatic toxicity of these regimen, although

frequently severe,does not usually prevent from their utili-
sation, and cardiac toxicity of AMSA seems lower than that
of anthracycline drugs.

3.- TREATMENT OF THE RESIDUAL DISEASE.
3.1.- Acute myelogenous leukemia.

Treatment of acute leukemia is usually divided
into induction, consolidation and maintenance phases. Two
major modifications have been recently introduced in this
classical schema.

a)- The distinction between induction and post-induction
phases does not need to be as stringent as in the past : the
total design of induction and consolidation courses could be
consequently applied whatever be the moment of the achievement of the complete remission (16). The major concept forming the basis of this treatment is that an intensive early
chemotherapy can reduce markedly the level of residual diseas

The protocol designed in St Bartholomew's Hospital
does not take into account the development of resistant subclones. This could be a concern for a minority of patients
if we extrapolate to AML what is known about Hodgkin's disease, where a mere repetition of the same protocol can cure
at least 50 % of patients. But this is far from being proven,
and the marked toxicity of chemotherapy in AML reduces the
ability to demonstrate this hypothesis.

Systematic introduction during early CR of new
combinations or dose schedules represents a second possibilit
Using this principle Mayer et al reported a 19 mth.med. dura
of CR using the VAPA intensive sequential protocol administered during a 15-month period. The consolidation was divide
into four sequences of drug combination, each sequence being
repeated four times : Adriamycin + Ara-C, Adriamycin + 5-
Azacytidine - an analog of cytosine which has some activity
in refractory AML (29)-, POMP regimen, and intermediate dos
of Ara-C. The good results of the VAPA experience could be
related in part to the young age of patients with 63 % less
17 yrs and no patient above 50 yrs. Another trial of intensi
ve sequential maintenance treatment led to more disappointin

results in Memorial Hospital, and raised controversies about the degree of intensity and the choice of drugs (1). This is a major debate since progress   in the chemotherapy could lead to competition with bone marrow allogenic transplant, the other major treatment for AML (23).

Most of the on-going or future chemotherapy trials in AML will be based on the above principles. In a recent pilot study from Wolff et al, 16 AML patients achieving a first CR received 1-2 courses of high dose Ara-C ($3g/m^2$ every 12 hrs during 6 days). 3 patients died of toxicity during this short intensive consolidation, 3 other relapsed, but 10 remain in CR 12 - 36 mths without further treatment (32). The AML 6 protocol from EORTC, after remission induction with daunomycin + Ara-C,   randomizes between 6 courses of Daunorubin-AraC or 6 courses of AMSA-5 Azacytidine alternating with AMSA-high dose Ara-C .

.2.- Acute lymphoblastic leukemia.

One of the regimens proposed during the last years according to the concept of intensive sequential maintenance treatment has been tested at the Memorial Hospital (1) : the L 10 protocol includes a consolidation phase using cell ycle specific drugs aimed at rapidly proliferating leukemia ells thought to be in high number at the beginning of the CR. During this phase 6 alternating cycles of methotrexate and cytosine arabinoside plus thioguanine are administered, along with intra-thecal methotrexate. Consolidation phase ends with L. Asparaginase and a bolus of cyclophosphamide ; it is followed by an eradication phase with 70 days cycles where cycle non-specific drugs - adriamycin, BCNU and Acti-mycin D - are administered, together with alternating cour-es of prednisone + vincristine and 6 MP + methotrexate. These consolidation and eradication phases are currently under study actually in the EORTC Hemopathy Working Party : patients entering CR are randomized for long or short (wi-out methotrexate and Ara-C + thioguanine courses) consoli-tion. Then all patients receive the L10 "eradication" sign, in outpatient clinics, for 6 cycles - 420 days -. his phase is followed by a more conventional maintenance treatment untill 3 years of CR.

While this trial is still open, the results of
our single institution are superior to the ones observed
previously in patients treated only with a conventional
6 MP + methotrexate maintenance treatment and periodic reen-
forcements with prednisone + vincristine with a significantly longer duration of CR.

The same difference was observed in the Memorial
Hospital when comparing the L 10 to the L2 protocol.

3.3.- In vitro combined with in vivo treatment of residual disease.

While this problem will be discussed in another
part of this symposium, it must be emphasized that in vitro
treatment of the bone marrow cells followed by autologous
transplantation is based on the same concepts and should
be tried as another method of intensive consolidation. Recently 8 AML patients in first CR have been treated by P.
Hervé and col. with a conditionning regimen by TACC and an
in vitro treatment by ASTA-Z-7557 (40-80 μ M). One patient
only relapsed, 2 died during the first days and the 5
others remain in CR after 2 - 12 months. 2 ALL patients in
second CR conditionned by TBI + cyclophosphamide and autografted after the same in vitro treatment remain in CR after
4 and 7 months ([11]).

REFERENCES

1.- Arlin ZA, Fried J, Clarkson BD. Therapeutic role of cell
    kinetics in acute leukeamia.
    Clinics in Haemat. 1978, 7 : 339 - 362
2.- Arlin ZA, Mertelsmann R., Kempin S, Gee T, Clarkson BD.
    Is further intensification of treatment warranted in
    acute non lymphoblastic leukemia ?
    Cancer Treat. Rep. 1982, 67 : 202
    (see replies from RJ Mayer et al and H. Preisler).
3.- Baker MA, Falk JA, Carter WH, Taur RN and the Toronto
    Leukemia Study Group.
    Early diagnosis of relapse in acute myeloblastic leuke-
    mia. Serologic detection of leukemia-associated anti-
    gens in human marrow.
    New. Eng. J. Med. 1979, 301 : 1353 - 1357

4.- Bhalla K, Stillman I, Grant S.
Selective eradication of Ara-C-resistant leukemic cells
utilizing combinations of thymidine and deoxycytidine
Blood 1982, 60, suppl. 1 : 152 a

5.- Bradstock KF, Janossy G, Tidman N et al.
Immunological monitoring of residual disease in treated
thymic acute lymphoblastic leukemia
Leuk. Res. 1981, 5 : 301 - 309

6.- Dahl GV, Kalwinsky DK, Murphy S et al.
Cytokinetically based induction chemotherapy and sple-
nectomy for childhood acute non lymphocytic leukemia.
Blood 1982, 60 : 856 - 863

7.- Gale RP, Foon KA, Cline MJ, Zighelboim J and the UCLA
Acute Leukemia Study Group
Intensive chemotherapy for acute myelogenous leukemia.
Ann. Int. Med. 1981, 94 : 753 - 757

8.- Greaves M, Paxton A, Janossy G, Pain C, Johnson S,
Lister TA
Acute lymphoblastic leukaemia associated antigen. III
Alterations in expression during treatment and in relapse
Leuk. Res. 1980, 4 : 1 - 14

9.- Hagenbeek A, Martens ACM.
Kinetics of minimal residual disease in a rat model for
human acute myelocytic leukemia in Experimental Hematology Today. SJ Baum, G.D. Ledney and DW van Bekkum
Editors. S. Karger. Basel 1980, p 215 - 221

0.- Hande KR, Stein RS, Mc Donough DA, Greco FA
Effects of high-dose cytarabine
Clin. Pharmacol. Therap. 1982, 31 : 669 - 674

1.- Hervé P.
Personnal communication.

2.- Hines JD, Oken MM, Mazza J, Keller A, Glick J
High dose cytosine arabinoside (Ara-C) and m-AMSA in
refractory acute non-lymphoblastic leukemia.
Blood 1981, 58, Suppl. 1 : 142 a

3.- Karanes C, Wolff SN, Herzig GP
High dose cytosine arabinoside in the treatment of
patients with refractory acute non-lymphocytic leukemia
Blood 1979, 54 supp 1 : 191 a

4.- Keating MJ, Smith TL, Gehan EA et al.
Factors related to the length of complete remission
in adult acute leukemia.
Cancer 1980, 45 : 2017 - 2029

5.- Legha SS, Keating MJ, Mc Credie KB, Bodey GP, Freireich EJ
Evaluation of AMSA in previously treated patients with
acute leukemia : Reseults of therapy in 109 adults
Blood 1982, 60 : 484 - 490

16.- Lister TA, Rohatiner AZS.
     The treatment of acute myelogenous leukemia in adults.
     Seminars Hemat. 1982, 19 : 172 - 192
17.- Mahoney D, Gonzales ET, Ferry GD et al.
     Childhood acute leukemia : a search for occult extra-
     medullary disease prior to discontinuation of chemo-
     therapy.
     Cancer 1981, 48 : 1964 - 1966
18.- Marie JP, Zittoun R, Thevenin D, Mathieu M, Viguie F.
     In-vitro culture of clonogenic leukaemic cells in acute
     myeloid leukaemia : growth pattern and drug sensitivity
     Br. J. Haemat. (to be published).
19.- Mathe G., de Jager R, Hulhoven R et al.
     L'aclacinomycin A dans les leucémies aigues et les
     lymphomes non-hodgkiniens leucémiques.
     Nouv. Presse Med. 1982, 11 : 25 - 28
20.- Mathe G, Schwarzenberg L, Mery AM et al.
     Extensive histological and cytological survey of
     patients with acute leukaemia in "complete remission".
     Br. Med. J. 1966, 1 : 640 - 642
21.- Mayer RJ, Weinstein HJ, Coral FS, Rosenthal DS, Frei E I
     The role of intensive post-induction chemotherapy in the
     management of patients with acute myelogenous leukemia
     Cancer Treat. Rep. 1982, 66 : 1455 - 1462
22.- Peterson BA, Bloomfield CD
     Re-induction of complete remissions in adults with
     acute non-lymphocytic leukemia.
     Leuk. Res. 1981, 5 : 81 - 88
23.- Preisler HD
     Therapy for patients with acute myelocytic leukemia who
     enter remission : bone marrow transplantation or che-
     motherapy ?
     Cancer Treat. Rep . 1982, 66 : 1467 - 1473
24.- Schabel FM Jr, Skipper HE, Trader MW et al.
     Drug control of Ara-C resistant tumor cells.
     Med. Pediatr. Oncol. 1982, Suppl. 1 : 125 - 148
25.- Schmid FA, Hutchison DJ, Otter GM, Stock CC
     Development of resistance to combinations of six anti-
     metabolites in mice with L1210 leukemia.
     Cancer Treat. Rep. 1976, 60 : 23 - 27
26.- Streifel JA, Howell SB
     Synergistic interaction between 1-β-D-arabinofuranosul-
     cytosine, thymidine, and hydroxyurea against human B
     cells and leukemia blasts in vitro.
     Proc. Natl. Acad. Sci. USA 1981, 78 : 5132 - 5136
27.- Stryckmans P, Debusscher L, Ronge-collard E, Socquet M,
     Zittoun R
     The labelling index of marrow myeloblasts : a predictive
     test for relapse of acute non-lymphoblastic leukemia
     Leuk. Res. 1980, 4 : 79 - 87
28.- Van Echo DA, Markus S, Wiernik PH
     A phase III trial of Arabinosyl-cytosine and thymidine
     (Ara-C + TdR) in adult relapsed acute leukemia (AL)
     Proceed 17th. Ann. Meet. Amer. Soc. Clin. Oncol. 1981,
     22 : 483

29.- Vogler WR, Miller DS, Keller JW (Writing Committe for
     the Southeastern Cancer Study Group).
     5-Azacytidine (NSC 102816). A new drug for the treat-
     ment of Myeloblastic Leukemia.
     Blood 1976, 48 : 331 - 337
30.- Whittaker JA, Reizenstein P, Callender ST et al.
     Long survival in acute myelogenous leukaemia : an in-
     ternational collaborative study.
     Br. Med. J. 1981, 282 : 692 - 695
31.- Willemze R, Zwaan FE, Colpin G, Keuning JJ
     High dose cytosine arabinoside in the management of
     refractory acute leukaemia.
     Scand. J. Haematol. 1982, 29 : 141 - 146
32.- Wolff SN, Marion J, Stein R, Flexner JM, Phillips GL,
     Herzig GP
     Therapy of acute non-lymphoblastic leukemia (ANLL) in
     first remission : Brief intensive consolidation with
     high-dose Ara-C (HDARAC).
     Blood 1982, 60 supplt. 1 : 159 a
33.- Yap B.S., Mc Credie KB, Keating MJ, Bodey GP, Freireich EJ
     Phase I - II study of 3-deazauridine in adults with
     acute leukemia.
     Cancer Treat. Rep. 1981, 65 : 521 - 524.
34. Zittoun R, Cadiou M, Bayle C, Suciu S, Solbu G, Hayat M,
     and the EORTC Leukemia and Hematosarcoma Group.
     Prognostic value of cytological parameters in acute
     myelogenous leukemia.
     Cancer (to be published).

. THE TREATMENT OF MINIMAL RESIDUAL DISEASE DURING REMISSION IN AML*

R.S. WEINER

1. INTRODUCTION

The challenge of treating acute myelogenous leukemia has shifted over the past decade from studies designed to increase the proportion of patients entering complete remission to studies aimed at prolonging the duration of complete remission. With the introduction of anthracycline antibiotics (1,2) and cytosine arabinoside (3,4), with the effective use of these drugs in combination, and with adequate access to platelets and more effective antibiotics, complete remission rates have risen to the range of 55-75% (5-7). Despite this marked improvement in remission induction, the median duration of remission for most large series reported in the literature averages less than a year (8-11). Disease-free survival of five years or more is nevertheless reported in 5-20% of patients who enter remission (12-15). Recent results from a few studies demonstrate that chemotherapy induced remissions can be durable for an even higher proportion of patients (16-17). Super-intensive chemotherapy and radiotherapy followed by allogeneic bone marrow transplantation in first emission appears to offer the highest probability of durable remissions without maintenance chemotherapy (18-20). While at least part of the durability of remission has been ascribed to the immune reaction of the graft against the leukemia cells as a concomitant of graft-versus-host disease (21,22), cytotoxic therapy alone has induced sustained remissions in patients receiving grafts from their identical twins (23). Some of the more successful chemotherapy regimens and the bone marrow transplantation experience share several features which may impact on curative therapy and which warrant further study.

Supported by grant R-10-CA-28143 from National Cancer Institute.

(1) The best results have been obtained when patients were treated intensively after they had achieved remission.

(2) Post remission therapy has included drugs or modalities that were different from those used to induce remission.

(3) The patients who did best were generally young.

(4) Sustained remissions were achieved without prolonged maintenance therapy.

As a first step in studying optimum post induction therapy, the Divisions of Medical Oncology and Hematology at the University of Florida undertook a pilot study of short term intensive therapy for patients with acute myelogenous leukemia (24). Based on the University of Florida Feasibility Pilot, the Southeastern Cancer Study Group then inaugurated a prospective clinical trial comparing four cytoreductive regimens after the induction of remission with a single intensive course of cytosine arabinoside and daunorubicin. The Southeastern Cancer Study Group trial compares intensive consolidation with the same drugs used for remission induction, intensive consolidation with drugs known to be effective in leukemias refractory to cytosine arabinoside and daunorubicin, less intensive consolidation therapy followed by maintenance therapy, and super-intensive cytoreductive therapy followed by allogeneic bone marrow transplantation.

2. METHODS

2.1 The University of Florida Feasibility Pilot

Twelve consecutive untreated patients with acute myelogenous leukemia who were below the age of 50 and who were treated at the Shands Teaching Hospital or the Gainesville Veterans Administration Hospital from December 1978 through July 1981 were entered into this study. One patient was 58 years of age and was accessioned in violation of the protocol but has been included in the analysis. Diagnosis of AML was based on morphological and histochemical examination of the bone marrow. The protocol prescribed four courses of intensive chemotherapy as outlined in Table 1. Cytosine arabinoside by continuous intravenous infusion at a dose of 200mg/m^2 per day for ten days with daunorubicin by intravenous bolus at a dose of 40mg/m^2 on days 1, 2 and 3 were used for induction of remission. For patients who entered remission, subsequent courses of chemotherapy were given when peripheral granulocytes were $\geq$ 2500/mm^3 and platelets were $\geq$ 100,000/mm^3 for a minimum of one week. The patients who

Table 1. University of Florida Feasibility Pilot for AML.

*Drugs	Course I	Course II & IV	Course III
DNR[1]	40mg/m2/d x 3d	40mg/m2/d x 3d	40mg/m2/d x 3d
ARA-C[2]	200mg/m2/d x 10d+	200mg/m2/d x 7d	
6-TG[3]		100mg/m2 bid x 5d	100mg/m2 bid x 5d
5-AZA[4]			150mg/m2/d x 7d

*DNR = Daunorubicin; ARA-C = Cytosine Arabinoside; 6-TG = 6-Thioguanine;
    5-AZA = 5-Azacytidine
+SEG AML 81-312 uses 100mg/m2/d x 10 during induction
[1] I.V. Bolus
[2] I.V. or S.C. continuous infusion
[3] P.O.
[4] I.V. continuous infusion

received courses two and four did so as outpatients with the cytosine
arabinoside being administered via an indwelling subcutaneous catheter and
a miniature constant infusion pump (Chroninfuser). Outpatients were
hospitalized when fever and granulocytopenia occured. After completion of
the fourth course of chemotherapy, no maintenance chemotherapy or
immunotherapy was administered. Central nervous system prophylaxis was
not given.

   A complete remission was defined as the absence of symptoms and
physical findings suggestive of leukemia, a normal peripheral hemogram
with the exception of anemia, and an M[1] bone marrow. After completion
of all chemotherapy and documentation of complete remission, patients were
followed at three to six month intervals. Each surviving patient had a
bone marrow examination at the date of last contact used to calculate the
Kaplan-Meier plots. For analysis, the duration of survival was measured
from the time of initial treatment and the duration of remission from the
time remission was documented by bone marrow examination.

.2 The Southeastern Cancer Study Group Prospective Clinical Trial
   SECSG AML 81-312 was activated July 20, 1981. The protocol remains
open and no interim analysis has been published. Patients are eligible if
they are 50 years of age or less and if they have previously untreated
acute myelogenous leukemia (FAB M1-5), or acute undifferentiated leukemia
and have failed an attempt at induction of remission with vincristine,

methotrexate and prednisone on SECSG ALL 78-333. Patients are ineligible
if they have had documented pancytopenia, refractory anemia, myeloprolif-
erative disorders, therapy-induced leukemia, prior exposure to any of the
study drugs, or medical contraindications to the use of daunorubicin. In
addition, patients less than 15 years of age are excluded from this
protocol.

Initially, the induction regimen was identical to the regimen used in
the University of Florida Feasibility Pilot (Table 1). However, of the
first 27 patients treated, nine had either severe or life-threatening
hemorrhagic enteritis. The dose of cytosine arabinoside during the ten
day infusion was therefore reduced to 100mg/m^2 per day with no further
reports of hemorrhagic enteritis in the subsequent 112 patients treated.
The dose of daunorubicin is 45mg/m^2 by bolus injection on days 1, 2 and
3 of the ten day induction course. The four regimens being compared for
post remission therapy are presented in Table 2. The intervals between
courses of therapy are determined by the rapidity of restoration of normal
peripheral blood counts in each patient. The absolute granulocyte count
must be $\geq$ 2500/mm^3 and platelet count must be $\geq$ 100,000/mm3 for at
least one week prior to the institution of the second and subsequent
courses of chemotherapy.

The bone marrow transplantation arm (Regimen D) is not yet activated.
For eligibility, patients will be 35 years of age or less, will have an
HLA-identical and MLC-non reactive sibling with no medical contraindications to serving as a bone marrow transplant donor, will have normal
cardiac function by radio-nucleotide scan, will have normal pulmonary
function tests including arterial blood gases, will consent to allogeneic
bone marrow transplantation, and will have adequate financial recources o
sponsorship to cover hospitalization expenses during the transplant
course. The patients transplanted will be compared to the cohort of
patients who are likewise less than 35 years of age and who have normal
cardiac function and normal pulmonary function at the time remission is
documented but who are not candidates for transplantation and are randoml
allocated among the other three post induction regimens.

The Southeastern Cancer Study Group protocol calls for stratification
by age, performance status, platelet count, and serum creatinine on
entry. At the time of documentation of remission, all patients 35 years
of age or younger will undergo family histocompatibility testing, radio-

TABLE 11   PROTOCOL AML 81-312:   Post-Induction Therapy Regimens.

Day	1	2	3	4	5	6	7	1	2	3	4	5	1	2	3	4	5	6	7
REGIMEN A Induction Drugs	CA	CA	CA	CA	CA	CA	CA												
	DN	DN	DN																
								Repeat for total of 3 courses, then no further therapy (NFT)											
REGIMEN B Non Cross Resistant Drugs	CA	CA	CA	CA	CA	CA	CA	AM	AM	AM	AM	AM	AZ	AZ	AZ	AZ	AZ	AZ	AZ
	DN	DN	DN										TG	TG	TG	TG	TG	TG	TG
													DN	DN	DN				⎫ NFT
REGIMEN C Maintenance	ca	ca	ca	ca	ca														
	TG	TG	TG	TG	TG														
	dn	dn	dn																
	Repeat for a total of 3 courses; rest for 3 months; then after 3 months rest, Ara-C 100mg/m2/d by continuous infusion for 5 days with DN 45mg/m2 on days 1 & 2 q 3 months for 1 year; NFT																		
REGIMEN D Allogeneic BMT (not yet activated)	ca	ca	ca	ca	ca														
	TG	TG	TG	TG	TG														
	dn	dn	dn																
	CY 60mg/kg/d on days -5 & -4; TBI 200 r BID on days -3, -2, & -1; MTX 12mg IT on days -6 & -3; Bone Marrow Transplant day 0; followed by intermittent MTX IV and IT during the first 100 days; then NFT.																		

CA = Cytosine Arabinoside 200mg/m2/d IV by continuous infusion days 1-7
DN = Daunorubicin 45mg/m2 IV bolus days 1-3
AM = m-AMSA 120mg/m2 IV by 2 hour infusion days 1-5
AZ = 5-Azacytidine 150mg/m2 IV by continuous infusion days 1-7
TG = 6-Thioguanine 100mg/m2 PO q 12h on days indicated
ca = Cytosine arabinoside 100mg/m2 IV bolus q 12h days 1-5
dn = Daunorubicin 10mg/m2 IV bolus days 1-5
CY = Cyclophosphamide
TBI = Total Body Irradiation
MTX = Methotrexate

nucleotide scan of the heart, and pulmonary function tests. Patients with a histocompatible and eligible donor and who fulfill the other criteria for transplantation will be allocated to the allogeneic transplant arm. Patients under 35 who are ineligible for allogeneic bone marrow transplantation will be stratified by cardiac and pulmonary status and randomly allocated to one of the other three post induction regimens. All patients between the ages of 35 and 50 will, as a separate cohort of patients, be randomly allocated to the other three post-induction regimens by the stratification criteria mentioned above.

3. RESULTS

3.1 University of Florida Feasibility Pilot Study

Nine men and three women with a median age of 34 (range 16 to 58) were entered on the protocol. One patient aged 58 represents an age-related protocol violation but has been included in all analyses. Five of the 12 patients were febrile on admission, but none had documented sepsis. The median leukocyte count was 8900/mm3 (range 1,500 to 395,000/mm3) and the median platelet count was 113,000/mm3 (range 2,000-284,000/mm3). Median performance status was 70% (range 40% to 100%).

Nine of the twelve patients (75%) attained a complete remission after one course of chemotherapy in a median of 28 days (range 24-36) after starting chemotherapy. Four of these nine patients received the three additional courses of chemotherapy per protocol. Of the remaining five patients, one suffered cardiac arrest and anthracycline-induced congestive heart failure during the first course. Her second course consisted of cytosine arabinoside alone and all chemotherapy was discontinued thereafter. This patient remains in continuous remission at four years. One patient was refractory to all transfused platelets and declined any therapy beyond course 2. This patient relapsed 13 months after remission and died. Another patient refused therapy after course 2 and remained in complete remission for 38 months, at which time he relapsed. He was successfully reinduced two months ago and is currently undergoing consolidation therapy. One patient relapsed after course 3 and died three months later. One patient had an HLA-identical sibling and underwent allogeneic bone marrow transplantation after course 2 in February 1981, and remains in complete remission. He was censored for purposes of analysis on the date of his transplant. Six of the 12 patients are alive and free of disease. Of these, four are in continuous complete remission 19 to 46 months after their last dose of chemotherapy.

Durations of remission and survival are depicted in Figures 1 and 2 as Kaplan-Meier plots.

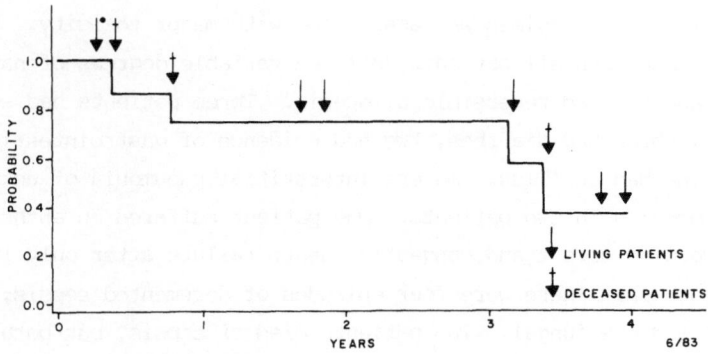

?IGURE 1. Kaplan-Meier plot of probability of remaining in complete re-nission for 9 patients who entered complete remission. One patient (·) vas censored at day 94 when he underwent allogeneic bone marrow transplan-:ation in February of 1981.

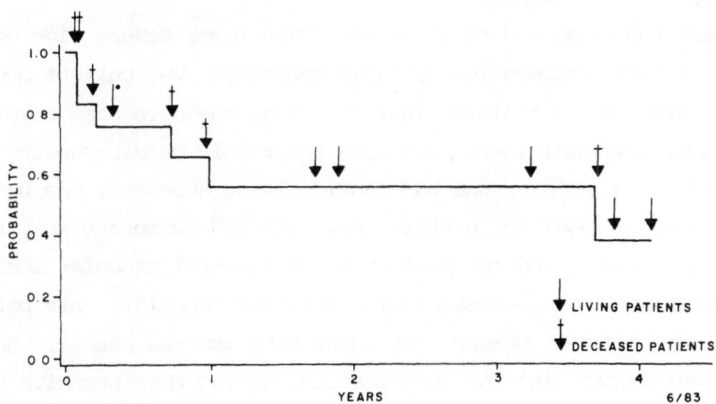

IGURE 2. Kaplan-Meier plot of probability of survival for all 12 atients who entered the University of Florida Feasibility Pilot for AML. ne patient (.) was censored at day 118 when he underwent allogeneic one marrow transplantation in February of 1981.

Follow-up for these patients is a minimum of 24 months and a maximum of 49 months from the date complete remission was documented. All patients in continuous complete remission are unmaintained, have a performance status of 100%, and are independent of medical care. Of the four patients who relapsed at 5, 11, 38 and 40 months after attaining complete remission, three have died. No patient has had evidence of central nervous system involvement with leukemia.

This intensive regimen was associated with major toxicity. During remission induction all patients suffered variable degrees of nausea and vomiting and all had reversible allopecia. Three patients had severe mucositis, three had diarrhea, two had evidence of gastrointestinal bleeding, and one had an ilius. Severe interstitial pneumonia of unknown etiology occured in two patients. One patient suffered an anthracycline induced cardiac arrest and congestive heart failure after only 120mg/m^2 of daunorubucin. There were four episodes of documented sepsis, three bacterial and one fungal. Two patients died of sepsis, but both had documented refractory leukemia. A third patient with refractory leukemia died of CMV pneumonitis and gastroenteritis. One patient developed uterine bleeding of sufficient severity to require hysterectomy. All patients had granulocytopenia (less than 200/mm^3) lasting a median of 24 days (range 9 to 28 days).

Courses 2 through 4 were associated with fewer severe side effects but nevertheless were accompanied by major toxicity. One patient had severe mucositis, one had gastrointestinal bleeding, one developed atypical mycobacterial pneumonia, one developed reversible cardiomyopathy after 480mg/m^2 of daunorubicin, one had candida liver abcesses, one had severe uterine bleeding requiring hysterectomy, one had pulmonary and intra-occular hemorrhages, and one patient had a cerebral vascular accident of unknown etiology, not associated with thrombocytopenia. This patient had residual impairment of memory, but motor function was normal. No patient died of chemotherapy-induced complications during the intensive consolidation therapy.

Intensive hematologic supportive care was required by this population of patients. Platelet transfusions were given prophylactically to maintain the platelet count above 20,000/mm^3. All patients required platelet transfusions during the first two courses. Three of five patients required platelet transfusions during course 3 and four of four patients required platelet transfusions during course 4. Granulocyte transfusions were used on six occasions during the course of the protocol.

3.2 Southeastern Cancer Study Group Protocol AML 81-312

As of March 1, 1983, 112 patients were entered on study. The Group-wide rate of remission induction is 70%. Sixty patients have thus far been randomized among arms A, B and C. Arm D is not yet active. Insufficient data has been analyzed to make even preliminary statements regarding duration of remission.

The hemorrhagic enteritis seen in 9 of the 27 patients treated with cytosine arabinoside at $200mg/m^2$ per day for 10 days and daunorubicin at $45mg/m^2$ per day on days 1, 2 and 3 during induction was severe and life-threatening. This complication was not seen among the 12 patients treated on the pilot protocol. Among the patients subsequently treated with cytosine arabinoside at $100mg/m^2$ per day for 10 days by continuous infusion, this complication was not observed. Likewise, cytosine arabinoside given at $200mg/m^2$ per day by continuous infusion for seven days in regimens A and B have not been associated with severe or life-threatening hemorrhage and the tolerance appears to be acceptable.

1. DISCUSSION

Our pilot study and several other studies using intensive post induction therapy are demonstrating that a high proportion of patients can have prolonged disease free survival with chemotherapy alone (16,17, 25-27). While this small cohort of patients has survived free of disease from 19 to 46 months since their last course of chemotherapy, the elements of therapy that have contributed to their durable remissions are undefined and are being studied in a large prospective clinical trial. The intensive induction regimen failed to rid the bone marrow of leukemic cells in three patients, indicating a primary resistance to the regimen as described by Preisler (28). Furthermore, the sustained administration of $100mg/m^2$ of cytosine arabinoside for 10 days proved unacceptably toxic when applied to a larger patient population. Hemorrhagic enteritis has been described with intensive cytosine arabinoside therapy (29). Neither the Feasibility Study nor the Southeastern Cancer Study Group clinical trial addresses the question of whether post induction chemotherapy pro-longs remission. Rather, the nature of the post induction therapy, its intensity, and duration are being studied. The pilot study prescribed three courses of post induction chemotherapy that were designed to use the maximum tolerated doses of the drugs used to induce remission as well as two additional drugs each of which had significant anti-leukemic activity in patients who were refractory to cytosine arabinoside and daunorubicin. The toxicity of the post induction therapy was significant but was not associated with mortality in any patient. Careful attention was paid to maximizing the hematologic and general health status of each patient prior to institution of the second and subsequent courses of chemotherapy in order to avoid treating patients in remission who had subclinical infections or compromised bone marrow. The use of intensive therapy early in remission when the numbers of residual tumor cells are low may minimize the emergence of resistant cells and relapse. The use of non-cross resistant drugs for intensive therapy may even be more effective in prolonging disease-free survival. The pilot study succeeded in demonstrating the feasibilty of administering intensive post induction chemotherapy and pointed out the toxicities and morbidity associated with such therapy.

The Southeastern Cancer Study Group clinical trial will involve 500 patients and will afford an opportunity to compare four post induction regimens, each representing a sound, but very different therapeutic approach and each based on sound experimental and clinical rationales. The rationale for repeating treatment with drugs that were successful in inducing remission is based upon the possibility that there exists a significant population of residual cells that are still sensitive to the drugs and for which repeated exposure to intensive doses may be effective in avoiding or delaying recurrent disease. This approach is supported by cytokinetic data accumulated from a variety of tumors (30,31) and is in conformity with the hypothesis for optimum treatment put forth by Norton and Simon (32). It denies, however, the hypothesis put forth by Goldie and Coldman which would require drugs with complementary modes of action and to which the leukemic cells are not likely to be cross-resistant for maximum therapy (33,34).

Early intensification may be more effective in prolonging disease-free survival if a series of non-cross reacting agents are employed to treat the residual leukemic cell population which may harbor cells that are resistant to the induction therapy. Regimen B of the Southeastern Cancer

Study Group protocol addresses this directly by adding m-AMSA,
5-Azacytidine and 6-Thioguanine to the cytosine arabinoside and
daunorubicin. All five of these agents have significant single agent
activity in acute myelogenous leukemia (1-4,35-40). The intensity of the
regimen combined with the introduction of the non-cross resistant drugs
applies the hypothesis of Norton and Simon as well as Goldie and Coldman
(32-34). Regimen C employs less intensive consolidation and intermittent
attenuated re-induction therapy for an additional year. This regimen has
been well tolerated in the preceding SECSG protocol for acute myelogenous
leukemia and was adopted as "conventional therapy".

Regimen D will provide an opportunity for prospective concurrent
comparison of allogeneic bone marrow transplantation early in first
remission with Regimens A, B and C for a cohort of patients between the
ages of 15 and 35. Allogeneic bone marrow transplantation will be carried
out at eight centers with established allogeneic bone marrow transplant
programs using a uniform preparative and post-graft regimen as well as
common supportive care guidelines.

Allogeneic bone marrow transplantation in a sense represents the
ultimate in intensive post remission induction therapy. The preparative
regimens utilizing combinations of drugs or drugs and radiotherapy are
designed without regard for preserving endogenous hematopoietic stem
cells. The intensity of the regimens are however severely limited by
extramedullary toxicity (41). The treatment-related mortality within the
first 100 days of transplantation is age dependent and ranges from 20 to
50%. On the other hand, young patients transplanted in first remission
who survive the early transplant period have an 80% chance of remaining
disease free for more than two years (18-20,42). Graft-versus-host
disease which is a major contributor to morbidity and mortality has also
been credited with contributing to the disease-free survival of patients
receiving allogeneic transplants for leukemia (21,22). Current efforts
aimed at decreasing mortality by modifying graft-versus-host disease may
or may not abrogate the salutory effects of graft-versus-host disease on
disease free survival. The role of allogeneic bone marrow transplantation
in the overall therapy of acute myelogenous leukemia is clearly not yet
established. While there is no doubt that allogeneic bone marrow
transplantation can result in prolonged disease free survival in patients
with acute myelogenous leukemia who are transplanted in first remission,

it is becoming apparent that chemotherapy with currently available drugs used with innovative strategies can also result in prolonged disease free survival.

Recent advances in drug development, immunogenetics and supportive care have contributed to increasingly successful treatment of residual disease. Options available today include long term maintenance chemotherapy, short term therapy with the same or different drugs, and super-intensive chemo-radiotherapy followed by allogeneic bone marrow transplantation. Small scale innovative clinical and laboratory investigations have and will continue to point the way towards advancement in the treatment of leukemia. It is appropriate, however, that well controlled large scale prospective clinical trials be performed to compare these options and to test the rationales on which they are based.

REFERENCES

1. Weil M, Glidewell OJ, Jacquillat C, et al. 1973. Daunorubicin in the therapy of acute granulocyte leukemia. Cancer Research, 33: 921-928.
2. Young CC, Ozols CF, Myers CE. 1981. The anthracycline antineoplastic drugs. New England Journal of Medicine, 305: 139-153.
3. Ellison RR, Holland JF, Weil M, et al. 1968. Arabinosyl cytosine: a useful agent in the treatment of acute leukemia in adults. Blood, 32: 507-523.
4. Southwest Oncology Group. 1974. Cytarabine for acute leukemia in adults: effects of schedule on therapeutic response. Archives of Internal Medicine, 133: 251-259.
5. Gale RP, Foon KA, Cline MJ, et al. 1981. Intensive chemotherapy for acute myelogenous leukemia. Annals of Internal Medicine, 94: 753-757.
6. Preisler HD, Rustum Y, Henderson ES, et al. 1979. Treatment of acute nonlymphocytic leukemia: use of anthracycline-cytosine arabinoside induction therapy and comparison of two maintenance regimens. Blood, 53: 455-464.
7. Yates JW, Wallace HJ, Jr., Ellison RR, et al. 1973. Cytosine arabinoside (NSC-63878) and daunorubicin (NSC-83142) therapy in acute nonlymphocytic leukemia. Cancer Chemotherapy Reports, 57: 485-488.
8. Bodey GP, Coltman CA, Hewlett JS, Freireich EJ. 1976. Progress in the treatment of adults with acute leukemia. Archives of Internal Medicine, 136: 1383-1403.
9. Freireich EJ, Bodey GP, McCredie KB, et al. 1976. Developmental therapy in adult acute leukemia. Archives of Internal Medicine, 136: 1417-1421.
10. Gale RP, Cline MJ for UCLA Acute Leukemia Study Group. 1977. High remission-induction rate in acute myeloid leukemia. Lancet, 1: 497-499.
11. Rosenthal DS, Moloney WC. 1972. The treatment of acute granulocytic leukemia in adults. New England Journal of Medicine, 286: 1176-1178.

12. Spiers ASD, Goldman JM, Catowsky D, et al. 1977. Prolonged remission maintenance in acute myeloid leukemia. British Journal of Medicine, 2: 544-547.
13. Peterson BA, Bloomfield CD. 1981. Long-term disease-free survival in acute nonlymphocytic leukemia. Blood, 57: 1144-1147.
14. Rai KR, Holland JF, Glidewell OJ, et al. 1981. Treatment of acute myelocytic leukemia: a study by Cancer and Leukemia Group B. Blood, 58: 1203-1212.
15. Keating MJ, Smith TL, McCredie KB, et al. 1981. A four-year experience with anthracycline, cytosine arabinoside, vincristine, and prednisone combination chemotherapy in 325 adults with acute leukemia. Cancer, 47: 2779-2788.
16. Weinstein HJ, Mayer RJ, Rosenthal DS, et al. 1983. Chemotherapy for acute myelogenous leukemia in children and adults: VAPA update. Blood, 62: 315-319.
17. Bell R, Rohatiner AZS, Slevin ML, et al. 1982. Short-term treatment of acute myelogenous leukemia. British Medicine Journal, 284: 1221-1224.
18. Thomas ED. 1983. Acute myelogenous leukemia. Journal of Cellular Biochemistry, 7: 44.
19. Gale RP, Kay HEM, Rimm AA, Bortin MM. 1982. Bone-marrow transplantation for acute leukaemia in first remission. Lancet, 2: 1006-1009.
20. Zwaan FE, Hermans J. 1983. Bone marrow transplantation for leukemia: European results of 487 cases. Experimental Hematology, 11: 180a.
21. Weiden PL, Flournoy N, Thomas ED, et al. 1979. Antileukemic effect of graft-versus-host disease in human recipients of allogeneic-marrow grafts. New England Journal of Medicine, 300: 1068-1073.
22. Weiden PL, Sullivan KM, Flournoy N, et al. 1981. Antileukemic effect of chronic graft-versus-host disease. Contribution to improved survival after allogeneic marrow transplantation. New England Journal of Medicine, 304: 1529-1533.
23. Fefer A, Einstein AB, Thomas ED, et al. 1974. Bone-marrow transplantation for hematologic neoplasia in 16 patients with identical twins. New England Journal of Medicine, 290: 1389-1393.
24. Weiner R, Oblon D, Kramer B, et al. 1982. Brief, intensive chemotherapy without maintenance therapy for acute myelogenous leukemia. IN: Current Chemotherapy and Immunotherapy: Proceedings of 12th International Congress of Chemotherapy. Washington, DC, ASM. pp. 1512-1514.
25. Sauter C, Alberto P, Buchtold W, et al. 1980. Three to five months remission induction treatment of AML followed by maintenance treatment or no maintenance treatment. Proceedings of ASCO/AACR, 21: 433.
26. Vaughan WP, Karls JE, Burke PJ. 1980. Long chemotherapy-free remissions after single-cycle times-sequential chemotherapy for acute myelocytic leukemia. Cancer, 45: 859-965.
27. Glucksberg H, Cheever MA, Farewell VT, et al. 1983. Intensification therapy for acute nonlymphoblastic leukemia in adults. Cancer, 52: 198-205.
28. Preisler HD. 1982. Treatment failure in AML. Blood Cells, 8: 585-602.
29. Slavin RE, Dias MA, Saral R. 1978. Cytosine arabinoside induced gastrointestinal toxic alterations in sequential chemotherapeutic protocols. A clinical-pathologic study of 33 patients. Cancer, 42: 1747-1759.

30. Skipper HE. 1978. Reasons for success and failure in treatment of murine leukemia with drugs now employed in treating human leukemias. IN: Cancer Chemotherapy, Vol. 1. Ann Arbor, MI, Monograph Publishers/University Microfilms International, pp. 1-166.

31. McCulloch EA, Buick RN, Curtis JE, et al. 1981. The heritable nature of clonal characteristics in acute myeloblastic leukemia. Blood, 58: 105-109.

32. Norton L, Simon R. 1977. Tumor size, sensitivity to therapy, and design of treatment schedules. Cancer Treatment Reports, 61: 1307-1317.

33. Goldie JH, Coldman AJ. 1979. A mathematic model for relating the drug sensitivity of tumors to their spontaneous mutation rate. Cancer Treatment Reports, 63: 1727-1733.

34. Goldie JH, Coldman AJ, Gudauskas GA. 1982. Rationale for the use of alternating non-cross-resistant chemotherapy. Cancer Treatment Reports, 66: 439-449.

35. Legha SI, Keating MJ, Zander A, et al. 1980. 4'-(acridinylamino) methanesulfon-m-anisidide (AMSA): a new drug effective in the treatment of adult acute leukemia. Annals of Internal Medicine, 93: 17-21.

36. Frei E III, Freireich EJ, Gehan G, et al. 1961. Studies of sequential and combination antimetabolite therapy in acute leukemia: 6-mercaptopurine and methotrexate. Blood, 18: 431-454.

37. Burchenal JH, Murphy ML, Ellison RR, et al. 1953. Clinical evaluation of a new antimetabolite, 6-mercaptopurine, in the treatment of leukemia and allied diseases. Blood, 8: 965-999.

38. Levi JA, Wiernik PH. 1976. A comparative clinical trial of 5-azacytidine and guanazole in previously treated adults with acute nonlymphocytic leukemia. Cancer, 38: 36-41.

39. Vogler WR, Miller DS, Keller JW. 1976. 5-Azacytidine (NSC 102816): a new drug for the treatment of myeloblastic leukemia. Blood, 48: 331-337.

40. Von Hoff DD, Slavik M, Muggia FM. 1976. 5-Azacytidine: a new anticancer drug with effectiveness in acute myelogenous leukemia. Annals of Internal Medicine, 85: 237-245.

41. Bortin MM, Gale RP, Kay HEM, et al. 1983. Bone marrow transplantation for acute myelogenous leukemia. Journal of American Medical Association, 249: 1166-1175.

42. Thomas ED, Clift RA, Buckner CD. 1982. Marrow transplantation for patients with acute nonlymphoblastic leukemia who achieve a first remission. Cancer Treatment Reports, 66: 1463-1466.

SHORT TERM CHEMOTHERAPY FOR ACUTE MYELOGENOUS LEUKAEMIA

T.A. Lister, W. Gregory, A.Z.S. Rohatiner, B. Birkhead, R. Biruls, M. Barnett, H.S. Dhaliwal, M.L. Slevin, J.A.L. Amess

INTRODUCTION

The use of increasingly intensive chemotherapy for the treatment of acute myelogenous leukaemia has led to an apparent improvement in the prognosis of younger patients. It has become possible to support them effectively through the inevitable myelosuppression and infection, thereby increasing the proportion achieving complete remission. In several series the duration of first remission has been prolonged (1,2,3).

This analysis has been undertaken to determine the impact of the introduction of short term intensive cyclical chemotherapy into the treatment of AML at St. Bartholomew's Hospital.

MATERIALS AND METHODS

1. _Treatment_ - It was intended that all patients should receive 6 cycles of one of three combinations comprising adriamycin, cytosine arabinoside and 6-thioguanine (Table 1).

Table 1 - Treatment Programmes

	BIX	BX	BXb
ADR	*50mg/m^2 day 1	25mg/m^2 days 1-3	40mg/m^2 day 1 35mg/m^2 day 2
ARA-C	100mg/m^2 BD days 1-5 (i/v inj)	100mg/m^2 BD days 1-7 (i/v inj)	200mg/m^2 days 1-7 (c.i/v inf)
6-TG	100mg/m^2 BD days 1-5	100mg/m^2 days 1-7	100mg/m^2 BD days 1-7
No of Pts	34	48	30

2. Patients - One hundred and twelve consecutive previously untreated younger adults with acute myelogenous leukaemia referred to St. Bartholomew's Hospital, between February, 1978 and December, 1981, form the basis of the analysis. Details of the patient population according to the treatment programme prescribed are shown in Table 2a and 2b and the numb of actual cycles of therapy received by them in Table 2c.

Table 2a- Patient Details

		Total	B-IX	B-X	B-Xb
Number of Patients		112	34	48	30
Male:Female		59:53	17:17	26:22	16:14
Age	Range	15-59	15-59	15-59	15-59
	Mean	41	43	42	40
	Median	44	43	44	44
Morphology	M1	40	10	13	17
	M2	23	9	11	3
	M3	11	1	6	4
	M4	26	9	13	4
	M5	6	2	2	2
	M6	6	3	3	-
Blast Count $(\times 10^9/1)$					
	0-9.9	6	18	28	14
	10-99	46	14	17	15
	100	6	2	3	1
Preleukaemic State					
	Yes	12	2	6	4
	No	100	100	42	26

Table 2b - Study Dates

Date	Study	No	Antibiotics Prophylactic	Antibiotics Therapeutic	Complete Remitters
Feb 1978	BIX	11	-------	T & C	6
June 1978	BXa	27	-------	T & C	11
April 1979	BIX	23	FRANCO	T & C	22
July 1980	BXb	30	FRANCO	T & C	15
Nov 1981	BXc	21	FRANCO	T & C	17

Table 2c - Total Cycles of Therapy Received

CYCLES	1	2	3	4	5	6	
STUDY							TOTAL
BIX	1	1	0	2	3	21	28
BX	1	1	4	1	4	17	28
BXb	1	1	2	5	1	5	15
TOTAL	3	3	6	8	8	43	71

3. Supportive Care - All patients were nursed in the open ward. Prophylactic bowel decontamination (4) was effected with oral framycitin, colistin, nystatin and amphoterocin B lozenges, fever was treated as a bacterial infection with appropriate broad spectrum antibiotics, and prophylactic platelet concentrations from single donors were given to maintain the platelet count above 20 $x10^9/1$.

RESULTS

Complete remission was achieved in 71/112 (63%) patients (Table 3). The duration of remission, disease free survival

Table 3 - Complete Remission Rates

STUDY	BIX	BX	BXb	
				TOTAL
	28/34	28/48	15/30	71/112
	(82%)	(58%)	(50%)	(63%)

nd survival of all patients receiving short term therapy are ompared with those treated in Barts Trials I-VIII, (5,6) each ith prolonged maintenance, in Figures I, II and III.

The duration of first complete remission was significantly onger for the group of patients receiving B-X than B-IX p < .01) (Figure IV). It was also significantly longer for atients entering complete remission with either B-IX or B-X but not X-b), for whom the mean intercycle time was less than 0 days than those for whom it was longer (p < .003) (Figure V). t was also significantly longer (p < .0002) (Figure VI) for hose patients treated with B-IX only who received more as

144

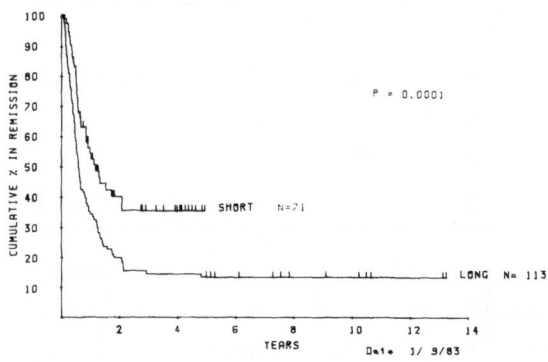

FIG I. ST. BARTHOLOMEW'S HOSPITAL AML STUDIES
REMISSION DURATION - SHORT TERM v LONG TERM THERAPY

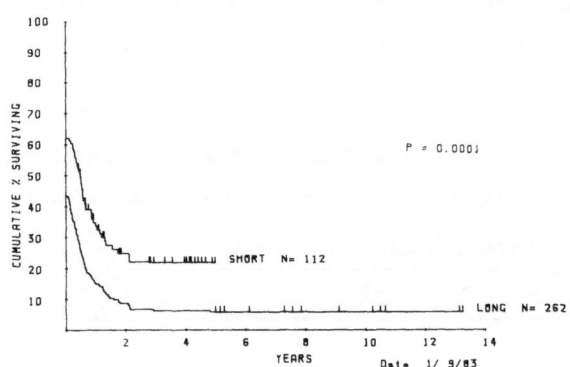

FIG II. ST. BARTHOLOMEW'S HOSPITAL AML STUDIES
DISEASE-FREE SURVIVAL - SHORT-TERM v LONG-TERM THERAPY

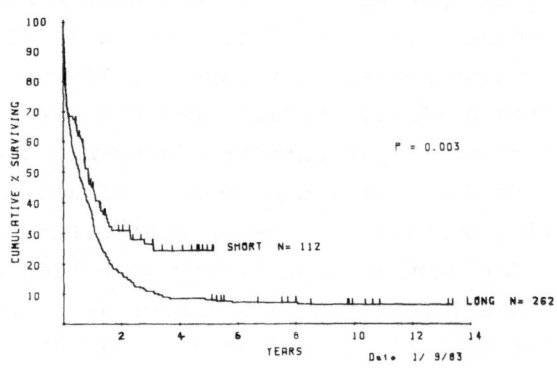

FIG III. ST. BARTHOLOMEW'S HOSPITAL AML STUDIES
SURVIVAL - SHORT-TERM v LONG-TERM THERAPY

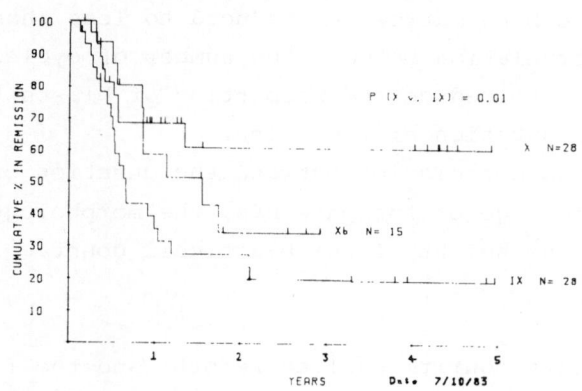

FIG IV. ST. BARTHOLOMEW'S HOSPITAL AML STUDIES
REMISSION DURATION BY TRIAL

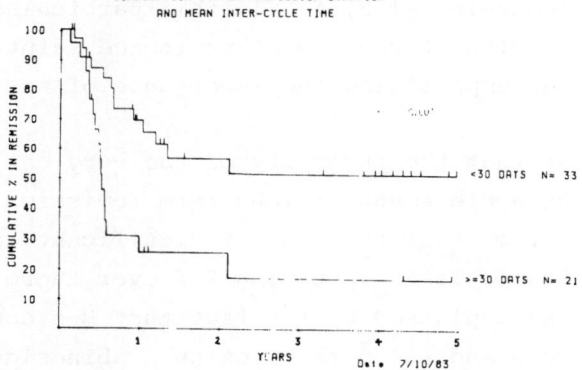

FIG V. ST. BARTHOLOMEW'S HOSPITAL AML STUDIES
CORRELATION BETWEEN REMISSION DURATION
AND MEAN INTER-CYCLE TIME

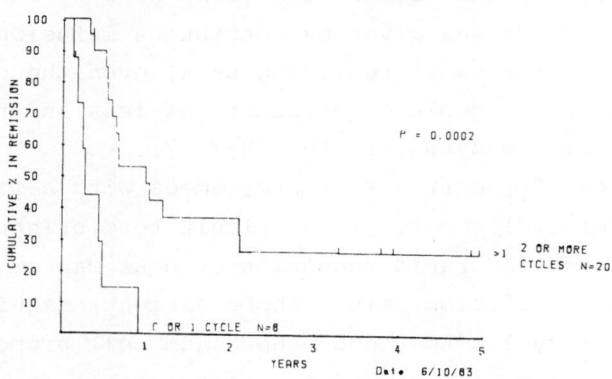

FIG VI. ST. BARTHOLOMEW'S HOSPITAL AML STUDIES
TRIAL IX - EFFECT OF CONSOLIDATION AFTER <5% BLASTS

opposed to less than one cycle of therapy after the proportion of blasts in the bone marrow was reduced to less than 5%. There was no correlation between the number of cycles of therapy required to reduce the proportion of blasts to less than 5% and the duration of remission.

There was no correlation between the duration of remission and the age of the pateints, the morphology of the blast cells or the height of the blast cell count.

DISCUSSION

These results confirm earlier reports and the finding of others that the intensification of the early therapy for younger adults has resulted in an increase in the duration of first complete remission (1,2,3). In this particular study, this was achieved without the use of prolonged maintenance treatment, further emphasising the importance of the initial therapy.

The argument that the intensity of the very early therapy is crucial to the achievement of long term remission is supported by the fact that there was a significant advantage in favour of those patients receiving B-X over those receiving B-IX. This may be explained by the fact that B-X contained 50% more adriamycin and 40% more cytosine arabinoside and 6-thioguanine in each of the first two cycles than B-IX. Against this lies the fact that the duration of remission for patients receiving B-Xb (almost identical to B-X, except that cytosine arabinoside was given by continuous infusion), was the same as that for those receiving B-IX, even though the number of cycles to complete remission was less and time to complete remission was shorter than B-X (7).

The design of the treatment programmes with a fixed total number of cycles makes it difficult to distinguish between the effect of rapid reduction of bone marrow infiltration and consolidation, since those patients requiring the least number of cycles to reduce the blast cell proportion to less than 5% will have received the most consolidation. Howe· in each of the three groups of patients, there was, for a

variety of reasons, a small number receiving <u>less</u> than six
cycles thereby making a tentative analysis possible. This
suggests, that for the least intensive of the three regimens
(b_IX), the more therapy given after remission, the greater
the probability of it being prolonged. It must, though, be
remembered that it is often difficult to distinguish the
difference between four, five and six per cent blast cell
infiltration of the marrow, and also that 'recovery blasts'
may be confused with persistent leukaemic infiltration. This
clearly makes the determination of the relevance of the quantity
of therapy given after remission difficult to assess.

The finding that the duration of complete remission
correlated closely with the mean intercycle time, those for
whom it was shorter having longer remissions than those for
whom it was longer, reinforces the argument that as much
therapy should be administered as quickly as possible. This
observation may partially explain why patients treated with
S-Xb, the most intensive regimen, did not have the best
remission duration, since their mean intercycle time was
significantly longer (7) than that of those patients receiving
S-X. In addition the number of patients receiving more than
a total of four cycles was small.

In conclusion these results support the further investigation of short term intensive cyclical combination chemotherapy
for younger adults with AML. They suggest that until such time
as a single cycle programme can be devised which effects cure
in most patients, that the intensity of each individual cycle
will be limited to that which allows re-treatment after a
relatively short interval.

REFERENCES

. Preisler HD, Brecher M, Browman G, et al. 198 . The
  treatment of acute myelocytic leukaemia in children and
  young adults.
. Weinstein HJ, Mayer RJ, Rosenthal DS, Coral FS, Camitta BM,
  Gelber RD. 1983. Chemotherapy for Acute myelogenous leukaemia
  in Children and Adults: VAPA update. Blood 62:2 p315
. Bell R, Rohatiner AZS, Slevin ML, Ford JM, Dhaliwal HS,
  Henry G, Birkhead BG, Amess JAL, Malpas JS, Lister TA.
  1982. Short-term treatment for acute myelogenous leukaemia

BMJ 284:1221
4. Schimpf SC, Grene WH, Young VM, Fratner CC, Jepson J,
   Cusack N. 1975. Infection prevention in acute non-
   lymphocytic leukaemia. Laminar air flow reverse isolation
   with oral non-absorbable antibiotics. Ann. Int. Med.
   36:770
5. Crowther D, Bateman CJT, Vartan CP etal. 1970. Combination
   chemotherapy using L-asparaginase, daunorubicin and
   cytosine arabinoside in adults with acute myelogenous
   leukaemia. Br. Med. J. 4:513
6. Lister TA, Whitehouse JMA, Oliver RTD, et al. 1980.
   Chemotherapy and immunotherapy for acute myelogenous
   leukaemia. Cancer 46:2142
7. Slevin ML, Rohatiner AZS, Dhaliwal HS, Henry GP, Lister TA
   1982. A comparison of two schedules of cytosine arabinoside
   used in combination with adriamycin or 6-thioguanine in
   the treatment of acute myelogenous leukaemia. Med & Pedia.
   Oncol. 10:1 p 185

FACTORS INFLUENCING DISEASE FREE INTERVAL AFTER ACHIEVING COMPLETE REMISSION
IN ACUTE LEUKEMIA
M.J. KEATING

The state which we term complete remission (CR) in acute leukemia is
a clinical diagnosis. No evidence of tumor can be detected by clinical
scrutiny or by examination of blood or bone marrow. However for many years
we have operated on the assumption that up to 100,000,000 leukemic blast
cells may be present at the time of complete remission and remain unidenti-
fied using current methodology (1). It was assumed that all patients had
minimal residual leukemia (MRL) at the time of CR and it is only recently
that there has been convincing evidence for a cured fraction in adult leukemia
2). The vast majority of patients received maintenance therapy after
achieving CR, a situation analogous to adjuvant treatment in solid tumors.
Instead of using surgery or radiation, the hematologist has used chemotherapy
as the modality to render the patient free of disease. Because of limitations of effective agents this same modality has had to be used in the
adjuvant setting. Bone marrow transplantation in CR is now an alternate
approach and is being used with increasing frequency in young patients (3).
    A key question which has been posed is whether maintenance therapy
is beneficial for some or all patients and clinical trials have been set
up to address this question. If maintenance therapy is useful, which
program is the best and what is the optimum duration of therapy? If some
patients have been helped by maintenance therapy, can we identify these
patients? If there are no patients being helped by maintenance treatment,
should we offer no treatment after achieving CR or should we try novel
approaches in the adjuvant setting. We have addressed these questions in
several studies at the M. D. Anderson Hospital and some of these studies
are reported below.
. LATE INTENSIFICATION
    Up until 1970, most patients who achieved CR were continued on the
same regimen which was used to induce remission. Relapse of the disease
occurred in almost all patients within two years, indeed less than one

year in more than half of the patients. The fundamental change in this pattern occurred in the late 1960's when cytosine arabinoside was introduc into remission induction and maintenance regimens (2). As an increasing proportion of patients were still free of disease at one year, most of whom had been induced into remission and maintained with ara-C containing regimens, a decision was made to administer a brief intensive course of treatment and then to discontinue chemotherapy. The drugs used in the late intensification study were selected for each patient on the basis of proven activity in AL and because the patients had not previously been exposed to them. The results were initially published in 1976 (4). Subsequently this study was updated and a prognostic factor analysis was performed to identify which patients were likely to remain disease free (5

Sixty-two patients who had been in CR for 8 to 45 months received three courses of late intensification; POMP (mercaptopurine, methotrexate vincristine and prednisone) were used in all except five patients. Forty-nine patients had acute myelogenous leukemia (AML), seven acute lymphobla: leukemia (ALL), and six acute undifferentiated leukemia (AUL). Twenty-five patients remain free of disease for more than five years since dis-continuation of chemotherapy. Twenty-two of the 37 relapses (59%) occurr within six months of starting treatment. The only factors related to probability of prolonged disease-free survival were a serum lactic dehy-drogenase level of < 400 mg/ml, a long duration of CR prior to initiation of late intensification and the dose received during late intensification (5).

This study illustrated that it was possible to discontinue treatment in adults with acute leukemia and that a significant proportion of these patients remain free of disease. All our studies since the late intensi-fication studies were completed have had a defined period of treatment after CR (9-24 months).

2. FACTORS ASSOCIATED WITH CR DURATION

In 1977 we analyzed the clinical and laboratory characteristics associated with remission duration in 202 patients who had achieved CR on regimen containing ara-C, vincristine and prednisone (OAP) combined with an anthracycline, either Adriamycin (Ad-OAP) or rubidazone (ROAP) (6). Most of these patients received OAP or cyclocytidine (an ara-C analogue) for remission maintenance. Several factors were associated with long CR duration. The CR duration of patients with AML was longer

than for ALL and those with AUL had a shorter CR duration. The only factor
which measured extent of tumor and which influenced CR duration was the
absolute blast cell in the blood (high value associated with short remission).
Liver, spleen and lymph node size had no effect on CR duration. While
the oldest group of patients (> 65 years of age) had the shortest CR
durations, no other age effect was noted. A high level of serum lactic
dehydrogenase (LDH) and high fibrinogen levels were associated with short
CR duration. A summary of the significant data is shown in Table A.

Table A.   Pretreatment Characteristics Related to Length of Complete Remission

Characteristic	Favorable Characteristic	Level of Significance
LDH	< 400 mU/ml	< .01
Blast cell count	< 10,000	< .05
Morphology	AML	< .01
Fibrinogen	Low	.01
Age	65 yrs.	10
Labelling Index	Intermediate value (9-13%)	.07

A number of events occurring during treatment influenced duration
of remission. Sensitivity to chemotherapy as measured by the number of
courses to remission and the rate of decrease of the leukemia burden in
bone marrow and blood was a favorable prognostic sign. In addition poor
tolerance of chemotherapy in the first three maintenance courses after
obtaining a CR was associated with a high relapse rate. Of interest was
the observation that most of the factors associated with probability of
obtaining a CR e.g. age, history of an antecedent hematologic disorder,
temperature at onset of treatment, liver size, renal function, etc. were
not strongly related to CR duration. Presumably, this is because these
factors measure probability of failing to achieve CR because of infection
and hemorrhage, rather than measuring characteristics of the tumor cells.
A rudimentry evaluation of the influence of cytogenetics on CR duration,
based on modal number and presence of metaphases did not show any strong
association with response.

Multivariate regression analytic techniques were used to develop a
Cox's regression model to determine the set of pretreatment characteristics
which best fits the observed CR duration data (6,7). This technique
identifies the factor most strongly related to CR duration, then the
factor which when added to the first factor best describes the data

and so on to third
fourth, fifth factors etc. until no other factor significantly adds to
the ability of the model to describe the observed data. Six factors adde
significant prognostic information as is shown in Table B.

Table B. Summary of Regression Analysis Relating Length of Response to
Patient Characteristics

Characteristic	Sig. Level of entry	Log-likelihood	Relative risk		
			Fav. *	Unf. +	Ratio
LDH	< .001	-437.506	.66	1.31	1.98
Fibrinogen	.001	-432.464	.71	1.52	2.14
Courses to CR	.004	-428.426	.79	1.80	2.28
AML	.081	-426.909	.83	1.54	1.86
Time to halving leukemic cells	.031	-424.570	.66	1.42	2.15
Age	.056	-422.749	.93	2.10	2.26

Cox's model relating length of CR to patient characteristics:

$$\ln \frac{\lambda(t)}{\lambda_0(t)} = .6840(LDH - 1.61) + .3788(Fibrinogen - 1.89)$$
$$+ .4103(Co.\ to\ CR - 1.57) - .6204(AML - .70)$$
$$+ .2567(Halv.Leuk.cells - 2.64) + .8139(Age - 1.09).$$

---

*Favorable characteristics: LDH≤ 400, fibrinogen < 250, 1 co. to CR,
AML, no leukemic cells day 1, age < 65.
+Unfavorable characteristics: LDH > 400, fibrinogen > 400, 3 co. to
CR, non-AML, leukemic cells halv. day 5, age ≥ 65.

ie fit of the model to the data from which it was derived is shown in
igure 1.

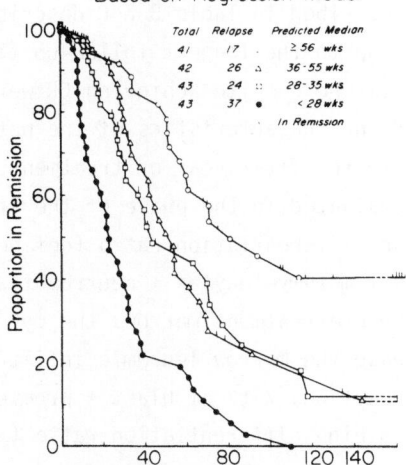

Length of CR By Predictions
Based on Regression Model

Total	Relapse	Predicted Median
41	17	≥ 56 wks
42	26	36-55 wks
43	24	28-35 wks
43	37	< 28 wks
		In Remission

[GURE 1. The fit of model to predict duration of remission; observed CR
iration according to predicted risk of relapse categories.

; AML was the predominant morphologic subtype a separate model was developed
or AML and a four-factor model resulted. The number of courses to CR was
ie strongest predictive factor for CR duration in AML (Table C).

ible C. Summary of Regression Analysis Relating Length of Response in
AML to Patient Characteristics

	Sig. level of entry	Log-likelihood	Relative risk		
			Fav.*	Unf.†	Ratio
ourses to CR	<.001	333.439	.66	2.30	3.48
)H	<.001	326.669	.61	1.41	2.31
ibrinogen	.004	322.625	.67	1.69	2.52
je	.08	321.092	.93	1.95	2.10

Cox's model relating length of CR to patient characteristics:

$$\ln \frac{\lambda(t)}{\lambda_0(t)} = .6223(\text{courses to CR} - 1.66)$$
$$+.8432(\text{LDH} - 1.59)$$
$$+.4648(\text{Fibrinogen} - 1.87)$$
$$+.7431(\text{Age} - 1.10)$$

*Favorable characteristics: 1 course to CR, LDH <400 mU/ml, fibrinogen
<250 mg/dl, age <65 yrs.
† Unfavorable characteristics: 3 courses to CR, LDH >400 mU/ml, fibrinogen
> 400 mg/dl, age > 65 yrs.

3. PREDICTING EARLY RELAPSE

The median CR duration of the 202 patients presented in the preceding section was one year. The models described in Table B & C described the risk of relapse from the time of CR up to the longest follow-up time. We were interested in detecting patients who despite achieving CR were at high risk of relapse. Thus we evaluated the characteristics of the patients which were associated with relapse in the first year of treatment. Addit. pretreatment characteristics were evaluated in the phase of the study, the most important of which were the differentiation ratio (defined as % blasts + promyelocytes/% myelocytes + metamyelocytes + neutrophils) and the percentage of eosinophils in the pretreatment marrow, the cytogenetic pattern and the time taken to decrease the marrow leukemic infiltrate (defined as (% cellularity on clot section) X (% of blast + promyelocytes in the smear differential) ÷ 100). A high differentiation ratio (> 15) is strongly associated with a low serum level of LDH and was found to predic for a high likelihood of staying in CR for more than one year. Patients with a translocation between chromosomes 8 and 21, t(8q;21q) and those with a single hyperdiploid clone with the addition of a single chromosome as the sole abnormality also had a high probability of staying in remissi for one year. Most of the patients did not have banding studies performe and in such patients the t(8q;21q) group was recognized by having a karyo of (-C,+D,+E,-G). The combination of factors which best fits the observe data were the cytogenetic pattern, differentiation ratio, a morphology with > 4% eosinophils or promyelocytic leukemia, less than 20 days to achieve cytoreduction to < 10 marrow infiltrate and the general morphologic subtype acute myelogenous leukemia. When the equation below is solved for an individual patient, a value for p between 0 and 1 will result. This value will be the chance of that patient staying in CR for

year (PCR 1). The model and the results when the model was tested in
he population from which it was derived is shown in Figure 2.

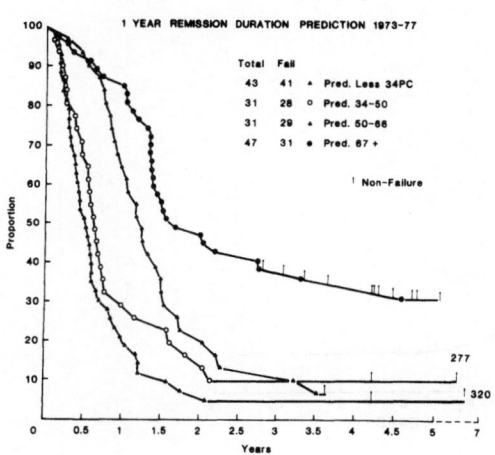

'IGURE 2. Fit of model to predict probability of staying in remission
'or one year; observed CR duration according to predicted probability of
.taying in CR for one year (PCR 1).

ighty   percent of the patients with the lowest PCR 1 (Pred. less 34)
ιad relapsed in one year. The patient with the highest PCR 1 values
Pred. 67+) had 84% still in CR at one year and most of the long term
·emission patients are in this group. This model was used to assign
atients to good and poor risk prognostic groups in protocol DT 79-95.
. IDENTIFICATION OF LONG TERM SURVIVORS IN AML
    In the mid 1970's it was becoming obvious that an increasing number
f patients with AML were remaining free of disease for more than 5 years
espite discontinuation of maintenance chemotherapy. A review of all
dults with AML who were treated at the M. D. Anderson Hospital between

1965 and 1976 was carried out (8). Forty-one (9%) of the 457 patients
have survived more than five years (Figure 3).

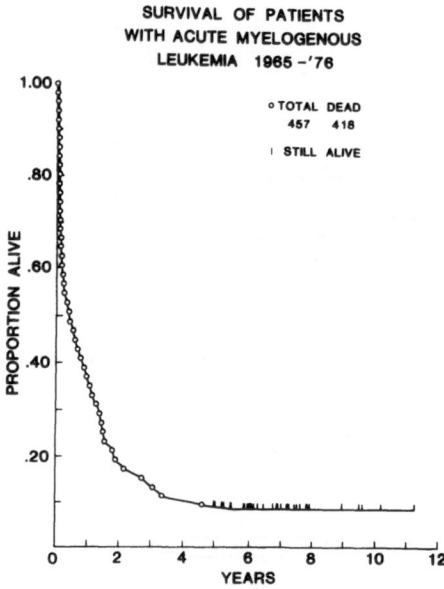

FIGURE 3. Survival of patients with AML treated between 1965 and 1976.
The proportion of long term survivors in various time periods were 1965-
1969, 1.8%; 1970-1972, 8.8%; and 1973-1976, 11.8%. The major factor
influencing probability of 5 year survival was whether or not patients
were treated with an anthracycline + ara-C combination or a full dose
ara-C regimen (Table D).

Table D. Overall Results and Five-Year Survival Rates According to
Chemotherapy Programs in AML (1965-1976)

Regimen	Total No. of Patients	No.(%) of 5-yr Survivors	No.(%) in Complete Remission	No.(%) in Continuous Complete Remission
Total	457	41(9)	207(45)	36(17)
Anthracycline-ara-C combination	223	29(13)	126(57)	25(20)
Ara-C	62	10(16)	24(39)	9(38)
Cyclophosphamide-ara-C combination	88	1(1)	31(35)	1(3)
Other	84	1(1)	26(31)	1(4)

Two hundred and seven (45%) of the 457 patients obtained a CR and could be considered as having achieved a condition of minimal residual leukemia. Apart from treatment, the factor associated with CR duration were similar to the factors described in sections 2 and 3. The five pre-treatment factors were serum LDH level, differentiation ratio, presence of eosinophils in the bone marrow, and a diagnosis of promyelocytic leukemia. Sensitivity of chemotherapy was related to remission duration as noted by the long duration of patients with the most rapid cytoreduction in blood and bone marrow (Table E).

Table E. Prognostic Factors Associated with CR Duration and 5 Year Remission

	207 Patients	
Factor	Complete Remission Duration	5-yr Continuous Complete Remission Rate
Pretreatment		
Antecedent hematologic disorder	> .10	> .10
Age	> .10	> .10
Temperature	> .10	> .10
Liver size	> .10	> .10
Auer's rods	> .10	> .10
Serum urea nitrogen level	> .10	> .10
Hemoglobin level	> .10	> .10
WBC count	.05-.10	.05-.10
Lactic dehydrogenase level	< .01	.01-.05
Differentiation ratio	< .01	.01-.05
Eosinophilia (marrow)	< .01	> .10
Promyelocytic leukemia	< .01	< .01
Treatment		
Hepatitis	< .01	.05-.10
Rate of cytoreduction		
Bone marrow	< .01	> .10
Blood	< .01	.05-.10

Additionally patients who developed SGOT elevation (> 2½ times normal) during maintenance therapy had longer CR durations than other patients. The major factor associated with 5 year CCR was the serum LDH level, differentiation ratio, and diagnosis of promyelocytic leukemia. The reason for the beneficial effect of "hepatitis" on CR duration and survival is not certain but has now been reported by at least three groups (8,9,10). A postulated mechanism is that the patients with hepatitis have gained normal immunocompetence and this is the reason for both enzyme elevation in response to a "hepatotropic" virus and prolonged remissions.

158

5. EFFECT OF TYPE AND DURATION OF MAINTENANCE REGIMENS

In 1976 we instituted a trial of rubidazone combined with ara-C, vincristine and prednisone (ROAP) for remission induction and consolidatic therapy (three courses after CR) in AML patients over 50 years of age (11) Maintenance was with cyclocytidine an analogue of ara-C and this was giver for two years. The results were compared with the historical experience with AdOAP induction and consolidation therapy (3 courses after CR) and OAP + BCG by scarification as maintenance therapy for nine months with POI late intensification (LI) in age-matched patients treated between 1973 & 1976. The results of remission induction therapy were 44/91 CRs for ROAP (48%) and 34/80 for AdOAP (43%). The median CR duration for the ROAP-cyclocytidine and ADOAP-OAP-LI groups were 37 weeks and 59 weeks respecti' (Figure 4).

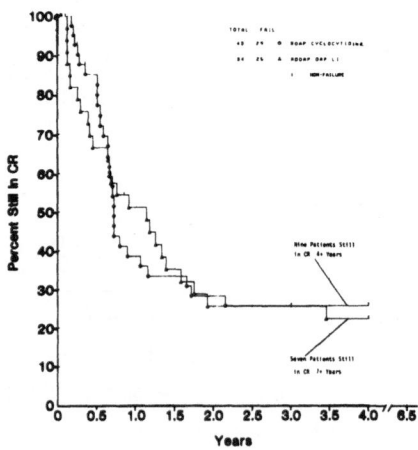

FIGURE 4. Remission duration of AML patients over 50 years of age mainta with cyclocytidine or OAP.

Seven (21) of the 34 AdOAP patients are still in CCR for more than sever years and nine (23) of the 44 ROAP patients are still in CCR for 4+ year One patient died in CR at 36 months from pancreatitis. Thus there was nc difference detected in two regimens in elderly patients with AML in which different maintenance regimens were used and in which treatment continued for varying time periods. It is notable that a substantial proportion of elderly patients was able to achieve prolonged remissions in AML.

In 1977, a program was initiated in patients less than 50 years of age with AML in which three regimens were given sequentially. AdOAP was given for 3 courses, ara-C + thioguanine (TG) for 3 courses and cyclophosphamide, rubidazone, vincristine and prednisone (CROP) for 3 courses. All treatment was then discontinued after 8-9 months of treatment. Thirty of 41 patients (73%) obtained a CR. Twenty-eight patients continued on the chemotherapy regimen. The median CR duration was 42 weeks. Eleven of the 21 patients who had treatment discontinued relapsed in the next six months. Only four of the 28 patients remain in CCR for more than four years. Two other patients are alive in prolonged second remission (Figure 5).

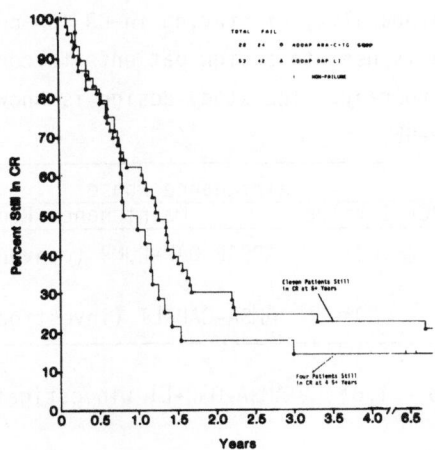

FIGURE 5. Remission duration of AML patients less than 50 years of age - nine months vs fifteen months maintenance treatment.

These 28 patients were compared with 53 matched control patients who had AdOAP induction therapy, OAP + BCG maintenance and POMP late intensification between 1973-1977. The median CR duration of the latter group was 65 weeks and 13 (24%) of these patients remain in continous complete remission for 6+ years. The overall CR duration and survival of the two groups was not significantly different. Shortening of the duration of maintenance therapy is associated with a shortening of median CR duration but this has not resulted in shortening of survival. There was however a slight reduction in the proportion of long term CCR patients.

The similar proportions of long term CCR patients in the reported studies (14-24%) suggest that a subset of patients exists who are very sensitive to chemotherapy or who have some other well defined biological characteristic which renders them curable with present conventional therapy whereas others are not curable with present regimens.

6. USE OF PROGNOSTIC INFORMATION IN CLINICAL TRIALS

The major purpose in studying prognostic factors in acute leukemia is to determine which patients benefit from conventional "best" treatment and which patients may benefit from a trial of innovative treatment approaches We have used two models to assign patients in our front-line leukemia protocol (DT 79-95). The first model assigns patients to conventional remission induction treatment, AdOAP, if the probability of obtaining a CR is > .60 and to investigational treatment with AMSA combined with ara-C, vincristine and prednisone, AMSA-OAP, if they have a predicted probability of response (P.P.R.) of < .60. Once patients achieve a CR, the model used to predict the probability of staying in CR for one year (PCR 1), described in section 3 is used to assign patients to conventional or investigational maintenance therapy. The study design is shown below:

Table F. Study Design in DT 79-95

Induction Phase			Maintenance Phase	
			PCR 1 Value	Maintenance Regimen
PPR ⩾.6, Receive ADOAP Rx (Conventional)	C R		⩾ .60*	ADOAP-OAP-POMP (conventional)
			< .60*	AMSA-OAP-LI (investigational)
PPR <.60, Receive AMSA-OAP Rx (Investigational)	C R		0 - 1.0*	AMSA-OAP-LI (investigational)

Using this technique, four maintenance groups are identified A: PPR ⩾.6 and PCR 1 ⩾ .6; B: PPR ⩾.6 and PCR 1 <.6; C: PPR <.6 and PCR 1 0-1.0; and D: Transplant group. Group A received conventional treatment. Grou D, the allogeneic transplant patients are compared with patients in the same age range and with the same PCR 1 values who do not have a suitable

*Patients < 30 yrs (all PCR 1 values) and 30-39 yrs with PCR 1 < .60 have allogeneic transplant if available donor.

donor. Groups A,B, and C are compared with their appropriate historical control groups in the 1973-77 population on which the models were derived, matched for PPR and PCR 1 values. The results are shown below:

Table G. Remission Duration in DT 79-95 According to PPR and PCR 1 Values Compared with Historical Control Groups

PPR	PCR 1	STUDY	PATIENTS	Median CR Duration (Wks)	
$\geqslant.6$	$\geqslant.6$	1973-77	53	78	P = .67
		DT 79-95	33	123	
$\geqslant.6$	$>.6$	1973-77	85	34	P = .08
		DT 79-95	48	50	
$<.6$	$\geqslant.6$	1973-77	22	88	P = .92
		DT 79-95	28	65	
$<.6$	$<.6$	1973-77	47	39	P = .94
		DT 79-95	32	31	

Thus no difference in the remission duration of the study groups compared with the control groups were detected. The transplant results are discussed by Dr. Dickie in this volume. This technique allows objective stratification of patients by predetermined characteristics. Appropriate matched control patients can be selected from well documented historical control patients. Using historical control groups, the need for concurrent randomized control groups is obviated. The patients who received conventional remission induction and maintenance regimens in the new study serve as a concurrent group as it is anticipated that they will match the historical group and this was so in the study DT 79-95. The PPR and PCR 1 values also give an objective estimate of the probability of response and CR duration for each patient within subsets of patients which the investigator may wish to evaluate. For example, if a new test has been performed only on a relatively small group of patients the PPR and PCR 1 values for these patients can be summed to give an expected CR rate and the proportion of patients expected to stay in remission for one year. These values can be compared with the observed outcomes.

. EFFECT OF CYTOGENETIC PATTERN ON CR DURATION

We have evaluated the cytogenetic pattern of 488 patients with AML treated between 1973 and 1982 (14). The CR rate was 276/488 (57%). The majority of patients from 1976 onwards had Giemsa banding studies performed. The median CR duration and proportion of patients projected to be in CR for one, two and three years is shown in Table H.

162

Table H. Duration of Complete Remission and Proportion of Patients in CR at Various Time Intervals According to Cytogenetic Category - AML 1975 - 82

Category	Pts.	CR Duration Median (wks)	Proportion in CR (Projected)		
			1yr	2yr	3yr
Translocation 8-21*	23	104+	.64	.52	.52
Translocation 15-17*	9	74	.74	.48	?
Hyperdiploid Simple	17	74	.79	.38	.38
Diploid	146	78	.60	.30	.26
Philadelphia (Ph+)	5	61	.75	?	?
46 XO Male	6	44	.50	.25	?
Hyperdiploid Complex	18	46	.38	.24	.19
Hypodiploid	4	44	.38	?	?
Pseudodiploid	11	42	.38	.14	.14
Karyotypic Instability	10	49	.50	.30	.10
Insufficient Metaphases	23	44	.36	.26	.25

The specific translocations t(8q;21q) and t(15q;17q) and those with a single hyperdiploid clone with only one additional chromosome appear to have a longer CR duration than the diploid patients whereas all other categories have inferior CR durations. No effect on CR duration was noted according to whether the patients with an abnormal karyotype had 100% abno cells (AA) or a mixture of abnormal and normal cells (AN) (Figure 6).

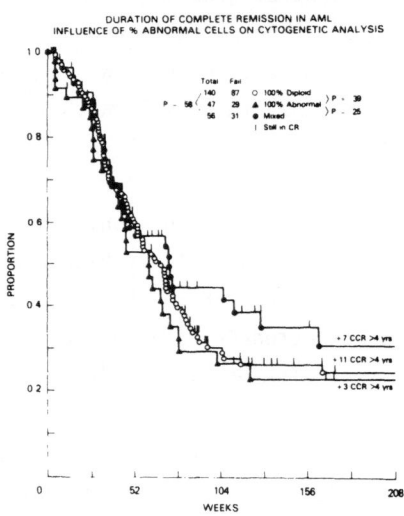

FIGURE 6. Remission duration according to proportion of abnormal cells on cytogenetic analysis

* Unbanded equivalent: t(8;21) = (-C+D+E-G), t(15;17) = Eq- + progranulocytic.

With the advent of banding techniques more specific translocations and
and other changes are being noted. Arthur and Bloomfield (15) have described
a change in the number 16 chromosome in association with eosinophilia.
As we have reported the favorable   of eosinophilia on CR, exploration
of the interaction of this specific abnormality and eosinophilia and the
effect on prognosis promises to delineate a syndrome similar to the
t(8q;21q) abnormality in young Auer rod positive patients and the t(15q;17q)
abnormality in acute promyelocytic leukemia. All three abnormalities
appear to be associated with long CR duration.

CONCLUSION

The outcome of patients who achieve a state of minimal residual
leukemia, CR, is extremely heterogeneous with present regimens used in
the maintenance of CR. Some patients relapse in 1-3 months whereas
others have stayed in remission off all treatment for more than 10 years
and are presumably cured. The first group of patients need new approaches
to treatment to give them a chance of long-term survival. The latter
patients could possibly have treatment discontinued at an earlier phase
than had been the custom. While the intensive analysis of clinical factors
has provided useful prognostic information which is already being applied
in the design and analysis of clinical trials, further progress in the area
awaits new discoveries in the fields of cytogenetics, cytokinetics, cellular
pharmacology and cell biology.

REFERENCES

1. Frei E, III., and Freireich EJ. Progress and perspectives in the
   chemotherapy of acute leukemia. Adv. in Chemother. 2:269-298, 1965.
2. Keating MJ: Early identification of potentially cured patients with
   acute myelogenous leukemia - A recent challenge. In: Adult leukemias
   1, C.I. Bloomfield (ed.), Martinus Nijhoff Publishers, The Hague/Boston/
   London, 1982, pp 228-263.
3. Thomas ED, Buckner CD, Clift RA, et al: Marrow transplantation for
   acute nonlymphoblastic leukemia in first remission. New Engl. of Med.
   301:597-599, 1979.
4. Bodey GP, Freireich EJ, Gehan E, et al: Late intensification therapy
   for acute leukemia in remission. JAMA 235:1021-1025, 1976.
5. Bodey GP, Freireich EJ, McCredie KB, et al: Prolonged remissions in
   adults with acute leukemia following late intensification chemotherapy
   and immunotherapy. CANCER 47:1937-1945, 1981.
6. Keating MJ, Smith TL, Gehan EA, et al: Factors related to length of
   complete remission in adult acute leukemia. CANCER 45:2017-2029,
   1980.
7. Cox DR. Analysis of binary data. London, Methuen, 1970.
8. Keating MJ, McCredie KB, Bodey GP, et al: Improved prospects for
   long-term survival in adults with acute myelogenous leukemia. JAMA
   248:2481-2486, 1982.

9. Barton JC, and Conrad ME. Beneficial effects of hepatitis in patients with acute myelogenous leukemia. Ann. Intern. Med. 90:188-190, 1979.
10. Wade JC, Wiernik PH, Schimpff SC, et al: Hepatitis prolongation of complete remission and survival in acute nonlymphocytic leukemia (ANLL) patients. Proc. Am. Soc. Clin. Oncol. 21:439, 1980 (Abstract C-474).
11. Keating MJ, McCredie KB, Benjamin RS, et al: Treatment of patients over 50 years of age with acute myelogenous leukemia with a combination of rubidazone and cytosine arabinoside, vincristine, and prednisone (ROAP). BLOOD 58:584-591, 1981.
12. Freireich EJ, Keating MJ, Smith T, et al: A method for evaluation of novel therapy in previously untreated patients: AMSA-OAP combination therapy in adult acute leukemia. Proc. Am. Soc. Clin. Oncol. 1:127, 1982 (Abstract C-493).
13. Winton EF, Martelo O, Hearn E, et al: Phase I-II study of 5-azacytidine (AZA) (NSC #102816) and Amsacrine (AMSA) (NSC #249992) in refracto adult acute leukemia. Proc. Am. Soc. Clin. Oncol. 174, 1983 (Abstract C-676).
14. Keating MJ, Cork A, Smith T, et al: A prognostically significant classification of cytogenetic patterns in acute myelogenous leukemia (A.M.L.). BLOOD 60:130a, 1982 (Abstract 449).
15. Arthur DC and Bloomfield CD. Partial deletion of the long arm of chromosome 16 and bone marrow eosinophilia in acute nonlymphocytic leukemia: A new association. BLOOD 61:994-998, 1983.

IN VITRO CHEMOTHERAPY AS A PRELUDE TO AUTOLOGOUS MARROW TRANSPLANTATION IN HEMATOLOGIC MALIGNANCY

GEORGE W. SANTOS AND HERBERT KAIZER

The successful application of autologous marrow transplantation to the treatment of neoplastic disease has three requirements: 1) It must be possible to obtain and viably store sufficient numbers of hematopoietic stem cells to insure recovery of hematologic and immunologic function; 2) Clonogenic tumor cells must be absent from the hematopoietic stem cell inoculum, and 3) The tumor remaining in the patient must be sensitive to an intensive pulse of pre-transplant therapy at doses that have acceptable extramedullary toxicity.

The long-term relapse free survival of a significant fraction of patients with acute leukemia (1) and non-Hodgkin's lymphoma (2, 3) who receive bone marrow transplants from identical twins suggest that cure of these diseases may be achieved by a supralethal pulse of cytoreductive therapy in the absence of graft-versus-tumor effects. Although few patients with these malignancies possess a monozygotic twin their autologous remission marrow is a source of syngeneic stem cells. The problem that prevents the more general use of cryopreserved autologous marrow is the presence of occult tumor cells in the remission marrow, particularly important in the case of acute leukemia. Although there may be some improvements to be made in the collection and cryopreservation of marrow, it would seem that focusing on these aspects of stem cell procurements, storage and recovery will probably be minimally productive, since the reported kinetics of hema-

Supported by PHS Grants CA-15396 and CAO-6973 awarded by the National Cancer Institute, DHHS

tologic reconstitution for autologous transplants with the use of total body irradiation (TBI) or equivalent marrow lethal therapy and widely varying approaches to processing storage and recovery variables have been remarkably similar (4). Thus, of the three requirements for successful application of autologous marrow transplantation for the treatment of hematologic malignancy two of the requirements have been at least partially solved but what remains is the problem of being able to give marrow that is free of clonogenic tumor cells.

In this communication we shall focus primarily on autologous transplantation in acute leukemia and lymphoma with particular attention paid to methods that might be used to purge marrow of putative tumor cells. We will give emphasis to chemical approaches.

ANIMAL AND IN VITRO MODELS FOR "PURGING"

"Purging" can be accomplished if some difference can be found between tumor cells and stem cells that will either allow the separation or destruction of one type in the presence of the other. In the course of such procedures the functional properties of the stem cells must, of course, be retained. There would seem to be three possible approaches to this problem: physical separation, immunological manipulation or pharmacologic treatment.

Physical separation methods have been most extensively studied by Dicke et al. (5-7). On the basis of information indicating the density of leukemic blasts may be different from that of normal stem cells (8) they have devised discontinuous albumin gradients for the separation of human marrow cells (5). Using electromicrographic and cytogenetic markers for leukemic cells that are more sensitive than light microscopy, they have shown a 1-log reduction in marker-positive leukemic cells in density fractions containing the bulk of stem cells as measured by CFU-c (7). Unfortunately, there are no critical animal models that have been presented using this technique. The applicability of this approach, therefore, must remain in question, particularly since a clinical trial was carried out in a limited number of patients and no advantage was seen if the remission marrow had been fractionated as described above or not (6).

A number of groups have focused on immunological approaches to the problem of in vitro elimination of tumor cells. We have previously reviewed the details of some of this work (9) in three animal models - a C3H mouse lymphoma (10), an AKR mouse leukemia (11), and a W/Fu rat acute non-lymphocytic leukemia (12) - incubation of marrow - tumor cell mixtures with heterologous cytotoxic antiserum to a tumor-associated antigen in the presence of complement resulted in the complete inactivation of clonogenic tumor as measured by the ability of such cell suspensions to rescue lethally irradiated animals without the development of tumor. In the C3H model (10) the antisera used was shown to have cytotoxic activity against marrow stem cells and lacked, therefore, absolute tumor specificity. This latter finding implys that arguments regarding the absolute specificity of tumor-associated antigens towards which the antiserum are directed are irrelevant. What is relevent is that the antiserum and conditions of incubation be such that sufficient numbers of stem cells survive under conditions where the tumor cells are destroyed. Subsequently, monoclonal antibody and complement or monoclonal antibody attached to a cellular toxin such as ricin have been shown to be effective in purging tumor marrow cell mixtures in animal models (13-15).

The feasibility of using in vitro pharmacologic treatment of marrow to eliminate all occult leukemic cells was first shown by our group using a metabolite of cyclophosphamide, 4-hydroperoxycyclophosphamide (4HC) which is cytotoxic in vitro (see reference 16 for a review of the properties of 4HC) was able to "purge" marrow tumor mixtures of tumor. A drug dose-dependent clearing of tumor cells from a normal marrow and tumor cells was demonstrated in a model of acute myelogenous leukemia in the Lewis-Brown Norway hybrid rat (17). Further increases of drug concentration resulted in increasing death rates due to marrow failure (18). It should be noted that in this system florid leukemia may be cured _in vivo_ if the animals are given otherwise lethal doses of Cyclophosphamide followed by the infusion of syngeneic marrow (19).

Recently ASTA-WERKE Laboratories have synthesized a stabilized oxazophosphorine derivative of 4HC (ASTA-Z-7557) that shows comparable _in vitro_ effects to 4HC. A Dutch group (20) reported that the _in vitro_ sensitivity of human leukemic clonogenic cells compared to normal hematopoietic progenitors was not different for ASTA-Z-7557. They used _in vitro_ cloning techniques for these assays. They concluded that preincubation of bone marrow with minimal residual leukemia for autologous marrow transplantation with this compound might not be effective. Previously Hagenbeek and Martens (21) reported on studies with 4HC in BN rat acute non-lymphocytic leukemia model. They reported that the clonogenic tumor cells were more sensitive than the hematopoietic CFUs with 4HC. Further reports by others were somewhat conflicting. Thus Gorin and his colleagues (22) using _in vitro_ clonogenic assays for human hematopoietic progenitors as well as leukemia colony formation reported a similar sensitivity by this assay to 4HC as well as the ASTA-Z-7557. Delforge _et al._ (23) on the other hand compared the cytotoxic effect of 4HC on the proliferation of human normal and leukemic CFUc. They concluded on the basis of the study that the results did not encourage the use of 4HC for specific elimination _in vitro_ of the leukemic cells contaminating the marrow of patients in complete remission. The studies were _in vitro_ studies.

In a less extensive study Stiff _et al._ (24) were able to demonstrate that the podophyllotoxin VP-16-213 was able to "purge" tumor cells from a mixture of normal C57B6 murine marrow and syngeneic EL-4 lymphoid tumor cells. Most recently a novel approach was used to purge marrow of tumor cells. The fluorescent dye merocyanine 540 (MC540) was proposed as a possible useful probe for developmentally regulated plasma membrane constituents on hematopoietic progenitor cells (25) since the dye reacts primarily with lipid bilayer of the plasma membrane. MC540 is a negatively charged fluorescent dye that binds preferentially fluid domains in the outer leaflet of the lipid bilayer of intact cells. Photoexcitation of membrane bound dye with green or white light causes increased dye uptake, impairment of the normal permeability properties of the plasma membrane and eventually cell death. Sieber et al. (26, 27) showed that with the use of dye that purging of leukemic cells from auto-logous marrow grafts in murine systems was possible. No clinical studies have as yet been performed with this method of purging, but it does show interesting possibilities.

AUTOLOGOUS MARROW TRANSPLANTATION IN LYMPHOMAS

The early data on autologous transplants in non-Hodgkin's lymphoma are in sharp contrast to the results seen in acute leukemia (vide infra). A number of prolonged disease-free survivors indicated potential cures (3, 28). These results suggested that tumor cell contamination of remission in mar-row is not an invariant feature in all lymphohematopoietic malignancies. Nevertheless some groups have begun to "purge" narrow in lymphomas. We shall first review the results of autologous marrow transplantation in lymphomas where the mar-row has not been "purged" of potential tumor cells.

To date, the best results with intensive combination chemotherapy in autologous bone marrow transplant have been achieved in non-Hodgkin's lymphoma. Appelbaum, for instance, reported 22 patients with refractory lymphoma treated with a combination of BCNU, cytosine arabinoside, cyclophosphamide and 6-thioguanine (BACT). Ten patients achieved complete re-mission and four patients (with Burkitt's lymphoma) remained free of disease for 1.5-4 years of follow-up (29). Kaizer et al. (30) reported three patients with non-Hodgkin's lymphoma treated with adriamycin, doxorubicin, cyclophosphamide and TBI. One patient (with Burkitt's lymphoma) achieved a com-plete remission and survives free of disease at the present writing of greater than 6.5 years. In 1980 Herzig (31) re-viewed the then existing data and pointed out that seven patients with Burkitt's lymphoma who were resistant to conventional therapy apparently were cured by the use of intensive combination of drugs or TBI with autologous marrow transplantation. This high rate of response and potential cures has continued with a later experience with Burkitt's lymphoma.

Subsequently, a number of reports have appeared that relatively long-term remissions with autologous bone marrow transplantation in bad prognosis non-Hodgkin's lymphoma may be obtained when these patients are prepared with intensive polychemotherapy (32-38) or high dose chemotherapy and TBI (34, 39-41). The Seattle group has one report to the contrary wherein eleven (previously heavily treated) patients were transplanted following preparation with cyclophosphamide and TBI. There was only one long-term survivor (42).

When patients were prepared for transplantation with minimal relapse or even early extensive relapse it appeared that the response rate for complete remission might approach 70-80%. The long-term survival, that is, of a year and greater appeared in most of the reports to be at the level of 40-60% of the patients. One cannot from these preliminary reports determine which preparative regimen has an advantage over the other or whether polychemotherapy has an advantage over regimens containing TBI. Data available scattered throughout these reports include some cases of refractory Hodgkin's disease that have been transplanted with encouraging results.

There have been few studies of the use of purged marrow in lymphomas. Baumgartner et al. (43) performed autologous marrow transplants for advanced abdominal Hodgkin's lymphoma after in vitro purging of marrow collected in a clinical remission with anti-Y29/55 monoclonal antibody and complement. Patients were prepared with vincristine, adriamycin, high doses of cyclophosphamide, and 600 rad TBI. In this preliminary report of four patients there was continuous complete remission for 1, 10, 12, and 17 months.

The Baltimore group (unpublished observations) has transplanted five patients with T-cell lymphoma and three patients with T-cell ALL in their second to fourth remissions. All the patients received cyclophosphamide (50 mg/kg i.v. on each of four successive days for a total dose of 200 mg/kg) followed by fractionated TBI over four days for a total dose of 1200 rad. The autologous marrow that was infused had been harvested in remission and treated with monoclonal anti-T-cell antiserum and complement. The antiserum was developed by Dr. R. Levy and his colleagues (44). The first patient with lymphoma received adriamycin in addition to the Cyclophosphamide before TBI. This patient has been previously reported (45) and survives in continuous complete remission for 35[+] months. Two other patients relapsed at 48 and 75 days after transplantation. The remaining two patients with T-cell lymphoma survive in continuous complete remission for 11[+] and 18[+] months following marrow transplantation. One of the T-cell leukemias died of hemorrhage at 16 days and the other two patients relapsed at 2 and 18 months following transplantation.

As part of a Phase I study of 4HC all patients in second or subsequent remissions were prepared with cyclophosphamide 50 mg/kg x 4 followed by 300 rad a day x 4 of TBI before receiving marrow that had been previously incubated with 4HC (40-100 ug/ml). Marrow was collected in a remission and one patient was transplanted in complete remission, two were transplanted in subsequent complete or partial remissions. Three patients relapsed, one at one month, and two at two months post-transplantation. Two patients survive continuously free of disease for 21[+] and 24[+] months following transplantation.

AUTOLOGOUS MARROW TRANSPLANTATION IN ACUTE LEUKEMIA

Early studies of marrow transplantation using marrow collected in a remission and then employed when the patient relapsed produced no real long-term cures. For example, when analysis of the actuarial leukemia free survival was made from data pooled from several centers a median duration of remission of from four to six months was found with no evidence of plateau of long-term disease-free survivals (46).

Dicke et al. (47) for example, reported 28 patients with relapsed acute leukemia treated with piperazinedione and TBI (750-950 rad single fraction or 1200 rad split fraction) followed by transplantation of autologous marrow that was cryopreserved during remission. Twelve patients or 43% entered complete remission with a median unmaintained duration of four months with a range of 2-14 months. For ten patients bone marrow was fractionated on albumin gradients to remove occult leukemic cells before cryopreservation. The fractionation procedure had no apparent effect on remission rate or duration. Herzig noted (31) that his group had treated 27 patients with acute leukemia at relapse with high dose cyclophosphamide and TBI (1,000 rad single fraction or 1200-1400 split fraction) followed by cryopreserved remission marrow. Nineteen patients or 69% achieved complete remission with a median duration of five months with a range of 2-16[+] months. Three patients in that series remain free of disease 8, 12, and 17 months post-transplant without further treatment. More recently Lucarelli et al. (48) reported a study in five patients using cyclophosphamide and TBI preparation regimen but they added a maintenance schedule with cytotoxic drugs. Three patients with acute lymphocytic leukemia (ALL) and two patients with acut non-lymphocytic leukemia (ANL) were transplanted in remission, three of these were in first remission, the others were in the second or third remission. Two relapses were seen at three and six months, the others survived for 5-10 months in complete unmaintained remission at the time of the report. Helbig et al. (49) reported on 12 patients with acute leukemia, five ALL and seven ANL. One was in relapse, eight were in first remission and three were in second remission. They were prepared with two days of cyclophosphamide 60 mg/kg x 2 and 600-760 rad of TBI given as a single dose. Of these 12 patients, relapses were seen at 30, 111, 145 and 281 days. Ten are alive from 13[+] - 583[+] days, but two of these patients did relapse at 271 and 244 days. Vellekoop (50) reported on 14 patients with adult ALL. These patients were begun on the protocol in their first re-

mission.   Chemotherapy consisted of cyclophosphamide, BCNU,
and VP-16-213.   Rescue bone marrow was fractionated over a
discontinuous albumin gradient to minimize possible contamination with leukemic cells.   The median total remission duration was 14 months.   Three patients relapsed after one course
of treatment, five patients relapsed after the second course.
Four patients died after the second course and two patients
remain alive and well in unmaintained remission with a total
remission duration of 42^+ and 47^+ months.   Stewart et al.
(51) reported on ten patients with ANL given autologous
transplants in their first remission.   They were prepared
with cyclophosphamide 60 mg/kg x 2 and 1000-1200 rad of TBI.
In addition, all patients were given a short course of
methotrexate following transplantation.   Four of these ten
patients survive for 4, 6, 26, and 31 months following the
autologous marrow transplant.

Netzel et al. (52) transplanted three children with refractory ALL in relapse.   All three marrows were incubated
with an IgG fraction purified from a rabbit anti-CALLA antiserum.   The first patient died on day seven of cardiac
failure, the second and third received complete remissions
but one of them relapsed at six months.   There is no report
of follow-up on the third patient.   In similar studies
Mitsuyasu et al. (53) reported on four patients with common
ALL antigen positive (CALLA) acute lymphoblastic leukemia in
second or subsequent remission or relapse.   The remission
marrow was incubated with a rabbit antiserum against the
CALLA antigen.   The patients received intensive chemotherapy
and TBI.   All patients had prompt engraftment.   At the time
of the report two patients survive in complete remission 1^+
and 16^+ months.   Sallan et al. (54) reported on nine patients
with ALL that were CALLA positive.   Remission marrows were
treated with an anti-CALLA monoclonal antibody (J-5) and
rabbit complement.   Patients were transplanted in second
remission employing VM-26 Ara-C, cyclophosphamide and 850 rad
TBI.   Seven of nine of these patients at the time of the
report remained in complete unmaintained remission from 1-22

months with a median of 5$^+$ months.

In 1980 the Baltimore group began a Phase I study employing 4HC as a tumor purging agent in patients with hematologic
malignancy, the preliminary results have been previously
reported (55). A total of 36 patients were included in the
study: 21 with ALL, 9 with ANL, 5 with non-Hodgkin's lymphoma
and 1 with neuroblastoma. In order to qualify for the study,
patients met the following criteria: 1) their expected two-
year disease free survival was less than 5%; 2) multiple samples of bone marrow prior to harvesting were microscopically
free of tumor (less than 5% blasts on marrow aspirate).

Eight patients with acute leukemia exhibited a partial
relapse with between 7-20% leukemic blasts in their marrow
during the time between the marrow harvesting and the start
of their preparative regimen. Except for two patients in
first remission for ALL and ANL, all patients were in their
second or subsequent remissions of leukemia or in partial
relapse.

The study was designed to escalate the concentration of
4HC used for in vitro treatment of the marrow by increments
of 20 ug/ml. Marrow collected from each patient was ali-
quoted into a treated and reserved fraction. Initially the
treated fraction was incubated with 40 ug/ml of 4HC and the
reserve marrow was untreated. In the next two groups of
patients the treated marrow was incubated at 60 and 80 ug/ml
and the reserve fraction was treated at 40 ug/ml. For the
subsequent two groups, experimental treatment was 100 and 120
ug/ml of 4HC while the reserve marrows were treated with 60
ug/ml. Patients with ALL and Non-Hodgkin's lymphoma were
prepared with 200 mg/kg of cyclophosphamide given over four
days and followed by 1200 rad given also over four days.
Patients with ANL received busulfan 16 mg/kg given over four
days followed by 200 mg/kg of cyclophosphamide over four
days. Marrow was infused 24-36 hours after the last dose of
cytoreductive therapy.

Overall analysis of the data revealed the following: 1)
incubation of marrow with 40-100 ug/ml of 4HC did not require

the use of reserve or "rescue" marrow since all patients showed evidence of engraftment. At 120 ug/ml 4/7 patients failed to show adequate engraftment and, therefore, this dose was considered too toxic; 2) a dose related inhibition of committed hematopoietic progenitor cells, measured in vitro was seen with complete inhibition at 80 ug/ml; 3) There appeared to be a slight dose related effect of 4HC when recovery curves for granulocytes, reticulocytes, and platelets were compared in patients whose marrows were incubated with 40 ug/ml, 60-100 ug/ml and 120 ug/ml.

Of the 21 patients with ALL two patients transplanted in their second remission survive in continuous remission for 16[+] and 18[+] months except for two patients at the 120 ug/ml dose who died too early to evaluate. All the other patients relapsed from 16-777 days after transplantation. The median days to relapse was 112 days following marrow transplantation.

Of the 9 patients with ANL two patients survive free of disease for 23[+] months (transplanted in third remission at 80 ug/ml) and 30[+] months (transplanted in first remission at 60 ug/ml). One patient transplanted in the sixth remission died of veno-occlusive disease 36 days after transplantation (80 ug/ml) and represented the only transplanted related death in patients whose marrow was incubated with 40-100 ug/ml of 4HC. Another patient died of sepsis on day 28 after failing to engraft following marrow incubation with 120 ug/ml of 4HC. The other five patients relapsed from 5-8.5 months following transplantation, the median relapse time was six months.

Herve et al. (56) reported on 22 patients (12 AML, 7 ANL, 3 CML) whose marrows were incubated with 60-80 ug/ml of STA-Z-7557. Nine of these patients were transplanted using this marrow while they were in complete remission (7 ANL, 2 ALL). There was a slight delay in engraftment time and one relapsed six months later. The other eight patients survive in continuous disease-free remission for 3[+] - 16[+] months. Unfortunately, the median time was not given.

SUMMARY AND CONCLUSIONS

The application of autologous bone marrow transplantation in lymphohematopoietic malignancies has only recently shown widespread interest and, therefore, conclusions must be interpreted with some caution. With this caveat, however, it appears that the procedure of high-dose polychemotherapy or high-dose chemotherapy and TBI followed by autologous marrow infusion in non-Hodgkin's lymphoma holds considerable promise. The choice of the most effective preparative regimen and whether or not marrow needs to be "purged" of occult tumor cells remains to be resolved by further clinical studies.

In acute leukemias where autologous marrow transplantation is performed in the second or subsequent remission, "purging" of the marrow would seem essential. At the moment, chemical or immunological methods to "purge" remission marrows would appear to hold considerable promise. The effectiveness of individual methods as well as their comparative effectiveness, however, remains to be defined. Even if an effective method is found, additional or changes in present anti-leukemic treatment will be needed since, on the basis of studies in syngeneic marrow transplants, one may still expect about a 50% relapse rate.

Although it would appear that autologous marrow transplantation makes the most biologic sense if performed in the first remission for high risk patients, such a study design poses some problems, since it has been estimated that 25 to 30% of patients may have very long complete remissions with chemotherapy alone. Furthermore, the data from syngeneic transplants indicate that the upper figure for long-term complete remissions for autologous transplants should not exceed 50%. How would one resolve the criticism that patients receiving autologous transplants in the first remission were those who were already "cured" of their disease at marrow harvest?

For these reasons we have embarked on a Phase II study of the use of 4HC to "purge" marrow in acute leukemia only in

the second remission. It is generally agreed that such
patients cannot usually be cured of their disease with chemotherapy. If our study shows a 30-50% disease-free survival,
then we will have at least indirect evidence that the marrow
"purging" was effective. A more direct approach would be to
randomize patients, but this poses problems with patient
acceptance and perhaps ethical problems.

REFERENCES

1. Santos GW. 1983, in press. Allogeneic and syngeneic marrow transplantation in acute leukemia with minimal residual disease. In B Lowenberg, A Hagenbeek (Eds.): Minimal
   Residual Disease in Acute Leukemia. Martinus Nijhoff
   Publishers BV, The Netherlands.
2. Appelbaum FR, Fefer A, Cheever MA et al. 1981. Treatment
   of non-Hodgkin's lymphoma with marrow transplantation in
   identical twins. Blood 58: 509.
3. Appelbaum FR and Thomas ED. 1983. Review of the use of
   marrow transplantation in the treatment of non-Hodgkin's
   lymphoma. J. Clin. Oncol. 1: 440.
4. Kaizer H and Santos GW. 1982. Autologous bone marrow
   transplantation in the treatment of leukemia, lymphomas,
   and other cancers. In I Ariel (Ed.): Progress in Clinical Cancer. Grune & Stratton, Inc. New York, pp. 31.
5. Dicke KA, McCredie KB, Stevens EE et al. 1977. Autologous
   bone marrow transplantation in a case of acute adult leukemia. Transplant. Proc. 9: 193.
6. Dicke KA, Zander A, Spitzer G et al. 1978. Autologous
   bone marrow transplantation in relapsed adult leukemia.
   Lancet 1: 514.
7. Dicke KA, Zander A, Spitzer G et al. 1979. Autologous
   bone marrow transplantation in relapsed adult leukemia.
   Exp. Hematol. 7: 170.
8. Moore MAS, Williams N, Metcalf D. 1973. In vitro colony
   formation by normal and leukemic human hematopoietic
   cells, interaction between colony forming and colony
   stimulating cells. J. Natl. Cancer Inst. 50: 591.
9. Kaizer H, Wharam MD, Johnson RJ et al. 1980. Requirements
   for the successful application of autologous bone marrow
   transplantation in the treatment of selected malignancies. Haematol. Blood Transf. 25: 285.
0. Economou JS, Shin HS, Kaizer H et al. 1978. Bone marrow
   transplantation in cancer therapy: Inactivation by antibody and complement of tumor cells in mouse syngeneic
   marrow transplants. Proc. Soc. Exp. Biol. Med. 158: 449.
1. Thierfelder S, Rodt H, Netzel B. 1977. Transplantation of
   syngeneic bone marrow incubated with leucocyte antibodies
   I. Suppression of lymphatic leukemia of syngeneic donor
   mice. Transplantation 23: 459.

178

12. Bast RC Jr, Feeny M, Greenberger JS et al. 1979. Elimination of leukemic cells from rat bone marrow using antibody and complement (C'). Proc. AACR ASCO 20 (abstr.): 239.
13. Vitetta ES, Krolick KA, Miyama-Inaba M et al. 1983. Immunotoxins: A new approach to cancer therapy. Science 219: 644.
14. Krolick KA, Uhr JW, Vitetta ES. 1982. Selective killing of leukaemia cells by antibody-toxin conjugates: Implications for autologous bone marrow transplantation. Nature 295: 604.
15. Thorpe PE, Detre SI, Mason AJ et al. 1983. Monoclonal antibody therapy: "Model" experiments with toxin-conjugated antibodies in mice and rats. Haematol. Blood Transf. 28. Modern Trends in Human Leukemia V. Neth, Gallo, Greaves, Moore and Winkler (Eds.). Springer-Verlag Berlin, Heidelberg.
16. Friedman OM, Miles A, and Colvin M. 1979. Cyclophosphamide and related phosphoramide mustards. In A Rosowsky (Ed.) Advances in Cancer Chemotherapy. Marcel Dekker, New York. pp. 143.
17. Sharkis SJ, Santos GW, and Colvin OM. 1980. Elimination of acute myelogenous leukemia cells from marrow and tumor suspensions in the rat with 4-hydroperoxycyclophosphamide. Blood 55: 521.
18. Kaizer H, Cote JP, Sharkis S et al. 1982. Autologous bone marrow transplantation in acute leukemia: The use of in vitro incubation of tumor-marrow mixtures with 4-hydroperoxycyclophosphamide (4HC) in a Wistar-Furth rat model of acute myelogenous leukemia (WF-AML). Proc. Am. Assoc. Cancer Res. 23: 194.
19. Santos GW and Sharkis SJ. 1978. Experience with syngeneic marrow transplantation in BN and WF rat models of acute myelogenous leukemia. In SJ Baum and GD Ledney (Eds.) Experimental Hematology Today. Springer-Verlag, New York, Inc. pp. 187.
20. Kluin-Nelemans JC, Martens ACM, Hagenbeek A et al. 1983. In vitro sensitivity of human leukemic clonogenic cells and normal hematopoietic progenitors to ASTA-Z-7557 is not different. Exp. Hematol. 11 (Suppl. 14) (abstr.): 9.
21. Hagenbeek A and Martens ACM. 1982. Autologous bone marrow transplantation in acute leukemia. Separation of hematopoietic stem cells from clonogenic leukemia cells by 4-hydroperoxycyclophosphamide. Exp. Hematol. 10 (Suppl. 11) (abstr.): 14.
22. Gorin NC, Douay L, Najman A et al. 1982. Study of the in vitro sensitivity of human leukemic cells and normal hematopoietic progenitors to 4-hydroperoxycyclophosphamide (4HC). The interest for the preparation of anti-leukemic autologous bone marrow transplantation. Exp. Hematol. 10 (Suppl. 11) (abstr.): 13.
23. Delforge A, Malarme M, Debusscher L et al. 1982. Comparison of the cytotoxic effect of 4 hydroperoxycyclophosphamide on the proliferation of human normal and leukemic CFU-C. Exp. Hematol. 10 (Suppl. 11) (abstr.): 14.

24. Stiff PJ, Wustrow T, DeRisi M et al. 1982. An in vivo murine model of bone marrow (BM) purification of tumor by VP-16-213. Blood 60 (Suppl. 1) (abstr.): 17a.

25. Sieber F, Meagher RC and Spivak JL. 1981. Differential sensitivity of mouse hematopoietic stem cells to merocyanine 540. Differentiation 19: 65.

26. Sieber F, Stuart RK, Sensenbrenner LL et al. 1982. Susceptibility to merocyanine 540-mediated photosensitization preferentially inhibits in vitro colony formation by two human leukemia cell lines. Clin. Res. 30 (abstr.): 331A.

27. Sieber F, Meagher RC, Sutcliffe AM et al.. 1983. Purging of leukemic cells from bone marrow grafts by merocyanine 540-mediated photosensitization. Clin. Res. 31 (abstr.): 412A.

28. Santos GW and Kaizer H. 1982. Bone marrow transplantation in acute leukemia. Sem. Hematol. 19: 227.

29. Appelbaum FR, Herzig G, Graw RG et al. 1979. Accelerated hematopoietic recovery following the infusion of cryopreserved autologous bone marrow in humans. Exp. Hematol. 7 (Suppl. 5): 297.

30. Kaizer H, Wharam MD, Johnson RJ et al. 1980. Requirements for the successful application of autologous bone marrow transplantation in the treatment of selected malignancies. Blut (Suppl. 25): 285.

31. Herzig GP. 1980. Autologous marrow transplantation in cancer therapy. In Progress in Hematology. EB Brown (Ed.) Vol. 12, pp. 1.

32. Philip T, Biron P, Herve P et al.. 1983. Massive cytoreductive regimen and autologous bone marrow transplantation in 32 cases of bad prognosis malignant lymphomas. Exp. Hematol. 11 (Suppl. 14) (abstr.): 69.

33. Gorin NC, Laporte JP, Douay L et al. 1983. Autologous bone marrow transplantation in the treatment of non-Hodgkin's lymphomas of high grade malignancy. Exp. Hematol. 11 (Suppl. 14) (abstr.): 70.

34. Philip T, Biron P, Maraninchi D et al. 1983. Experience of massive cytoreductive regimen and autologous bone marrow transplantation in 22 cases of bad prognosis malignant lymphomas. Proc. Am. Soc. Clin. Oncol. 2 (abstr.): 207.

35. Ricci P, Gabbi M, Bandini G et al. 1983. Autologous bone marrow transplant (ABMT) following superintensive chemotherapy in untreated non-Hodgkin's lymphoma (NHL). Exp. Hematol. 11 (Suppl. 13) (abstr.): 161.

36. Philip I, Philip T and Lenoir GM. 1983. In vitro outgrowth of Burkitt's lymphoma cell clones following cultivation of cytogenetically normal bone marrow: Application to autologous bone marrow transplantation. Exp. Hematol. 11 (Suppl. 13) (abstr.): 169.

37. Tannir N, Spitzer G, Zander A et al. 1983. High-dose cytoreductive therapy and bone marrow transplants in patients with refractory lymphoma. J. Cell. Biochem. Suppl. 7A (abstr.): 61.

180

38. Hartmann O, Pein F, Beaujean F et al. 1983, in press. The effects of high-dose polychemotherapy with autologous bone marrow transplantation in children with relapsed lymphomas. Med. Ped. Oncol.

39. Philips GL, Herzig RH, Wolf SN et al. 1983. Cyclophosphamide - Total body irradiation with and without boost radiotherapy in autologous bone marrow transplantation for relapsed lymphoma. Exp. Hematol. 11 (Suppl. 14) (abstr.): 69.

40. Barbasch A, Higby D, Brass C et al.. 1983. Autologous bone marrow transplantation (ABMT) in advanced malignancies. Proc. Am. Soc. Clin. Oncol. 2 (abstr.): 242.

41. Gulati S, Langleben A, Jain K et al.. 1983. Autologous stem cell transplantation (ASCT) after total body irradiation (TBI) and high dose cytoxan for poor prognosis lymphoma. Proc. Am. Soc. Clin. Oncol. 2 (abstr.): 218.

42. Bensinger W, Buckner CD, Stewart P et al. 1983. Autologous bone marrow transplantation in end stage lymphomas. J. Cell. Biochem. Suppl. 7A (abstr.): 58.

43. Baumgartner C, Brun del Re G, Forster HK et al. 1983. Autologous bone marrow transplantation (ABMT) for advanced abdominal non-Hodgkin's lymphoma (NHL) after in vitro purging with anti-Y29/55 monoclonal antibody and complement. Exp. Hematol. 11 (Suppl. 14) (abstr.): 6.

44. Engleman EG, Warnke R, Fox RI et al. 1981. Studies of a human T lymphocyte antigen recognized by a monoclonal antibody. Pro. Nat. Acad. Sci. 78: 1791.

45. Kaizer H, Levy R, Brovall et al. 1982. Autologous bone marrow transplantation in T-cell malignancies: A case report involving in vitro treatment of marrow with a pan T-cell monoclonal antibody. J. Biol. Resp. Modif. 1: 233.

46. Gale RP. 1980. Bone marrow transplantation in leukemia. J. Supramol. Struct. Suppl. 4: 3.

47. Dicke KA, Zander AR, Spitzer G et al. 1979. Autologous bone marrow transplantation in relapsed adult acute leukemia. Exp. Hematol. 7 (Suppl. 5): 170.

48. Lucarelli G, Porcellini A, Izzi T et al. 1983. Autologous bone marrow transplantation (ABMT) in acute leukemia in remission. Exp. Hematol. 11 (Suppl. 14) (abstr.): 68.

49. Helbig W, Kubel M, Schutze W et al. 1983. Autologous bone marrow transplantation in acute leukemia (AL). Exp. Hematol. 11 (Suppl. 14) (abstr.): 68.

50. Vellekoop L, Dicke KA, Zander AR et al. 1983, in press. Repeated high dose cyclophosphamide, BCNU and VP-16-213 and autologous bone marrow transplantation in adult lymphocytic leukemia in first remission. Europ. J. Cancer and Clin. Oncol.

51. Stewart P, Buckner CD and Thomas ED. 1983. Autologous marrow transplantation (AMT) in patients with acute non-lymphocytic leukemia (ANL) during first remission. J. Cell. Biochem. Suppl. 7A (abstr.): 57.

52. Netzel B, Rodt H, Haas RJ et al. 1981. Autologous marrow transplantation in childhood acute lymphoblastic leukemia: Elimination of leukemic cells from the graft by antileukemia antibodies. Exp. Hematol. 9 (Suppl. 9): 142.

53. Mitsuyasu R, Champlin R, Wells J et al. 1983. Autologous bone marrow transplantation after in vitro marrow treatment with anti-calla heteroantiserum and complement. Proc. Am. Soc. Clin. Oncol. 2 (abstr.): 184.

54. Sallan S, Bast R, Lipton J et al. 1983. Autologous bone marrow transplantation in childhood acute lymphoblastic leukemia. Blood 60 (Suppl. 1) (abstr.): 172a.

55. Kaizer H, Stuart RK, Fuller DJ et al. 1982. Autologous bone marrow transplantation in acute leukemia: Progress report on a Phase I study of 4-hydroperoxycyclophosphamide (4HC) incubation of marrow prior to cryopreservation. Amer. Soc. Clin. Onc. 1 (abstr.): 131.

56. Herve P, Tamyo E, Lamy B et al. 1983. In vitro treatment of autologous marrow cells collected in leukaemia patients using cyclophosphamide derivative. Exp. Hematol. 11 (Suppl. 14) (abstr.): 10.

IN VIVO AND IN VITRO PHARMACOLOGIC PURIFICATION OF BONE MARROW CONTAMINATED
WITH TUMOR CELLS USING VP16-213 AND NITROGEN MUSTARD

PATRICK J. STIFF , THOMAS P.U. WUSTROW , ALAN R. KOESTER , MICHAEL F. DERISI
AND BAYARD D. CLARKSON [3]

INTRODUCTION

When used as a therapeutic modality for patients with acute leukemia in
remission, supralethal chemo-radiotherapy and an allogeneic or syngeneic
bone marrow(BM) transplant appears to be superior to conventional
therapy(1). Selected patients with an acute non-lymphocytic leukemia in
first remission, who have a HLA-matched donor for example, can now expect a
two year or longer disease-free survival probability of 60-70%(2).
Unfortunately, only about one in three eligible patients have a suitable
HLA-matched donor. A variety of methods are being explored to expand this
form of therapy to those patients without suitably matched donors.
Autologous BM, obtained during a period of remission, has been tried as the
graft for patients without a suitable donor, but no long term remissions
have been achieved when the same anti-leukemic therapy that is given with
allogeneic or syngeneic transplants was administered(3). As would be
predicted on the basis of cell kinetic data(4), BM removed after the
attainment of a complete remission, when used as an autologous graft in a
patient with leukemia still does contain sufficient neoplastic cells to
engraft successfully and eventually lead to a clinical relapse.

Pharmacologic(5-7) and immunologic(2,8,9) methods of bone marrow
purification are beginning to be explored in hope of eliminating
contaminating tumor cells in remission marrows. This would allow for
reconsideration of autologous transplantation for patients without a
HLA-matched donor. Sharkis et al(5) used an active congener of
cyclophosphamide, 4-hydroperoxycyclophosphamide(4-HC), to purify, in vitro,
a rat BM of 1.6% contaminating tumor cells obtained from an acute
myelogenous leukemia cell line. Lethally irradiated transplant recipients

survived without any evidence of tumor engraftment, when the tumor/BM cell mixture was incubated with 60 nM of 4-HC and used as the transplant source Having demonstrated activity in this and a second animal model(6) they hav begun to treat human bone marrows in patients with acute leukemia in secor or subsequent remission(7). Other groups have begun to use monoclonal antibodies to purify BM specimens particularly those raised against surfac antigens of the lymphocytes of acute lymphocytic leukemia(8,9).

The effectiveness of these two methods remains to be determined. The major potential advantage of using pharmacologic agents as marrow purifyir agents would be their nonselective antitumor activity against a variety o usually heterogenous human tumors, while the advantage for monoclonal antibodies would be their apparent lack of inhibition of normal hematopoietic stem cells. The greatest antitumor effect may ultimately l in combinations of antibodies, pharmacologic agents, or a combination of both modalities.

Because of the effectiveness of 4-HC, we decided to investigate VP16-213(VP-16), a semisynthetic derivative of podophyllotoxin, and nitro mustard(HN$_2$), a second alkylating agent. VP-16 is an active agent for th treatment of a variety of malignant human tumors including both acute lymphocytic and nonlymphocytic leukemia, small cell undifferentiated carcinoma of the lung, diffuse lymphomas, testicular carcinoma and neuroblastoma(10). HN$_2$ is reported to be similar in activity to 4-HC in preliminary studies against two human B-cell lymphoma cell lines(11). Because of the spectrum of these two agents and the fact that they do not require in vivo activation for their activity, we decided to investigate them in an animal model of marrow purification utilizing a murine T cell leukemia-lymphoma, EL-4, a syngeneic tumor of the C57B6 mouse. If active this model, VP-16 and HN$_2$ would then deserve consideration as additional agents to be used for marrow purification in future human studies.

In hopes of establishing dosage guidelines for possible future human use, we determined as well the normal hematopoietic stem cell damage caus by these drugs. This was measured both in vivo, using the survival of mi transplanted with the treated BM as an endpoint, and in vitro, using bott committed(CFU-C;Colony Forming Unit-Culture) and pluripotent(CFU-S;Colony Forming Unit-Spleen) stem cell assays.

MATERIALS AND METHODS

Animals

Male C57B6 mice(Harlan Spraque-Dawley Inc. and Jackson Labs), nine to twelve weeks were used for all studies. They were housed in sterile cages in a laminar air flow hocd(Envirico) and fed sterile water and lab chow(Purina Labs) ad libatum.

Tumor

EL-4, a syngeneic T-cell lymphoma of the C57B6 mouse(12), was maintained in suspension in the log phase of growth, in a 5% CO_2 atmosphere at 37° C(Forma Labs). The doubling time was determined to be 12.2 ± 0.2 hours. The culture media used was RPMI-1640(M A Bioproducts) supplemented with fetal bovine serum(Sterile Systems) at a concentration of 20%(20% RPMI).

Drugs

VP16-213 was supplied in five ml ampules at a concentration of 20 mg/ml(Bristol Labs) in an organic solvent(13). Dilutions for studies were made with RPMI-1640, immediately prior to each experiment. HN_2 was provided as the powder in 10 mg vials(Mustargen;Merck Sharp and Dohme Company). It was reconstituted and diluted immediately before use with a 0.9% NaCl solution.

Purging Studies

Initially, in vitro clonageneic assays were done to determine the relative sensitivity of normal marrow and tumor stem cells. Bone marrow for all studies was removed from the tibias, humeri and femurs of the normal donor mice. The cells were washed twice and then suspended in 20% RPMI at a concentration of 5×10^6 cells/ml for the drug incubations. EL-4 cells were concentrated to 5×10^6 cells/ml in the same media. Dose response curves were established by independent incubations with VP-16 and HN_2 at various concentrations from 5.0 to 55.0 ug/ml for VP-16 and 0.025 to 0.30 ug/ml for HN_2 for 60 minutes at 37° C. After incubation the cells were centrifuged at room temperature at 200 x g for ten minutes and the supernatant fluid removed. The cells were additionally washed twice with 20% RPMI and re-suspended in fetal bovine serum for the stem cell assays.

Incubations for subsequent in vivo studies were similarly done. Based on the in vitro data showing its superiority, only VP-16 was studied in this group of experiments. Each mixture of 20-25 $\times 10^6$ BM cells and either 1 x 10^7, 5×10^6 or 1 x 10^6 EL-4 cells was incubated for 60 minutes with a concentration of 40 ug/ml of VP-16. This concentration was determined by the in vitro assays as described below. After washing, the mixtures were suspended in 0.2 ml aliquots in preparation for transplantation.

Recipient mice received total body irradiation to a total dose of 10! rads from a cesium source(137Cs) at a rate of 266.96 rads/minute using a small animal irradiator(J. L. Shepherd Co.) Immediately following irradiation, the mice were inoculated with the cell mixture via the orbit plexus or tail vein. The mice were followed for survival, with all death investigated by a postmortem examination and histologic evaluations of t spleen, liver, lung and kidneys, where appropriate.

Stem Cell Assays

CFU-C(Colony Forming Unit-Culture) and CFU-S(Colony Forming Unit-Spleen) hematopoietic stem cell assays were performed as previously described(14,15), with minor modifications. Briefly, the BM cells were cloned as are normal human BM cells, in 1% methylcellulose at a concentration of 1×10^5 cells/plate for the CFU-C assays, using a feeder layer of 1×10^6 human peripheral blood leukocytes, immobilized in 0.5% a as the source of colony stimulating activity. Colonies were scored after seven days of incubation at 37° C in a 5% CO_2 atmosphere. Quadruplicate assays were performed on each specimen, and the plates were counted using inverted microscope(Leitz). A colony was considered as an aggregate of 5 or more cells.

CFU-S assays were done using various BM cell inocula, depending on t concentrations of VP-16 and HN$_2$ incubated with the cells. For example BM cells that were untreated and those treated with 10 ug/ml of VP-16, the inoculum was 1×10^5 cells. For cells exposed to 20 and 30 ug/ml the inoculum was 2×10^5, for cells exposed to 40 ug/ml the inoculum was 5×1 and for cells exposed to 55 ug/ml the inoculum was 7.5×10^5. A similar escalating inocula schema was used for the HN$_2$. The mice were lethally irradiated and inoculated with the cells as described above. They were sacrificed ten days after inoculation and the splenic colonies were count after the spleens were immersed in Bouin's solution, using a dissecting microscope(Wild Heerbrug).

Tumor stem cell assays were similar to the CFU-C assays except for omission of the white cell feeder layer. Quadruplicate assays were coun after seven days in culture with a colony containing 20 or more cells.

Human Bone Marrow and Tumor Cell Line Studies

Normal human BM was obtained after written informed consent from either normal volunteers or patients with neoplastic diseases undergoing a BM aspiration for staging purposes. The BM was histologically normal in all cases. The BM and two human B-cell lymphoma cell lines, SK-DHL-2 and Raji, were incubated for one hour with VP-16 identically to the murine BM and EL-4 described above. The CFU-C and tumor CFUs were plated and incubated as above. The tumor CFUs were counted on day seven for the SK-DHL-2 and day ten for the Raji, while the CFU-C were counted on day ten. A tumor colony consisted of 20 or more cells and a CFU-C consisted of 40 or more cells.

Statistics

The two sample t-test was used in this study to select differences among proportions .

RESULTS

The results of the normal BM and EL-4 clonageneic cell assay inhibition are shown in Figures #1 and #2 for VP-16 and HN respectively. The baseline cloning efficiencies were for the CFU-C and EL-4 CFUs, .127±.027 and 19.3 ±3.0(S.D.)% . A striking difference in clonageneic cell kill was noted at each concentration of VP-16 with approximately the same one log of inhibition of clonageneic cells occurring at 40 ug/ml of VP-16 for the BM CFU-C but at only 1.25 ug/ml for the tumor cell colonies. No tumor colonies were present at VP-16 concentrations greater than 20ug/ml, while the difference in the inhibition between the CFU-C and tumor CFUs at 20 ug/ml was approximately 3 logs. Also shown in Figure #1 is the simultaneously obtained CFU-S cell kill. Although the CFU-C cell kill caused by VP-16 was less than that for the CFU-S cells at 10 ug/ml($p < .05$), no differences between these cells were seen at all the higher doses tested.

As shown in Figure #2, the greatest differential BM CFU-C and El-4 CFU cell kill caused by HN_2 was approximately 1.5 logs occurring at a dose of 0.2 ug/ml. At no dose of HN_2, ranging from 0.025 to 0.30 ug/ml was there any difference between the degree of BM CFU-C and CFU-S cell killing.

All lethally irradiated mice receiving BM transplants that were incubated with various concentrations of VP-16 up to and including 40 ug/ml(n=12) survived with obvious prompt hematopoietic reconstitution. The 40 ug/ml dose was used for the mixing studies because of the degree of CFU-C and CFU-S inhibition at this concentration and the marked differential

188

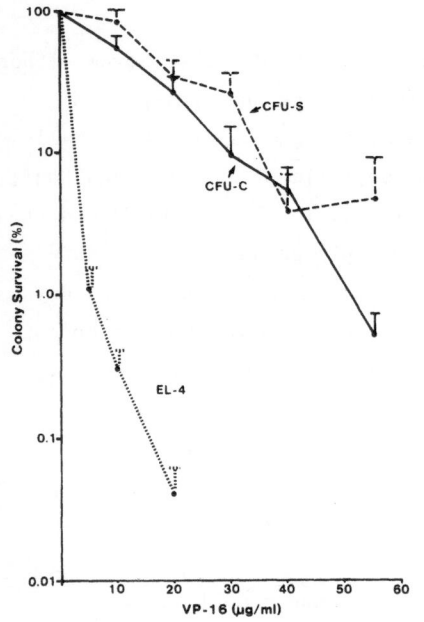

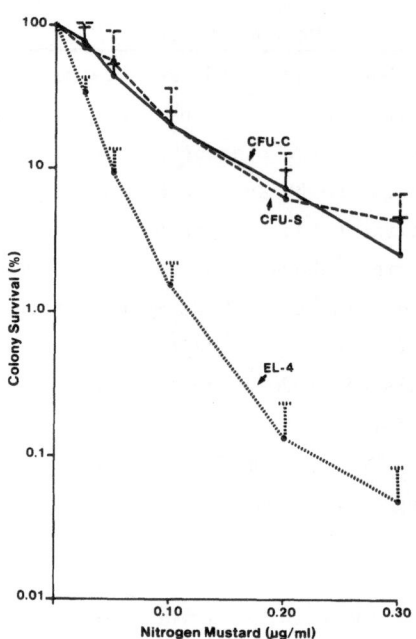

FIGURE 1. C57B6 murine BM CFU-C, CFU-S and EL-4 CFU inhibition after a 1 hour exposure to VP-16 at $37^{\circ}C(+SD)$.

FIGURE 2. C57B6 murine BM CFU-C CFU-S and EL-4 CFU inhibition after a 1 hour exposure to HN_2 at $37^{\circ}C(+SD)$.

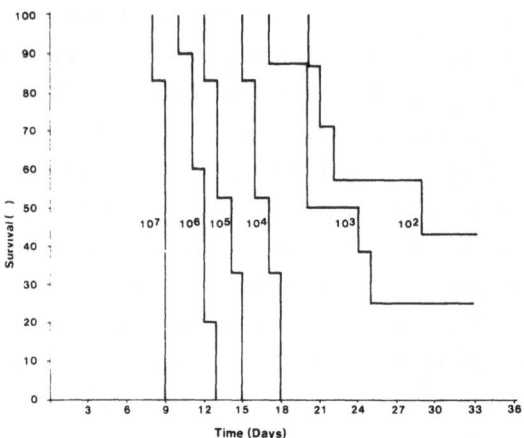

FIGURE 3. Survival of healthy C57B6 mice inoculated with varying numbers of viable EL-4 Leukemia cells in the log phase of growth.

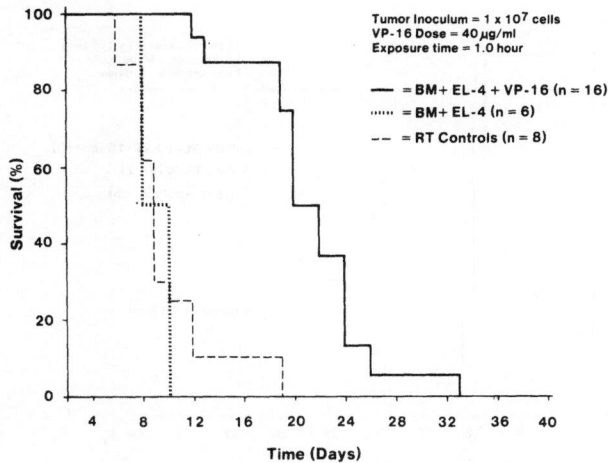

'IGURE 4. Survival of lethally irradiated C57B6 mice inoculated with a
umor/BM cell mixture treated in vitro with 40 ug/ml of VP-16 for 1 hour
t 37°C. The tumor cell inoculum was approximately 30% of the total.

ensitivities of the tumor and normal BM stem cells. Reconstitution using
M treated with concentrations of VP-16 greater than 40 ug/ml was not
ttempted.

As shown in Figure #3, a viable EL-4 cell inoculum of 10^4 cells led to
he death of all healthy mice with a median survival of 17 days. No healthy
ouse dying from a smaller number of tumor cells survived greater than 29
ays. All animals receiving transplants of BM and tumor treated with drug
ere thus followed for three times as long(90 days) to verify the absence of
umor cell engraftment.

In the first series of tumor/BM cell/VP-16 mixing studies, the
ioculum contained 1 x 10^7 EL-4 cells(approximately 1/3 of the total
ioculum). Compared to controls(Figure #4) receiving the mixture without
icubation with VP-16, those receiving the 'purged' sample lived
ignificantly longer, with a median survival of 22 vs. 9 days(p<.01). All
iimals receiving the VP-16 treated mixture did however, ultimately die as a
:sult of tumor cell engraftment.

In the second series, 1 x 10^6 or approximately 3% of the total inoculum
re tumor cells. As shown in Figure #5, in contrast to mice receiving 1 x
i^7 cells, all animals receiving these 'purged' mixtures survived 90+ days,
cept for a single animal who died at 13 days after transplantation.
wever, this animal had no tumor seen at the time of autopsy.

190

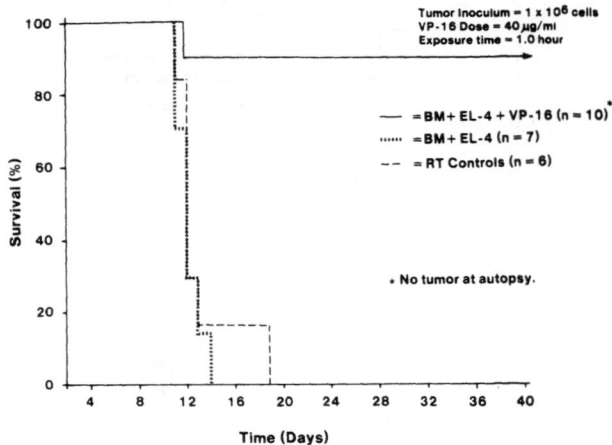

FIGURE 5. Survival of lethally irradiated C57B6 mice inoculated with a tumor/BM cell mixture treated in vitro with 40 ug/ml of VP-16 for 1 hour at 37°C. The tumor cell inoculum was approximately 3% of the total.

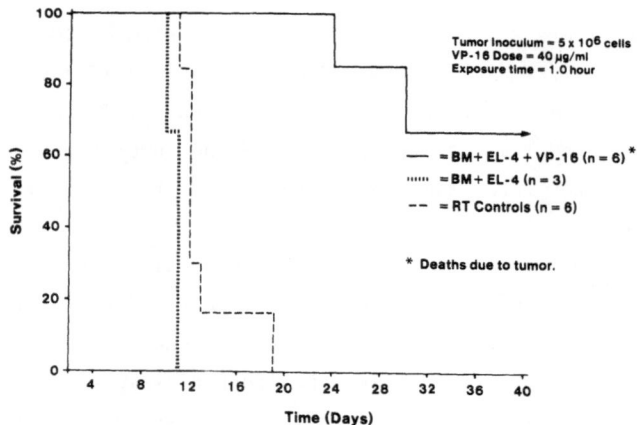

FIGURE 6. Survival of lethally irradiated C57B6 mice inoculated with a tumor/BM cell mixture treated in vitro with 40 ug/ml of VP-16 for 1 hour at 37°C. The tumor cell inoculum was approximately 15% of the total.

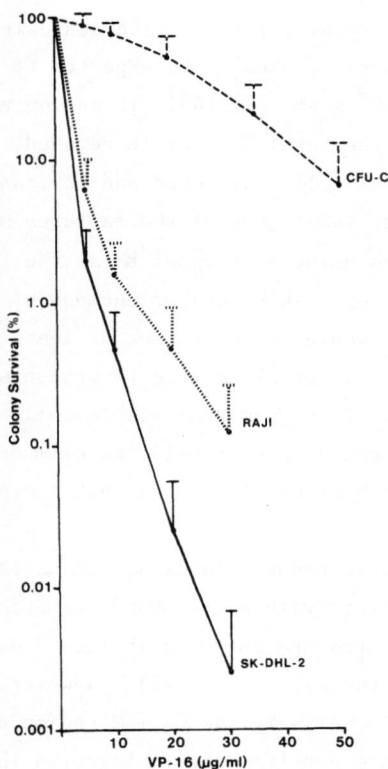

FIGURE 7. Human BM CFU-C, and SK-DHL-2 and Raji B-cell lymphoma CFU inhibition after a 1 hour exposure to VP-16 at 37°C(+SD).

In the final series of in vivo mixing experiments, 5×10^6 tumor cells(15% of the inoculum) were mixed with the usual BM dose. While two did die at 24 and 29 days of disseminated tumor, the other four survived 90+ days, without tumor engraftment(Figure #6).

Incubating VP-16 with human BM demonstrated an inhibition of CFU-C similar to that for the murine CFU-C and CFU-S(Figure #7). Against two human B-cell lymphoma cell lines(Raji and SK-DHL-2) we demonstrated almost a 4 log differential cell kill at 30 ug/ml of the VP-16 for the SK-DHL-2 line with 51.3±19.6% CFU-C and 0.024±0.031% tumor CFUs surviving at this concentration. There was slightly less inhibition of the Raji line at all concentrations tested with the maximum differential of approximately 2 logs occurring at 30 ug/ml of VP-16.

DISCUSSION

Based on cell kinetic data, a patient with acute leukemia in remissio
after induction chemotherapy can usually be expected to have a minimum
residual tumor burden of 10^8 stem cells(4). If during an autologous BM
transplant one percent of the total BM pool is removed, there would be a
minimum of 10^6 leukemic stem cells collected and re-transfused. This
undoubtedly accounts for at least some of the failures seen in the
previously reported studies using autologous BM as the transplant source f
patients with an acute leukemia in second or subsequent remission(3). If
this were not a cause, one would expect to see at least the 10-20% long te
remissions seen when syngeneic or allogeneic BM transplants are done for
this group of patients(2). These residual viable cells then, if sensitive
to an exogenous agent(s), could theoretically be eliminated from the BM
specimen permitting the same clinical results that a syngeneic transplant
would provide.

VP-16 is a semisynthetic podophyllotoxin, but unlike the parent
compound it does not interfere with microtubule formation(12). Cell lines
exposed to this agent in vitro are arrested in late S or G2 phase with a
resultant accumulation of the cells in G2(12). However, Look et al(16)
demonstrated no increase in cells in the G2 + M region of the DNA histogra
in eight patients with acute non-lymphocytic leukemia in relapse undergoir
treatment with this agent, although they noted a G2 phase arrest of cell
cycle progression. Because of this and a decreased percentage of cells ir
active DNA synthesis after treatment, they postulated that there was a
selective cell killing in the G2 and S phases. Accompanying these findin;
was a marked marrow blast cytoreduction of 84% in the first 24 hours afte
single dose of VP-16 of 200 mg/m^2 given IV. Although a G2 arrest of tumo
cells exposed to VP-16 has been repeatedly demonstrated, the degree of th
arrest has recently not been shown to correlate with drug dosage(17). DN
scission was however found to be dose dependent in this study and it is
postulated that VP-16 causes the DNA strand breakage in the same manner a
does ionizing radiation. The lethally damaged cells appear however to be
able to enter and complete DNA synthesis allowing them to enter G2, but a
unable to proceed to chromosome condensation and ultimately are unable to
divide. This would then account for the G2 arrest. As this DNA strand
breakage was demonstrated to be dose related, it may explain why there wa
no preferential killing of the more committed(CFU-C) but presumably

kinetically more active stem cells compared to CFU-S cells, at VP-16 doses greater than 10 ug/ml in our study. The lack of a differential cell killing of more committed stem cells(CFU-C) due to HN_2 was not unexpected as other alkylating agents such as L-phenylalanine mustard and busulfan have been known not to exert a differential effect(18).

Pre-clinical activity of VP-16 was established in a number of animal systems as well as in human tumor cell lines(19-21). Against the T1 lymphoma cell line it was found to be the second most active agent(21). Because of these findings and its in vivo activity against the human tumors most likely to be successfully treated by supralethal therapy with BM transplantation especially the above mentioned data on relapsed acute leukemia, we tested it in vitro as a BM purging agent.

After demonstrating a marked differential sensitivity of the tumor and normal hematopoietic stem cells in vitro to VP-16, we successfully eliminated as many as 15% contaminating tumor cells from BM/tumor cell mixtures using VP-16, without impairing our ability to successfully restore hematopoiesis after lethal irradiation. This occurred despite the fact that approximately one log of the pluripotent hematopoietic stem cells transplanted were destroyed at the 40 ug/ml dose of VP-16 used for the in vivo studies. This would appear to suggest that the CFU-C/S assays are not predictive of hematopoietic reconstitution when BM, treated with VP-16 is used as the transplant source for lethally irradiated mice. This would concur with the data of Kaizer et al who have demonstrated prompt hematopoietic reconstitution for transplanted patients when 90% or greater of the CFU-C in their BM have been destroyed by 4-HC(7). Why this occurs is unknown. One possibility is that the other critical component of the transplant i.e. the stromal cells(histiocytes, fat cells and reticulum cells) is resistant to the VP-16 drug treatment. These undamaged cells given in relatively normal numbers with a pharmacologically-treated transplant may then be more critical to rapid reconstitution than are what is presently felt to be more important, an 'adequate' CFU-S number. The other possibility is that even with a log killing of CFU-S, there are still sufficient numbers of these cells to lead to hematopoietic reconstitution. There is no doubt that the cell dose given to the mice in this study is in excess of the minimum dose of 0.8×10^8 cells/kg body weight to insure reconstitution(22); yet again considering the cell inoculum, the weight of the animals and the degree of CFU-S killing demonstrated here, universal

survival would not have been predicted. Transplants using a higher dose o
VP-16 may help resolve the question, and are planned. For the present
however, it does not appear that surviving CFU-C or CFU-S numbers are
predictive of reconstitution when pharmacologically treated BM is used as
the transplant source.

It should be noted that the 40 ug/ml VP-16 concentration used here is
substantial, being approximately four-fold higher than the peak serum leve
obtained after an IV dose of 100 mg/m^2 of this drug(23). Based on this,
preliminary studies demonstrating a degree of inhibition of human BM CFU-C
and BFU-E similar to that of murine marrow(24), and our data on the two
human B-cell lymphoma cell lines presented here, VP-16 should be considere
as a purging agent for tumors such as the lymphomas, the acute leukemias a
small cell lung carcinoma which are known to be responsive at this
conventional dose.

The demonstration of the activity of HN_2 in this study may be
significant, even though it did not appear to be as active in the in vitro
murine assays as VP-16. As combination chemotherapy for the leukemias anc
lymphomas is superior to single agents, and because we optimized the
conditions of this group of experiments, it is reasonable to expect that a
one pharmacologic agent would not be sufficient to totally purify a BM of
residual leukemia or lymphoma cells. Thus as in clinical applications of
combination chemotherapy, depending on the agents tested, a mixture of dru
such as VP-16 and HN_2, or a drug(s) and monoclonal antibodies might effect
greater tumor cell kill without an increase in normal hematopoietic stem
cell damage. In vitro studies to test this hypothesis using combinations
pharmacologic agents are planned.

SUMMARY

Alternatives to allogeneic or syngeneic BM transplantation for patie
with an acute leukemia without a HLA-matched donor include the use of
autologous BM, purified of tumor cells in vitro by pharmacologic agents.
vitro and in vivo testing of this technique in a murine model using VP-16
and in vitro testing with HN_2 have been successfully completed. After
demonstrating a marked differential sensitivity for EL-4 leukemia
clonageneic cells over that for both BM CFU-C and CFU-S cells for
VP-16(maximum differential approximately 3 logs) and HN_2 (maximum
differential 1 1/2 logs), in vivo testing with VP-16 was done. Mixing 2C

x 10^6 normal BM cells, and varying numbers of viable EL-4 cells with a 40 ug/ml concentration of VP-16 for one hour and using this as the BM transplant for lethally irradiated syngeneic C57B6 mice, we demonstrated survival without tumor development when tumor cell concentrations as high as 15% were used. Using VP-16 on two human B-cell tumor cell lines(SK-DHL-2 and Raji), we again demonstrated a marked differential kill of up to 4 logs over that for human CFU-C. VP-16 and HN_2 are potentially useful BM purifying agents for sensitive tumors that originate or frequently metastasize to it.

ACKNOWLEDGEMENT

This work was supported in part by a Central Research Committee Grant #17-83 from the Southern Illinois University School of Medicine.

REFERENCES

1. Appelbaum FR, Cheever MA, Fefer A, Greenberg PD, Glucksberg H, Buckner CD, Thomas ED: A prospective study of the value of maintenance therapy or bone marrow transplantation in adult acute leukemia. Blood 60(Supp 1):163a, 1982.
2. Santos GW, Kaizer H: Bone marrow transplantation in acute leukemia. Semin Hematol 19:227,1982.
3. Gale RP: Bone marrow transplantation in leukemia. J Supramol Struct (Supp 4):3,1980.
4. Clarkson BD, Fried J: Changing concepts of treatment in acute leukemia. Med Clin NA 55:561,1971.
5. Sharkis SJ, Santos GW, Colvin M: Elimination of acute myelogenous leukemic cells from marrow and tumor suspensions in the rat with 4-hydroperoxycyclophosphamide. Blood 55:521,1980.
6. Kaizer H, Cote JP, Sharkis S, Stuart RK, Santos GW: Autologous bone marrow transplantation in acute leukemia: The use of in vitro incubation of tumor-marrow mixtures with 4-hydroperoxycyclophosphamide in a Wistar-Furth rat model of acute myelogenous leukemia. Proc Amer Assoc Can Res 23:194,1982.
7. Kaizer H, Stuart RK, Fuller DJ, Braine HG, Saral R, Colvin M, Wharam MD, Santos GW: Autologous bone marrow transplantation in acute leukemia: Progress report on a phase I study of 4-hydroperoxycyclophosphamide incubation of marrow prior to cryopreservation. Proc Amer Soc Clin Oncol 1:131,1982.
8. Champlin RE, Territo MC, Ho WG, Wells J, Gale RP, Billing R: Prolonged remission following autologous bone marrow transplantation for acute lymphoblastic leukemia utilizing in vitro treatment with anti-CALLA antiserum. Blood 60(Supp 1):165a,1982.
9. Bast RC, Ritz J, Lipton JM, Feeney M, Sallan SE, Nathan DG, Schlossman SF: Elimination of leukemic cells from human bone marrow using monoclonal antibody and complement. Cancer Res 43:1389,1983.
10. Cavalli F: VP-16-213(Etoposide): A critical review of its activity. Cancer Chemother Pharmacol 7:81,1982.
11. Jain K, Langleben A, Gulati S, DeRisi M, Yopp J, Colvin M, Clarkson B:

In vitro chemopurification of bone marrow. Proc Amer Assoc Cancer Res 24:316,1983.

12. Ghose T, Guclu A, Tai J, Mammen M, Norvell ST: Immunoprophylaxis and immunotherapy of EL-4 lymphoma. Eur J Cancer 13:925,1977.

13. Issel BF: The podophyllotoxin derivatives VP16-213 and VM-26. Cancer Chemother Pharmacol 7:73,1982.

14. Pike BL, Robinson WA: Human bone marrow colony growth in agar-gel. J Cell Physiol 76:77,1970.

15. Till JE, McCulloch EA: A direct measurement of the radiation sensitivit of normal mouse bone marrow cells. Radiat Res 14:213,1961.

16. Look AT, Dahl GV, Rivera G, Mauer AM: Clinical and cell kinetic studies of the effects of the epipodophyllotoxin VP16-213 during therapy of refractory acute nonlymphocytic leukemia. Cancer Chemother Pharmacol 7:161,1982.

17. Kalwinsky DK, Look AT, Ducore J, Fridland A: Effects of the epipodophyllotoxin VP-16-213 on cell cycle traverse, DNA synthesis, and DNA strand size in cultures of human leukemic lymphoblasts. Cancer Res 43:1592,1983.

18. Botnick LE, Hannon EC, Hellman S: Limited proliferation of stem cells surviving alkylating agents. Nature 262:68,1976.

19. Sieber SM, Mead JAR, Adamson A: Pharmacology of antitumor agents from higher plants. Cancer Treat Rep 60:1127,1976.

20. Stahelin H: Activity of a new glycosidic lignan derivative(VP16-213) related to podophyllotoxin in experimental tumors. Europ J Cancer 9:215 1973.

21. Drewinko B, Barlogie B: Survival and cycle-progression delay of human lymphoma cells in vitro exposed to VP-16-213. Cancer Treat Rep 60:1295, 1976.

22. Urso P, Congdon CC: The effect of the amount of isologous bone marrow injected on the recovery of hematopoietic organs, survival and body weight after lethal irradiation injury in mice. Blood 12:251,1957.

23. D'Incalci M, Farina P, Sessa C, Mangioni C, Conter V, Masera G, Rocchetti M, Bromhilla Pisoni M, Piazza E, Beer M, Cavalli F: Pharmacokinetics of VP16-213 given by different administration methods. Cancer Chemother Pharmacol 7:141,1982.

24. Stiff PJ, Wustrow T, DeRisi M, Koester A, Lanzotti V, Clarkson B: An ir vivo murine model of bone marrow purification of tumor by VP16-213. Blood 60(Supp 1):173a,1982.

AML CELL HETEROGENEITY. IMPLICATIONS FOR LEUKEMIA CELL SEPARATION FROM AUTOLOGOUS BONE MARROW GRAFTS.

Bob Löwenberg and Jan Bauman.

1. SUMMARY

For tumor cell purging of autologous marrow transplants it is critical to separate out the neoplastic stem or precursor cells. The biologic meaning of tumor cell heterogeneity is therefore of direct importance to the application and evaluation of purification methods. We have phenotyped AML blasts of a single case of AML in detail and studied the clonogenic capacities of AML subpopulations with varying phenotypes by the abilities to form colonies in vitro. AML colony forming cells were characterized and selected with complement dependent cytotoxicity of a number of monoclonal antibodies and fluorescence actived cell sorting. Several conclusions can be made. The variable cellular composition of human AML reflects a systematic organization of maturation stages. Colony forming cells are precursors with specific phenotypes while colony end cells have lost the clonogenic properties and express more mature markers on their surface. Thus, AML precursors as normal myeloid progenitors, can differentiate along the myeloid pathway, although to a restricted level. Various cases of AML seem to have L-CFU with distinct phenotypes. It may be important to characterize L-CFU in AML in individual patients before cleaning their marrow autografts in order to monitor and achieve efficient cell kill and to avoid the selective removal of non-clonogenic AML blasts by a laborious procedure, which does not contribute a therapeutic effect.

2. INTRODUCTION

If cell separation methods are applied to clean autologous marrow transplants (ABMT) from residual tumor cells, a detaile knowledge of the biologic relationships of tumor cell hetero- geneity is required. Cell separation approaches should particu larly be directed towards the subset of the malignancy which i responsible for tumor cell growth and expansion, and effective selective tumor cell removal should include therefore the tumc stem- and precursor cells. We have previously reported a color assay for AML progenitor cells with a high plating efficiency which may permit the specific characterization of AML clonoger cells (1;2).

Here we present a series of experiments in a patient with untreated AML with the objective to analyse the cellular relat ships between the mixture of AML cells and disclose the proper of the AML stem cells relative to the other cellular subpopula tions of the neoplasm. Whole and clonogenic AML blasts were ty employing colony cultures and applying a selected panel of monoclonal antibodies directed against a number of antigens normally expressed on the cell surface of human blood cell tyj

3. MATERIALS AND METHODS

Preparation of cells

Leukemic blasts were separated from the bone marrow of a patient with newly diagnosed AML (French-American-British cytologic subtype: M2) in a discontinuous albumin gradient (2 depleted of E-rosette forming cells as described (3). The AML blast cells from three other patients were also used in the complement lysis test.

Colony assay

AML colonies were grown in the PHA-leukocyte feeder system reported in detail (4). On day 7, the day of maximal colony growth, colonies of 50 cells or more were counted with an inv microscope (Zeiss). Colony cells were also picked from the pl with a Pasteur pipette, suspended, washed twice in Hanks Bala

Salt Solution (HBSS) and then used in indirect immunofluorescence.
In some experiments AML blasts were also plated in the double agar
layer with a leukocyte feeder (10;2) and in agar gel with human
placental conditional medium as the stimulus.

Monoclonal antibodies (McAb)

McAb anti-Ia was purchased from Ortho Pharmaceutical
Corporation, Raritan, New Jersey (OKIa) and used in titers of
1:20. AT1 was a generous gift by Dr A. Hekman (Netherlands Cancer
Institute, Amsterdam). It detects an antigen identical or closely
related to T10 and was used in titers of 1:50. McAb's S3-13,
S16-144, S4-7 and S17-25 were kindly disposed to us by Dr G.
Rovera, The Wistar Institute, Philadelphia. The properties and
specificities have been described (5-8). S3-13 is an IgM which
reacts with 100% of myeloblasts but not with other granulocytic
cells, with 30% of blood monocytes and 40% of T-lymphocytes and
was used in a titer of 1:50. McAb S4-7, an IgM, reacts with an
antigen on monocytes (60% positivity in indirect immunofluorescence) and with myeloblasts, granulocytes and cell
intermediate stages of the granulocytic series. The McAb has been
used in a 1:500 concentration.
The S16-144, an IgM McAb in ascites, reacts with myeloblasts,
promyelocytes, myelocytes and metamyelocytes as well as with
monocytes (100%). In FACS analysis it was applied in 1:50 titer.
Finally, the S17-25 McAb is an IgG2B which demonstrates an antigen
expressed on myeloblasts (40%), monocytes (75%) and T-lymphocytes
(100%). A 1:10 concentration was utilized in complement mediated
lysis experiments. The B4.3 McAb was provided by Dr P. Lansdorp,
Central Laboratory of the Blood Transfusion Service, Amsterdam.
B4.3 (IgM) reacts with granulocytic cells and not with other
peripheral blood cells. It was used in concentrations of 1:500 (in
indirect immunofluorescence) and 1:250 (in complement cytotoxicity
tests). The anti T-6 McAb was the OKT6 from Ortho Pharmaceutical
Corporation and used in 1:20 concentration. The WT1 McAb is
reactive with E-positive blood lymphocytes and human thymus cells
and a small proportion of granulocytes and was used at 1:100 (9).

Indirect immunofluorescence

Cells were fixed with paraformaldehyde (0.04%) washed with HBSS, incubated with the McAb in relevant concentrations for 3 min. on ice. The cells were then washed and incubated for anot 30 min. with GAM-Ig-FITC (1:40), purchased from Nordic Immunol gical Reagents, The Netherlands. 200 cells were scored for positive and negative staining with a Zeiss fluorescence microscope.

Fluorescence actived cell sorting (FACS)

A FACS II (fluorescence actived cell sorter) from Becton Dickinson was used to measure immunofluorescence intensity as expression of the antigen density on the cell surface of AML blasts and to collect subpopulations of positively (with varyi intensity) and negatively fluorescent cells for colony growth vitro.

Complement mediated cytotoxicity of L-CFU

AML blasts ($1-2 \times 10^6$ cells) were incubated in 1-2 ml HBSS wi the appropriate concentration of the monoclonal antibody for 3 min. at $0^{\circ}C$ and then centrifuged. To the cell pellet rabbit complement (40% in HBSS) was added and the resuspended cells w subsequently incubated in a 1 ml volume for 30 min. at $37^{\circ}C$. 1 the cells were washed twice and reconstituted in HBSS and usec cell plating. Comparative incubations without complement, complement alone, and HBSS without complement or McAb were rur controls. Colonies from each incubation were scored in triplic cultures. Percentage kill of L-CFU was expressed relative to t complement control, which was set at 100%.

4. RESULTS

Here we present the results of typing of AML colony forming cells in a patient with AML which was studied as a model case. Purified AML blasts were phenotyped in indirect immunofluoresc with a number of monoclonal antibodies prior to culture and ac following outgrowth to colonies in culture. This comparative analysis revealed marked changes in the phenotype following culture. The expression of certain antigens increased or appeared on the cell surface of the cells, while the reactivity with other monoclonals decreased (table 1).

Table 1

Immunologic phenotypes of pure AML blasts before and after colony culture.

		% positive immunofluorescence	
McAb	no. of exp.	before culture	after colony culture
anti Ia	3	67	66
AT1	2	65	26
T6	3	0	42
WT1	2	34	0
B4.3	5	11	38
S4.7	1	23	49

Immunofluorescence was also done with McAb T3, T4, T8, T11, BA-1, antiplatelet McAb C2 and C13, and anti-glycophorin McAb IVB but the cells were negative before and after culture. They were also negative on E-rosette testing. Values indicate mean percentages of positively fluorescing cells.

These results were consistent with the development of more mature cell stages along the myeloid pathway. Immunologic maturation was associated with consistently blastic morphologic features and occasionally an increase in aspecific α-naphtyl esterase or myeloperoxidase staining. This information suggested that the heterogeneous make up of AML cells as they circulate in vivo, may be an expression of the residual differentiation capacities of the cells and that the cellular heterogeneity in fact is a reflection of a diversity of maturation steps.
L-CFU were then characterized with FACS cell sorting and the cells

Table 2

FACS cell sorting of AML blasts with McAb S3-13

fractions (channel no.)	S3-13 fluorescence	no. of cells recovered ($\times 10^3$)	no. of colonies		
			PHA-l.f.assay	HPCM	leukocyte feeder
0-100	-	4883	<1	17	43
100-115	÷	17697	15	66	43
115-130	++	19981	115	339	213
130-300	+++	8608	0	14	9
	total recovery	51169 (102%)			

500×10^3 cells were labelled with McAb S3-13, analysed for fluorescence intensity (relative to the unstained control) and sorted in four fractions. The fractions were assayed for L-CFU content in three colony assays.

No. of colonies are expressed per 1×10^5 cells.

collected on the basis of fluorescence intensity (labelled relative to the unstained control cells as: -; +; ++; +++). An example
of an experiment with McAb S3-13 in which the cells were plated in
three parallel colony assays is given in table 2. In particular,
the cells with ++ positive expression of S3-13 appeared to possess
colony forming capacities, while the negative (-) and strongly
reactive (+++) subpopulations of AML blast cells lacked colony
forming potential. A summary of the analysis of L-CFU with FACS
sorting and a variety of McAb's is given in table 3.

Table 3

Phenotypes of AML colony forming cells (1-CFU) and non-colony
forming cells as assessed with FACS analysis in one case of AML.

marked with McAb	L-CFU	non-L-CFU
Ia	+	-/+/++
AT1	+	-/+/++
NT1	-	-/+
34.3	-	-/+
34.7	+	-/+
T6	-	-/+

L-CFU were characterized in McAb dependent complement mediated
lysis by evaluating the reduction in colony forming cells
following the incubation. This was done with the two McAb's, anti
Ia and B4.3, and employing the AML blast cells from 4 newly
diagnosed patients. It is evident from the results presented in
table 4 that there is inter-individual variability as to the
phenotype of L-CFU. In patient no. 1 L-CFU are Ia and B4.3
positive, in patient no. 2 L-CFU are Ia positive but B4.3 negative
and in patients no. 3 and no. 4 L-CFU appear negative for Ia as
well as B4.3.

Table 4

Complement mediated cytotoxicity of two monoclonal antibodies
L-CFU.

		Reduction of L-CFU following exposure to the monoclonal antibody	
Patient			
no.	FAB class	anti-Ia	B4.3
1	M2	+	+
2	M1	+	-
3	M1	-	-
4	M2	-	-

5. DISCUSSION

If immunologic principles are applied to separate out leuke
cells from autologous bone marrow grafts, the biologic meaning
tumor cell heterogeneity should be well understood in terms of
clonogenic potential of the various populations. We have prese
data to indicate that subpopulations of AML cells with diverse
phenotypes can be distinguished and ranked according to maturi
(clonogenic versus non-clonogenic). L-CFU with an immature
phenotype differ in the expression of cell surface markers fro
the progeny which they generate in colony culture. On the basi
antigen density more subtle distinctions and characterizations
L-CFU can be made. Thus, AML cells do not represent a fixed
differentiation block but can proceed along the pathway of
maturation to a variable extent. This leads to a number of
conclusions: 1) it is not possible to directly derive from the
presenting phenotype of AML the analogous normal precursor cel
stage at which transformation has taken place; 2) L-CFU should
distinguished with specific markers among the whole tumor mass
the phenotypes of L-CFU in different patients may vary; 3) sir
most likely maturation and proliferation is associated with
expanding cell numbers, L-CFU phenotypes may represent minorit

this implies that diagnostic approaches for residual leukemia and separation techniques of autologous marrow grafts should specifically monitor for L-CFU. It is possible that current separation methods in marrow autografts miss a crucial AML subset, i.e., the L-CFU, since they are usually directed towards the dominant phenotype of the neoplasm. In a certain McAb positive AML (e.g. B4.3) it was found that the positive tumor subset represented the non-clonogenic compartment and thus this McAb would have been a misleading guide for cleaning autografts.
It has become clear from these investigations that AML cells although to a limited extent share the capacities of myeloid differentiation with normal precursors.
A selective diagnosis of residual AML cells and the selective removal of residual AML blasts can probably not take advantage of unique antigens on the cell surface. It is possible however that the expression of antigens of specific density may give a clue to the selectivity of these methods.

Acknowledgements
This work was supported by the Netherlands Cancer Society "The Queen Wilhelmina Fund".

5. REFERENCES

1. Löwenberg B., Hagemeijer A. and Swart K.: Karyotypically distinct subpopulations in acute leukemia with specific growth requirements.
   Blood 59: 641-645, 1982.

2. Swart K., Hagemeijer A. and Löwenberg B.: Acute myeloid colony growth in vitro: differences of colony-forming cells in PHA-supplemented and standard leukocyte feeder cultures.
   Blood 59: 816-821, 1982.

206

3. Wouters R. and Löwenberg B.: On the maturation order of AML
   cells: a distinction on the basis of self-renewal propertie
   and immunologic phenotypes.
   Blood, 1984, in press.

4. Swart K., Hagemeijer A. and Löwenberg B.: Studies on chroni
   myeloid leukemia cell populations with colony-forming
   abilities in PHA-leukocyte feeder and Robinson assays.
   Leukemia Res. 6: 55-62, 1982.

5. Pessano S., Bottero L., Faust J., Trucco M., Palumbo A.,
   Pegoraro L., Lange B., Brezim C., Borst J., Terhorst C. and
   Rovera G.: Differentiation antigens of human hemopoietic
   cells: patterns of reactivity of two monoclonal antibodies.
   Cancer Research, in press.

6. Pagliardi G.L., Pessano S., Palumbo A., Levis A., Bottero
   L., Ferrero D., Lange B. and Rovera G.: Differentiation,
   maldifferentiation or arrested differentiation in human
   acute myelogenous leukemias.
   Symposia of 13th International Cancer Congress. E.A. Miranc
   (ed). A.R. Liss, New York, in press, 1982.

7. Ferrero D., Pagliardi G.L., Broxmeyer H.E., Venuta S., Lanç
   B., Pessano S. and Rovera G.: Two antigenically distinct
   subpopulations of myeloid progenitor cells (CFU-GM) are
   present in human peripheral blood and marrow.
   Proc.Natl.Acad.Sci. 80: 4114-4118, 1983.

8. Pessano S., Ferrero D., Palumbo A., Bottero L., Hubbell H.,
   Lange B. and Rovera G.: Differentiation antigens of normal
   and leukemic myelomonocytic cells in normal and neoplastic
   hematopoiesis. UCLA symposium on molecular and cellular
   biology, vol. 9, Alan R. Liss, Inc. NY, NY, 1983.

9. Tax W.J.M., Willems H.W. Kibbelaar, M.D.A., de Groot J. et al: Monoclonal antibodies against human thymocytes and T-lymphocytes.
In: Prohides of the Biological Fluids. 29th Colloquium 1981 (Ed. H. Peeters) pp. 701-704, Pergamon Press, Oxford.

0. Pike B.L., and Robinson W.A.: Human bone marrow colony growth in agar gel.
J.Cell.Physiol. 1970, <u>76</u>, 77.

ELIMINATION OF LEUKEMIC CELLS FROM REMISSION MARROW SUSPENSIONS BY AN IMMUNOMAGNETIC PROCEDURE

Karel A. Dicke, M.D., Ph.D., Christopher H. Poynton, M.D. and Christoher L. Reading, Ph.D.

INTRODUCTION

A large number of early observations on immunity by Paul Ehrlich (1854-1911) allowed him to anticipate the great therapeutic potential that could be derived from manipulation of the immune system.[1,2] The advent of monoclonal antibodies[3] has brought such possibilities much closer to realization giving us a considerable armamentarium. Although we now have available a vast variety of mouse monoclonal antibodies and a few human monoclonals, a major problem still exists - how can these antibodies be used to kill or remove cancer cells? This has an important application in clinical bone marrow transplantation since one of the main obstacles in autologous bone marrow transplantation is the potential contamination of tumor cells in the marrow cell suspension to be grafted.

It may not be sufficient merely to expose the tumor cells to a monoclonal antibody[4]. One of the ways to use monoclonal antibodies (MCA), is to lyse the MCA-coated cells with complement. Although theoretically appealing, this approach has considerable problems. Firstly, only some subclasses of mouse MCA fix complement and secondly, low cell concentrations of not more than 3×10^7 cell/ml are required, together with large amounts of complement, usually resulting in only partial complement lysis.

Several agents with therapeutic potential have been conjugated to monoclonal antibodies including drugs and lymphokines. Previous efforts to target drugs have included incorporation into liposomes[5,6,7], albumin microspheres[8,9,10], magnetic microspheres[11], incorporation with other macromolecules[12] and covalently linked antibody-drug complexes[13,14]. A number of established chemotherapeutic agents such as methotrexate[15], adriamycin and daunomycin[16,17] chlorambucil[18,19] have been used conjugated to antibody, and while considerable progress has been made in this field, clinical trials have not yet been conducted.

Monoclonal antibodies conjugated to various plant toxins have attracted considerable interest. Over 50 plants have now been identified as containing toxins[20] of which the toxin ricin from the castor bean Ricinus communis has received the most attention. Toxins, such as diptheria toxin[21] and ricin consist of two chains. The A (toxic) chain acts inside the cell by inhibiting protein synthesis on the 60S subunit of ribosomes[22]. The B chain acts at the surface like a monovalent lectin, binding to galactose and N-acetylgalactosamine residues on the cell, and anchors the toxin to the membrane. The B chain is therefore capable of binding to practically all mammalian cells. Thus, the idea came about to use a monoclonal antibody for binding to the cell instead of the B chain, so that monoclonal-A chain toxic conjugates could then be used.

A number of problems have been associated with this approach (i) variable steric hindrance of the antibody specificity can occur with A chain conjugation[23]. In addition, antibodies with only moderate affinity for cell surface antigens substantially reduce A chain penetration[24]. With this system, immunotoxins compare favorably with complement-mediated lysis with MCA and are able to achieve 100% cytotoxicity in some cell lines[25]. The use of Fab fragments which contain the antibody binding site of antibodies (MW 80,000) linked to toxin may be of further value, due to greater organ penetration. Since the B chain has such an important role in A chain penetration, a number of ways of blocking the lectin specific B chain binding have been tried so that the whole ricin (A+B chain) could be conjugated to MCA. Chemical modification of the galactose/N-acetyl galactosamine receptor on the B chain is under investigation, but more success has been achieved by competitively inhibiting the binding by including 100mM lactose or galactose in the medium. In this way several patients have had their bone marrows treated, purging them of residual leukemic cells followed by autologous transplantation, with suitable prior cytoreductive therapy[26].

The idea of physically removing unwanted cells selectively from a

:ell suspension has been studied by a large number of groups. Physical 'emoval of cells circumvents the numerous problems of using toxins, hemotherapeutic agents, and complement, but has the limitation that it an only be used in vitro. Density gradient separations have been used o remove lymphocytes from bone marrow cells.[27] Also density radients were used to eliminate leukemic cells from marrow cell uspensions. A biological effect, even with removal of up to 90% of the eukemic cell population as obtained by gradient centrifugation has not een been demonstrated[28,29]. More recently, we have attempted to emove leukemic cells by increasing their density, using colloidal gold articles (40-100 nm) with antibodies attached (immunogold)[30] with nitial promising results. We have now designed a simpler separation ased on the use of immunomagnetic colloidal particles and a magnetic eparation.[31]

ATERIALS AND METHODS

. Preparation Of The Colloid

The basis of the formation of our magnetic colloids is the chemical eduction of very dilute cobalt (II) chloride with sodium borohydride (aBH$_4$). For cobalt, some of the reaction products are undoubtedly the rides Co_2B and CoB which are also paramagnetic. The reaction can also : used for the reduction of iron (II) and (III) chloride, with greater rmation of metallic iron[32]. In forming a colloid with a uniform rticle size, first a nucleation reaction has to take place, and then e colloid grows on the nuclei. It is the number of nuclei first rmed that determines the size of the colloid, given a finite amount of actants[33,34]. Hence, it is possible by controlled nucleation and owth to make colloids of a variety of sizes. Once formed, the tallic cobalt or iron colloid, if left alone, dissolves over a few urs in solution, so it is necessary to passivate the surface. This n be done in a variety of ways, but treatment with 1mM-5mM potassium chromate is effective. The excess passivating agent is removed by alysis or ultrafiltration eith prior to or after protein binding. oteins (antibodies, lectins, etc.) can be bound to the colloid at the ropriate pH (just above the isoelectric point of the protein), in the e way as with colloid gold. These colloids will pass easily through fillipore filter (0.22 or 0.45 micron pore size), which will sterilize m for clinical use. The colloid can be washed magnetically, which will agrregate it, by centrifugation after stabilization with polyethylene glycol (PEG) 20,000 MW, or best of all by controlled ultrafiltration to remove the excess protein. Nonspecific protein absorption to the colloid is blocked with excess proteins (5% fetal bovine serum, FBS). There is some evidence that bovine serum albumin (BSA) may not be the most appropriate material to use, since impurities in it can bind quite strongly to the surface of certain cells. We have coated the colloid with an affinity purified IgG fraction of goat antimouse immunoglobulins.

B. The Magnet

As the development of the colloid took place, it became apparent that we would need a fairly powerful magnet. The magnet used for our first clinical separation with the colloidal cobalt was an electromagnet. It had 1,500 turns of wire, generated between 0.1 - 0.2 TELSA (1000-2000 gauss). The cell suspension after incubation with immunocobalt was passed through the magnetic field in a siliconized glass tube with galvanized iron wire in the tube, which maximized the magnetic gradient inside the tube. However the electromagnet had a severe heating problem after about 20 minutes, which we were unable to resolve satisfactorally since it produced about 2 kilowatts as heat. In addition, the coil of siliconized galvanised iron wire in the center of the tubes would quickly deteriorate after several separations, and needed repeated time consuming replacement. These problems were overcome by switching to a permanent magnet and the most powerful ones available are made of cobalt with a rare earth element, usually europium or samarium. At their pole face, a gradient of 8,500 gauss/oersteds (0.85T) is claimed.

For our test separations usually on a small scale (10^8 cells), a small cobalt/samarium magnet (2 1/2" x 1/2" x 1/2") applied to the side of a polystyrene test tube was used, with good recoveries and cell removal A large cobalt/samarium magnet was made up for our clinical separations to fit the bottom of a tissue culture flask, which would be exposed to one pole of the magnet. The supernatant containing the nonadherent cells is then decanted. Such a static system has proved to have a major disadvantage when scaled up for large bone marrow separations; great care is required in decanting, so as not to allow any adherent cells to come off leading to rather lower total cell recoveries

(about 50%) than is possible in a smaller system in a tube, where the
cells are adherent in a more compact fashion.

We are currently improving our permanent magnet system to optimize
the magnetic gradients at intervals along a continuous flow through
system in a glass tube again, similar to the design of the original
electromagnet, but without the leaking problem. Magnetic stainless
steel wire of the 300 series (3oz or 312 are probably best) can be
incorporated in the tube to further enhance the magnetic gradient.

2. Separation

1. Test Separation

Our basic test system uses a concentration of 10^8 cells/ml and
before separation the antibody-reactive fraction varies from 1 to 60% of
the cells. With the cells at 4^0C throughout the whole procedure
prevents immunomodulation, the cells are incubated with the monoclonal
antibody for 60 minutes in a 250 ml tissue culture flask and then the
immunocobalt colloid, with goat anti-mouse immunoglobulins bound to it,
is added and the cells reincubated for a further 60 minutes. Separation
is performed either with the magnets (cobalt/samarium) over about an
hour in a tissue culture flask followed by decanting , or by flowing the
cell suspension through a magnetic field in which the magnetic gradients
are maximized in various ways to give a so called high gradient magnetic
separation.

2. Clinical Separation

The clinical separation procedure consists of the following steps:

1. Collection of 1000ml marrow cells from the donor by multiple
   aspirations from the iliac crest under general anesthesia.
2. Passage through a Haemonetic cell separator or gradient
   centrifugation to remove most granulocytes and red cells.
3. Incubation of the remaining cells with mouse monoclonal
   antibody reactive with the leukemic cells of the patient for 45
   minutes at 4^0C. These antibodies are selected when the patient
   is untreated or in relapse.
4. Three washes by centrifugation with Hepes buffered Hanks
   balanced salt solution at 500g.
5. After resuspension of the cells, incubation with immunocobalt
   coated with affinity purified IgG fraction goat anti-mouse
   antibody for 60 minutes at 4^0C.

6. Magnetic separation with permanent magnet for 60 minutes at 4^0C followed by decanting the negative cells or by continuous flow in a high gradient magnetic separation to remove antibody colloid coated cells.

7. One wash with Hepes buffered Hanks balanced salt solution.

8. Filtration (glass filter, pore size 40-80 micron) and washing with Hanks balanced salt solution.

.9. Sampling for in vitro progenitor testing and measurement of separation efficiency.

10. The cell suspension is then frozen and stored in liquid nitrogen. (Cryopreservation).

RESULTS

1. Several test systems to evaluate the efficacy of separation of the immunomagnetic procedure have been used.

a. Rh positive red blood cells. Rh positive red blood cells coated with human anti-D (Rhesus) can be used for elementary testing using a goat-anti human colloid. This system has been useful in trying to reduce non-specific trapping of cells in the magnetic aggregates, and demonstrates the importance of thoroughly washing unbound antibody from the colloid prior to use. In such simple systems where all the cells are antibody reactive, we have achieved six logs of removal. However, cross linking with the second antibody, particularly if the colloid is not fully washed, leads to a lot of cellular aggregation, and the system is not a useful model for selective cell removal.

b. Removal of sheep rosette receptor positive T lymphocytes from peripheral blood and bone marrow. We attempted to remove ER positive cells with the immunomagnetic procedure. For this purpose the T-11 MCA was used. The results are shown in Table 1. The indirect immunofluorescence technique was used to detect T-11 positive cells before and after magnetic separation. The background of this assay is 0-2% in our laboratory. ACT-1 is a monoclonal antibody prepared by Centecor using PHA stimulated human lymphocytes as immunogen. Only a subpopulation of unstimulated lymphocytes are positive in peripheral blood and bone marrow. Separation results of two experiments have also been listed in Table 1.

TABLE 1
EFFICIENCY OF REMOVAL OF ANTIBODY REACTIVE CELLS
WITH THE IMMUNOMAGNETIC PROCEDURE

		% Antibody Reactive Cells	
SOURCE	ANTIBODY	BEFORE SEPARATION	AFTER SEPARATION
BM	T11	9	2.5
PB	T11	19	3.5
PB	T11	55	2
BM	ACT-1	7.0	0.7
BM	ACT-1	3.8	0

BACKGROUND IMMUNOFLUORESCENCE RANGE FROM 0-2%)

. Removal of K562 leukemic cells from a mixture of marrow cells by the immunomagnetic procedure. We have mixed K562 cells and normal bone marrow cells in a 1:10 ratio. K562 cells (a human leukemic cell line) are clonogenic in vitro. The plating efficiency is between 30-50% e.g., 200 colonies per 500 cells plated. K562 cells form colonies in agar without addition of HPCM or any other colony stimulating factor. There is a direct relationship between the number of cells plated and the number of colonies in the plate. We have attempted to determine the efficacy of K562 removal from a mixture of 10×10^6 K562 cells and 90×10^6 normal bone marrow cells. ACT-1 MCA was used since it reacts with 100% of the K562 cells. The results of a separation experiment have been listed in Table 2. In this experiment a 2-3 log reduction was achieved.

Table 2
ELIMINATION OF K562 LEUKEMIC ELLS FROM BONE MARROW CELL SUSPENSIONS
MIXED WITH K562 CELLS,* USING THE IMMUNO COLLOID**

	Number Of Cells Plated	Number Of Colonies
BEFORE SEPARATION K562+BM	5,000	217
AFTER SEPARATION K562+BM	5,000	1
	50,000	7.3
	100,000	10

NCLUSION: Degree of elimination is between 2 and 3 logs (0.5%). Number of colonies in 5×10^3 cells before separation is approximately equivalent to that in 2×10^6 cells after separation.

*Ratio Bone Marrow/K562 10:1.
*ACT-1 MCA (Centocor Inc., Philadelphia).

Clinical Separations. Four bone marrows have so far been treated r clinical purposes with the immunocobalt colloid. All are patients th common acute lymphoblastic leukemia antigen positive leukemia ALL) in remission that had J5 antibody positive leukemic cells (90%)

when in relapse. Four of these bone marrows have been reinfused after the patients received high dose cytoreductive therapy.

The effect of the separation procedure on the hemopoietic progenitors in vitro was evaluated and the results are listed in Table 3. It can be noted that there is no adverse side effect of the procedure on the hemopoietic progenitor cells in vitro.

TABLE 3
EFFECT OF SEPARATION ON NORMAL HEMOPOIETIC PROGENITORS
WITH J5 ANTIBODY

	agar*	methyl cellulose*		
	GM-CFC	GM-CFC	BFU-e	MCFC
Before separation	18.3	59.5	17.5	2
After separation (i)	23	103.5	31.6	6
(ii)	17	77.5	30	2.5
Before separation	11.7	15.5	3	0
After separation (i)	7.7	13	1	0
(ii)	32.7	78.5	3.5	0
Before separation	6	20	0	0
After separation	91	148	8.5	0

*colonies per 10^5 cells plated

The results of removal of J5 positive cells from the normal cell suspension have been documented in Table 4. After separation the number of J5 positive cells dropped except in the first patient. In that patient we divided the marrow cell suspension in three equal parts and ran these portions sequentially through the magnetc field. The separation of the first part was not successful whereas J5 positive cells could not be documented in the other two portions after separation. Detection of J5 positive cells was done by the indirect immunoflourscence technique. In Table 5 the hemopoietic recovery data of three patients have been listed. No adverse effects were observed on engraftment by the immunomagnetic procedure. Patient 1 stayed in remission for three months. This marrow was collected in second remission and transplantation was performed in CR 2. The preconditioning regimen consisted of CBV (Cyclophosphamide 6 g/m^2 , BCNU

300 g/m^2 and VP-16 600 g/m^2)[35]. The bone marrow in patient 2 was collected in third remission. Transplantation occurred in CR 3 and eukemia recurred three months after transplantation. Patient 3 was transplanted in CR 2 with marrow cells collected in second remission. She is still in remission 5+ months after transplant. No additional toxicity in the patients was observed which could have been attributed o exposing the cells to the immunomagnetic procedure. The fourth atient died early after transplant (day 17) due to persistent infection lready present before transplantation.

Table 4
RECOVERY DATA FROM CLINICAL SEPARATIONS

atient*	%J5 +ve cells** Before	After	% recovery of total number of cells after separation
#1	4	4	74
	4	0	29
	4	0	35
#2	8	1	54
	8	1	30
#3	12.2	1.6	43.6
	12.2	1.8	43.3

In patient 1, the bone marrow suspension was divided into three equal irts and sequentially separated. In patients 2 and 3 the bone marrow ell suspension was divided into two equal parts.

3 - 5 positive cells were detected by the indirect immunofluorescent echnique.

TABLE 5
HEMOPOIETIC RECOVERY IN PATIENTS AFTER IMMUNOMAGNETIC
BONE MARROW SEPARATION

unts in peripheral blood	Patient #1	Patient #2	Patient #3
atelets 50 x 10^9/liter	Day 20	Day 33	Day 27
atelets 100 x 10^9/liter	Day 23	Day 35	Day 30
anulocytes 0.5 x 10^9/liter	Day 20	Day 36	Day 26
anulocytes 1.0 x 10^9/liter	Day 22	Day 40	Day 28

SCUSSION

The clinical studies described in this manuscript were primarily ied at testing the effect of the immunomagnetic procedure on stem cell toxicity and on unknown adverse side effects in the patients. Certainly, on theorectical grounds a biological effect of the separation procedure might be expected providing that the leukemic cell population in the patient is sufficiently sensitive to the high dose chemotherapy regimen. The leukemic stage of the patients enroled in this program was far advanced and the remissions preceeding transplantation were short. This indicated a leukemic cell population resistent to chemotherapy.

Despite this, the remission in the third patient exceeds the duration of remission proceeding transplantation. We are currently making improvements in:

(a) The magnetic susceptibility of the colloid: incorporating more iron or reducing the amount of boride formed by using a hypophosphite ion instead of the borohydride ion as the reducing agent are being investigated. A high iron containing colloid has been made.

(b) The passivation, to avoid dichromate. This would be theoretically very appealing with Al_2O_3, which forms a thin hard impermeable coat on cobalt.

(c) Quantification of protein binding with, for example radiolabelled antibody. This is already in progress with ^{75}S labelled mouse monoclonal MDA001.

(d) The sizing of the colloid by transmission EM, light scattering techniques, and scanning EM. This will lead to greater ability to control the size of the cobalt colloid.

(e) Isoelectric focussing of each protein prior to binding to the colloid which is now established as standard procedure in colloidal gold systems. This will lead to better protein binding through more accurate knowledge of the pI of the protein being bound.

(f) The magnetic gradients by changing the design of the magnet With colloids of greater magnetic susceptibility this may not prove to be such a limiting factor.

(g) The surfactants for the colloid. We are investigating those that irreversibly coat the surface of cobalt and are able to covalently bind antibody.

Colloidal cobalt suspensions may have applications beyond bone marrow transplantation. In biological systems, it may have a role in magnetic immunoassays, radiolabelling and boron neutron capture for the high boride containing colloids. These and other uses remain to be explored.

REFERENCES
1. Ehrlich P. 1906 In: The collected papers of Paul Ehrlich. Vol II: Immunology and Cancer Research (Edit. by F. Himmelweit, M. Marquardt and H. Dale), pp. 442-447. Pergamon Press, Oxford 1957.
2. Ehrlich P. 1907 In: The collected papers of Paul Ehrlich. Vol III: Chemotehrapy. (Edit. by F. Himmelweit, M. Marquardt and H. Dale), pp. 106-129. Pergamon Press, Oxford 1957.
3. Kohler G, Milstein C. 1975. Continuous culture of fused cells secreting antibody of predifined specificity. Nature 256:495-497.
4. Baldwin RW, Embleton MJ, Price MR. 1981. Monoclonal antibodies specifying human tumor associated antigens and their potential for therapy. Molec. Aspets Med. 4:329-368.
5. Gregoriadis G. 1977. Targeting of drugs. Nature 265:407-411.
6. Kataoka T, Kobayashi T. 1978. Enhancement of chemotherapeutic effect by entrapping 1-beta-D-arabinofuranosyl cytosine in lipid vesicles and its mode of action. Ann. N.Y. Acad. Sci., 308:387-394.
7. Mayhew E, Papahadjopoulos D, Rustum YM, Dave C. 1978. Use of liposomes for the enhancement of the cytotoxic effects of cytosine arabinoside. Ann. N.Y. Acad. Sci., 308:371-386.
8. Gregoriadis G, Neerunjun ED. 1975. Homing of liposomes to target cells. Biochem. Biophys. Res. Comm., 65:537-544.
9. Kramer PA. 1974. Albumin microspheres as vehicles for achieving specificity in drug delivery. J. Pharm. Sci., 63:1646-1647.
10. Rahman Y, Cerny EA, Tollaksen SL, Wright B, Nance SL, Thomson JR. 1974. Liposome-enapsulated Actinomycin D: Potential in cancer chemotehrapy. Proc. Soc. Exp. Biol. Med., 146:1173-1176.
11. Widder KJ, Senyei AE, Scorpelli DG. 1978. Magnetic mirospheres: A model system for site specific drug delivery in vivo. Proc. Soc. Exp. Biol. Med. 158:141-146.
12. Szekerke M, Driscoll JS. 1977. The use of macromolecules as carriers of antitumor drugs. Eur. J. Cancer 13:529-537.
13. Arnon R, Sela M. 1982. In vitro and in vivo efficacy of conjugates of daunomycin with antitumor antibodies. Immunol. Rev., 62:5-27.
14. Flechner I. 1973. The cure and concomitant immunization of mice bearing Ehrlich ascites tumors by treatment with an antibody-alkylating agent complex. Eur. J. Cancer 9:741-745.
15. Mathe G, Loc TB, Bernard J. 1958. Effet sur la leucemie L1210 de la souris d'une combination par diazotation d'A-methopterine et de gamma globulines de hamsters porteurs de cette leucemie par heterogreffe. C.R. Acad. Sci., (Paris) 246:1626-1632.
16. Hurwitz ER, Levy R, Maron M, Wilchek M, Arnon R, Sela M. 1975. The covalent binding of daunomycin and adriamycin to antibodies with retention of both drug and antibody activities. Cancer Res., 35:1175-1181.
17. Levy R, Hurwitz ER, Maron R, Arnon R, Sela M. 1975. The specific cytotoxic effects of daunomycin conjugated to antitumor antibodies. Cancer Res., 35:1182-1185.
18. Davies DAL, O'Neil GJ. 1973. In vitro and in vitro effects of human specific antibodies with chlorambucil. Biol. J. Cancer, 28(Suppl 1):285-298.

19. Dullens HFT, DeWeger RA, Vennegoor C, Den Omer W. 1979. Anti-tumor effect of chlorambucil-antibody complexes in a murine melanoma system. Eur. J. Cancer 15:69-75.
20. Barbieri L, Stirpe F. 1982. Ribosome-inactivating proteins from plants: Properties and possible uses. Cancer Surveys 1:489-520.
21. Pappenheimer AM. 1977. Diphtheria toxin. Ann. Rev. Biochem., 46:69-94.
22. Olsnes S, Pihl A. 1982. Cytotoxic proteins with intracellular site of action: Mechanism of action and anticancer properties. Cancer Surveys 1:467-487.
23. Jansen FK, Blythman HE, Carriere D, Casellas P, Gros P, Paolueci F, Pan B, Pancelet P, Richer G, Vidal H. 1981. Replacement of the B chain of nicin with specific conventional or monoclonal antibodies. In receptor-mediated binding and internalization of toxins and hormones. (Ed. JL Middlebrook and Kohn LD). Academic Press, New York, p. 351.
24. Pau B, Blythman HE, Casellas P, Gros O, Gros P, Jansen FK, Paolucci F, Vidal H, Voisin GA. 1980. Conjugates between a toxin subunit and monoclonal antibodies (immunotoxins) with high specific cytotoxicity. In Protides of the Biological Fluids (ed. Peeters H), Pergamon Press, Oxford, p. 497.
25. Jansen FK, Blythman HE, Carriere D, Casellas P, Gros O, Gros P, Laurent JC, Paolucci F, Pau B, Poncelet P, Richer G, Vidal H, Voisin G. 1982. Immunotoxins: Hybrid molecules combining high specificity and potent cytotoxicity. Immunol. Rev., 62:186-216.
26. Filipovich AH, Quinones R, Valera D, Kersey JH. 1983. T lymphocyte depletion of human bone marrow in vitro for prevention of graft vs host disease (GVHD) in allogeneic bone marrow transplantatio (BMT). Twelfth Annual Meeting of the International Society for Experimental Hematology held in London, July 10-14, p. 188.
27. Dicke KA, Spitzer G, Peters L, Stevens EE, Hendriks W, McCredie KB. 1978. Approaches to graft-versus-host disease following bone marrow transplantation in monkeys and man. Transplant. Proc., 10:217-221.
28. Dicke KA, Spitzer G, Peters L, et al. 1979. Autologous bone-marrow transplantation in relapsed adult acute leukemia. Lancet, March, pp. 514-517.
29. Vellekoop L, Thomson S, Stewart D, et al. 1979. Separation of human leukemic cells and normal demopoietic stem cells by density centrifugation on a discontinuous albumin gradient. Eighth Annual Meeting of the Internation Society for Experimental Hematology held in Rotterdam, The Netherlands, August 20-24, p. 101.
30. Vellekoop L, Reading C, Chandran M, Tindle S, Dicke KA, Verma DS. 1982. Cell separation on the basis of immunogold-coupled monoclonal antibodies. Blood, 60(Suppl)174A.
31. Poynton CH, Reading CL. 1983. Monoclonal antibodies: The possibilities for cancer therapy. In Press. Revue canadienne de biologie.
32. James BD, Wallbridge MGH. 1970. Reactions of alkali metal tetraborohydrates. Prog. Inorg. Chem., 11:141-204.
33. Frens G. 1973. Controlled nucleation for the regulation of the particle size in monodisperse gold suspensions. Nature 241:20-22.
34. Frens G. 1972. Particle size and sol stability in metal colloids. Kolloid zu Polymere 250:736-741.
35. Rahman Y, Cerny EA, Tollaksen SL, Wright B, Nance SL, Thomson JR.

1974. Liposome-encapsulated actinomycin D: Potential in cancer chemotherapy. Proc. Soc. Exp. Biol. Med., 146:1173-1176.

THE USE OF IMMUNOTOXINS TO KILL NEOPLASTIC B CELLS

ELLEN S. VITETTA AND JONATHAN W. UHR

1. INTRODUCTION

Paul Ehrlich first discussed the potential use of anti-bodies as carriers of pharmacologic agents (1). During the last 10 years there have been many attempts to apply this concept to the elimination of neoplastic and other target cells using antibodies coupled to toxic agents. A cell-binding antibody conjugated to a plant or bacterial toxin has been termed an "immunotoxin". One such toxin, ricin, like most toxic proteins produced by bacteria and plants, has a toxic polypeptide (A chain) attached to a cell binding polypeptide (B chain) (2). The B chain is a lectin that binds to galactose-containing glycoproteins or glycolipids on the cell surface. By mechanisms that are not yet well understood, the A chain of the cell bound ricin gains access to the cell cytoplasm presumably by receptor-mediated endocytosis and penetration of the membrane of the endocytic vesicle (3). There is evidence that the B chain can also facilitate the translocation of the A chain through the membrane of the endocytic vesicle, possibly by forming a pore (4-7). In the cytoplasm, the A chain of ricin inhibits protein synthesis by enzymatically inactivating the EF-2 binding portion of the 60S ribosomal subunit. It is thought that one molecule of A chain in the cytoplasm of a susceptible cell can kill it (3).

The A and B chains of ricin can be separated, purified and covalently linked to antibodies derivatized with the thiol-containing cross-linker, SPDP. In the case of A chain containing immunotoxins, the antibody portion substitutes for the lectin

portion (B chain) thus allowing the specific targeting of th
toxic A chain to the relevant target cells.

2. THE MURINE BCL_1 MODEL

This disease bears a close resemblance to the prolymphc
cytic form of chronic lymphocytic leukemia in the human i.e
splenomegaly and severe leukemia (8,9). Injection of one BCl
cell into a normal BALB/c mouse results in leukemia in approxi
mately one-half of the recipients 12 weeks later (10). Tumc
bearing mice usually survive for 3-4 months after receivir
10^5 - 10^6 tumor cells. The BCL_1 tumor cells bear large amount
of cell surface IgMλ and traces of IgDλ, both of which have th
same idiotype.

3. ELIMINATION OF BCL_1 CELLS FROM BONE MARROW

In initial experiments, immunotoxins containing anti-idic
typic antibody directed against the tumor-derived Ig we:
incubated with populations of BCL_1 tumor cells and contro
cells. The specific immunotoxin decreased protein synthesis :
the populations containing tumor cells by 70-80%; the percen
age of tumor cells in these populations was also 70-80%
Control immunotoxins containing irrelevant antibodies had i
effect on BCL_1 cells nor did specific immunotoxins have .
effect on normal splenocytes, on T cell tumors, or on another
cell tumor bearing a different idiotype (Fig. 1). Anti-idic
type antibody by itself did not affect protein synthesis
BCL_1 cells. These results indicate that immunotoxin-mediat
killing of neoplastic B cells in a mixed population is specif
(11).

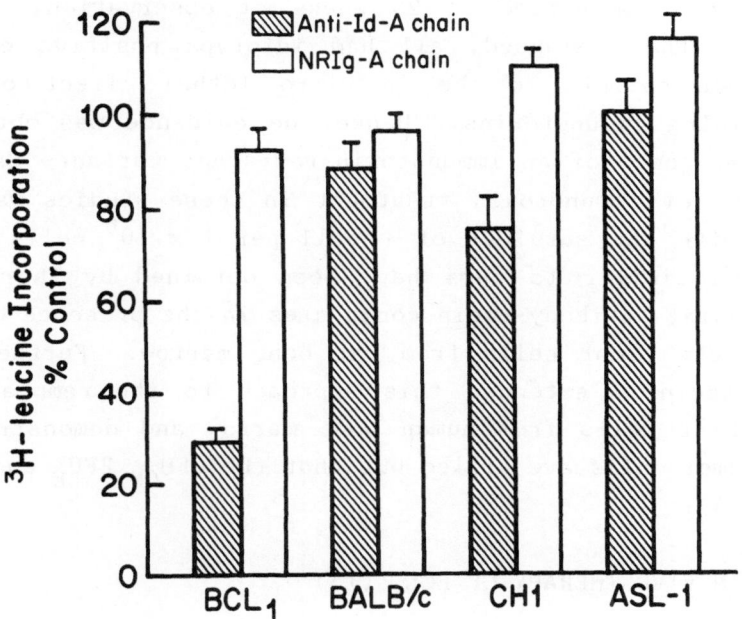

Figure 1. Effect of anti-Id-A chain on protein synthesis in BCL_1 cells, normal BALB/c splenocytes, ASL-1 tumor cells, and CH1 tumor cells. Anti-Id-A chain was used at 0.2 µg/ml. The CH1 cell express IgMλ on their surface but lack the BCL_1 idiotype. Hatched bars, anti-Id-A chain; empty bars, NRIg-A chain.

Similar studies were performed using a tumor infiltrated bone marrow (12) (containing 15% BCL_1 cells) because of the clinical implications of removing tumor cells from marrow. In addition, it was possible to evaluate the nonspecific killing of stem cells by adoptively transferring the treated cells into lethally irradiated recipients. In these studies, anti-Ig immunotoxin was used since, the only requirement for the specificity of the immunotoxin was that it kill all the tumor cells but not the stem cells. Thus, it was possible to use a polyvalent antibody against Ig rather than an anti-idiotypic antibody. The results of these experiments (Fig. 2) indicate that) the hematopoietic system of all the animals was reconstituted

because all lethally irradiated mice survived.   2) 15 of 2(
mice treated with tumor reactive immunotoxin did not develo]
tumor over a period of 25 weeks of observation.   Of the :
animals that relapsed, all had idiotype positive cells tha
were susceptible to the in vitro lethal effect of anti-I,
containing immunotoxins.   Hence, no evidence was obtained fo
the emergence of an immunotoxin-resistant variant. Rather, th
results of immunotoxin treatment in these studies was consis
tent with the survival of 1 cell per 1×10^6 cells injected
Results similar to ours have been obtained by Thorpe et al
(13) using antibody-ricin conjugates in the presence of lactos
to delete tumor cells from rat bone marrow.   Furthermore, w
have recently extended this approach to the removal of neo
plastic B cells from human bone marrow and demonstrated tha
the tumor cells are killed but that the CFU_{GM} BFU_E and CFU_E ar
not (14).

4.   IN VIVO THERAPY OF BCL_1 (15)

For these experiments, mice bearing massive tumor burden
(20% of body weight or approximately 10^{10} tumor cells) wer
employed. The strategy was to reduce the tumor burden by a
least 95% using nonspecific cytoreduction and to eliminate th
remaining tumor cells with immunotoxins directed against eithe
the idiotype or the δ chain of sIgD on the BCL_1 cells.   Th
rationale for using anti-δ is that sIgD is present on a larg
proportion of B cell tumors and, therefore, would present
more practical reagent for clinical therapy.   Furthermore
after cytoreductive therapy, there are virtually no sIg[
positive normal B cells or serum IgD to bind the immunotoxir
Normal B cells can also be regenerated from sIgD⁻ cells.   I
these experiments, nonspecific cytoreduction was accomplishe
with a combination of splenectomy and fractionated total lyn
phoid irradiation (TLI).   Animals receiving no further treat
ment other than TLI and splenectomy were dead within 8 weel
(Fig. 3). The injection of these cytoreduced mice with contr(

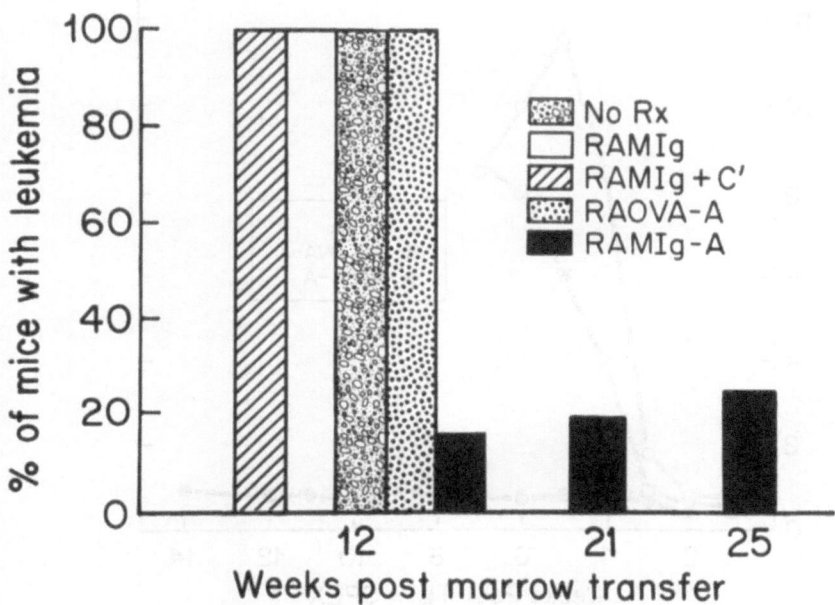

Figure 2. Adoptive transfer into lethally irradiated recipients of BCL$_1$-containing bone marrow cells treated with rabbit antibody (Ab) to mouse Ig conjugated with A chain. Bone marrow cells containing 10 to 15 percent tumor cells were injected into groups of 20 mice at 10^6 marrow cells per mouse. Every two weeks after adoptive transfer the mice were examined for leukemia. At 25 weeks, all surviving mice were killed and 10^6 spleen cells were adoptively transferred into normal recipients. The spleen cells from one of the mice caused a tumor in these recipients 10 weeks later. Thus, this mouse is scored as leukemic at 25 weeks.

228

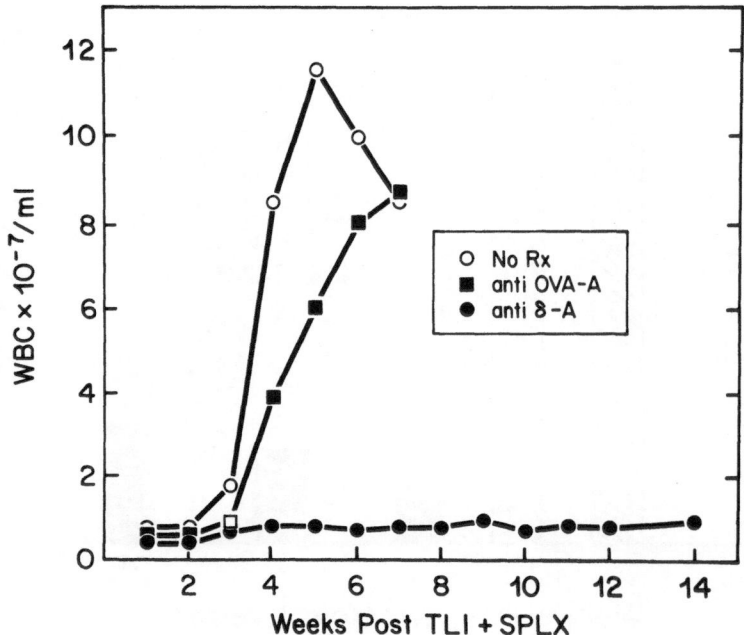

Figure 3. Effect of TLI, splenectomy, and administration of immunotoxin on leukemic relapse of BCL_1-bearing mice. Aft‹ nine doses of TLI and splenectomy, mice were injected with t‹ doses of 20 µg of anti-δ or control immunotoxin or were n‹ injected. There were nine mice per group. Leukemic relap‹ was monitored by determining the number of white cells in t‹ blood of the treated mice. The control mice were all dead at wk after TLI. The rabbit anti-mouse δ-A chain-treated gro‹ was monitored for a period of 14 wk post-TLI, at which poi‹ the experiment was terminated.

immunotoxins or antibody alone did not prolong their survival. In contrast, animals receiving anti-δ immunotoxins appeared disease-free as judged by the absence of detectable idiotype-positive cells 12 to 18 weeks later in 3 of 4 experiments. In one experiment, treated mice relapsed at 8-10 weeks after immunotoxin therapy. It should also be noted that 14 weeks after such immunotoxin treatment, mice in remission had normal or above normal levels of sIgD-bearing B lymphocytes. Hence, stem cells, pre-B cells or sIgD⁻ lymphocytes had fully restored the virgin B cell compartment.

These results suggest that 1) either remaining tumor cells had been eradicated in the animals that appeared tumor-free or that some viable tumor cells remained but were "held in check" by host resistance mechanisms. 2) Immunotoxin to a normal tissue component, in this case sIgD, can be used to render animals disease-free and the host can survive the effects of such cross-reactivity and can reconstitute the B cell compartment. To determine whether the animals were disease-free, tissues were then transferred from disease-free animals 25 weeks after treatments. All animals adoptively transferred tumor into normal mice indicating that the animals were not tumor-free and suggesting that host resistance had developed.

The partial success of these experiments was probably due to the fact that nonspecific cytoreduction was successful in reducing the number of remaining tumor cells to a level which could be effectively killed by a non-lethal dose of the immunotoxin. In addition, the immunotoxins in this instance did not kill all the remaining tumor cells yet prolonged remissions occurred. Presumably, the remaining viable tumor cells did not produce progressive disease because of a tumor-specific immune response.

.   USE OF B CHAIN-CONTAINING IMMUNOTOXINS TO POTENTIATE A
    CHAIN-CONTAINING IMMUNOTOXINS

It is known that in many cases ricin conjugates are signi-icantly more toxic than antibody-A chain conjugates (4-7). In

addition, free B chains can syngerize in vitro with A chain-co
taining immunotoxins in specifically killing target cells (5)
It is postulated, therefore, that the greater toxicity of rici
containing immunotoxins as compared to A chain-containin
immunotoxins is due to the capacity of the B chain to facili
tate the entry of A chain into the cytoplasm (reviewed in 5)
It would be desirable to develop a strategy in which the puta
tive transport role of the B chain could be preserved whil
eliminating and minimizing its function as a lectin. On
approach would be to utilize two types of immunotoxins. Tumc
reactive antibodies could be conjugated to either ricin A chai
or ricin B chain. Affinity purification of the immunotoxins c
their respective antigens would be used to remove free A and
chains. Using the two immunotoxins, the two subunits of th
ricin toxin could thereby be delivered independently to th
same target cell.

As seen in the upper panel of Figure 4 (16), when Dauc
cells were treated with either a low dose of rabbit anti-huma
Ig-A chain (RAHIg-A) or a variety of doses of rabbit anti-huma
Ig-B chain (RAHIg-B), no toxicity was observed. However, whe
the RAHIg-A was mixed with various concentrations of RAHIg·
there was significant cytotoxicity. It is of interest tha
this treatment of the Daudi cells with the mixture of immunc
toxins was performed in medium lacking galactose. As shown :
the bottom panel of Figure 4, when Daudi cells were treate
with a low dose of RAHIg-A, a variety of doses of rabbit ant:
ovalbumin-B (RAOVA-B) or mixtures of the two, no toxicity wa
observed except at the highest dose of the RAOVA-B . The:
results indicate that the target cell specificity of the ant:
body combining site of the immunotoxin is essential for syner;

The precise events that underlie the synergy are unclea:
One possibility is that the two immunotoxins that bind to tl
same target cell are endocytosed together and are present
the same endosome. Therein, interchain disulfide bonds may
split and free ricin may be formed in the endocytic vesicl
The B chain would then facilitate translocation of the A cha

into the cytoplasm with resultant cell death. These results represent a new strategy for utilizing the potential toxic property of the A chain and the pore-forming ability of the B chain in a manner which retains the specific toxicity conferred by the antibody.

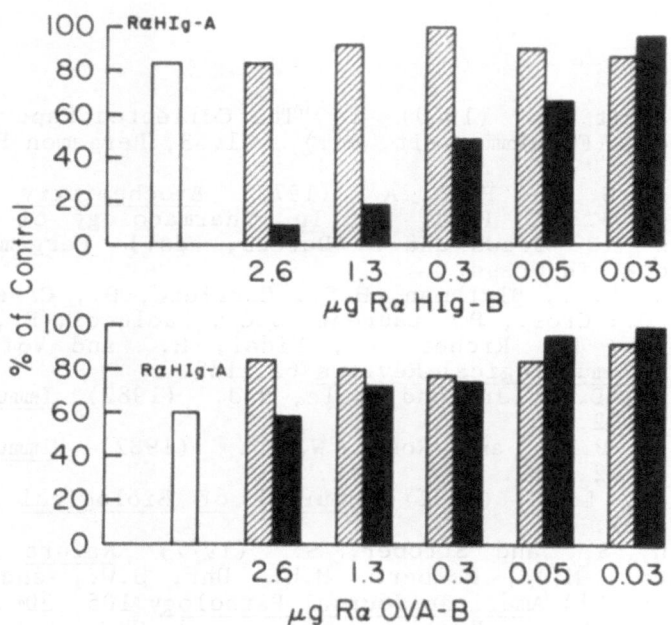

Figure 4. The use of mixtures of A chain and B chain containing immunotoxins to kill Daudi cells in vitro. Daudi cells were cultured with a nontoxic concentration of either RαHIg-A □, or nontoxic doses of either RαHIg-B (upper panel) ▨ , or RαOVA-B (lower panel) ▨. The solid bars ■ , represent mixtures of the single dose of the RαHIg-A plus different concentrations of either RαHIg-B (upper panel), or RαOVA-B (lower panel). Cells were treated with immunotoxin for 15 minutes at 4°C, washed, and cultured for 16 hours at 37°C in medium containing immuno-toxin. Cells were labeled for 4 hours with ^{3}H-leucine and harvested. The controls were not treated with immunotoxins but were incubated and labeled in the same manner.

232

6. ACKNOWLEDGEMENTS

We thank our colleagues, Drs. Krolick, Villemez, Isakson and Cushley who collaborated with us on these studies, our technicians, Ms. C. Bockhold, Mr. Y. Chinn, Ms. K. Gorman, Ms R. Baylis, Mr. J. Hudson, Ms. L. Trahan and Mr. T. Tucker, and Ms. D. Tucker for secretarial assistance. These studies were supported by CA-28149 from the NIH.

REFERENCES

1. Himmelweit, F. (1960) In "The Collected Papers of Pau Ehrlich" (F. Himmelweit, ed.), Vol. 3, Pergamon Press, New York.
2. Olsnes, S. and Pihl, A. (1973) Biochemistry 12, 3121
3. Olsnes, S. and Pihl, A. In "Pharmacology of Bacteria Toxins" (J. Drews and F. Dornes, eds.) Pergamon Press New York, in press.
4. Jansen, F.K., Blythman, H.E., Carriére, D., Casellas, P. Gros, O., Gros., P., Laurent, J.C., Paolucci, F., Pau, B. Poncelet, P., Richer, G., Vidal, H., and Voisin, G.A (1982) Immunological Reviews 62, 185.
5. Neville, D.M., Jr. and Youle, R.J. (1982) Immunologica Reviews 62, 75.
6. Thorpe, P.E., and Ross, W.C.J. (1982) Immunologica Reviews 62, 119.
7. Houston, L.L. (1982) Journal of Biological Chemistr 257, 1532.
8. Slavin, S., and Strober, S. (1977) Nature 272, 624
9. Muirhead, M.J., Holbert, M.H., Uhr, J.W., and Vitetta E.S. (1981) American Journal Pathology 105, 306.
10. Vitetta, E.S., Krolick, K.A., and Uhr, J.W. (1982 Immunological Reviews 62, 159.
11. Krolick, K.A., Villemez, C., Isakson, P., Uhr, J.W. an Vitetta, E.S. (1980) Proceedings National Academy Scienc U.S.A. 77, 5419.
12. Krolick, K.A., Uhr, J.W., Slavin, S., and Vitetta, E.S (1982a) Journal Experimental Medicine 155, 1797.
13. Thorpe, P.E., Mason, D.W., Brown, A.N.F., Simmonds, S.J. Ross, W.C.J., Cumber, A.J., and Forrester, J.A. (1982 Nature 297, 594.
14. Muirhead, M.J., Martin, P.J., Torok-Storb, B., Uhr, J.W. and Vitetta, E.S. Blood, in press, 1983.
15. Krolick, K.A., Uhr, J.W. and Vitetta, E.S. (1982b Nature 295, 604.
16. Vitetta, E.S., Cushley, W., and Uhr, J.W. Proceedings National Academy Science U.S.A., in press, 1983.

MONOCLONAL ANTIBODIES FOR PURGING BONE MARROW OF ACUTE LYMPHOBLASTIC LEUKEMIA OR GRAFT VERSUS HOST PRODUCING CELLS:ANTIBODY PLUS COMPLEMENT OR IMMUNOTOXINS.

J. Kersey, D. Vallera, N. Ramsay, L. Filipovich, R. Stong, T. LeBien
R. Youle, D. Neville
P. Beverley

INTRODUCTION

A major goal of marrow transplantation is to remove unwanted marrow cells and infuse only those stem cells which are responsible for engraftment. Positive selection for stem cells is possible. Attempts at this approach have to date been largely thwarted by the lack of unique markers for stem cells in humans. The process of positive selection for stem cells is also complicated by the relatively large number of cells which are necessary for prompt marrow engraftment in humans. An alternative to positive selection of marrow stem cells is to perform negative selection to remove unwanted cells from the marrow inoculum. Two major types of cells can be removed in this process. First, in patients with malignant processes involving marrow, e.g. leukemia, the leukemic cells can be removed prior to autologous marrow rescue. Second, T lymphocytes that produce graft versus host disease (GVHD) can be removed by marrow purging prior to allogeneic transplantation.

At the University of Minnesota our approach to the problem of purging marrow of unwanted leukemic cells or GVHD producing cells is to use monoclonal antibodies. Monoclonal antibodies have the advantage over heteroantisera in that they can be produced in a very homogeneous manner in large quantities. Monoclonal antibodies have an advantage over chemical means of purging the marrow in that these antibodies are highly

---

supported in part by the following grants from the NIH: CA 21737, CA 5097 and CA 31685.

specific for individual cell surface determinants. Our approach is to use antibodies which are well characterized both with respect to binding to normal lymphohemopoietic cells as well as the unwanted cells in the marrow. Our current studies involve methods for optimization of killing of the unwanted cells before infusion into the recipient. Previous studies by our group suggested that reliance on in vivo mechanisms (e.g. complement or antibody-mediated cellular cytotoxicity) was not likely to be effective in the removal of antibody coated cells (1). Our recent studies have focused on ex vivo killing using rabbit serum as a complement source or the use of conjugates of antibody to the toxic lectin ricin. Both the complement and ricin methods are potentially useful, and each is currently in use for different purposes in our human marrow transplantation program at Minnesota.

REMOVAL OF ALL CELLS USING BA-1, BA-2, AND BA-3

BA-1, BA-2, and BA-3 are three antibodies produced in Minnesota; the major features of each of these antibodies is summarized in Table 1. BA-1 binds to about 85% of cases of ALL of probable B lineage (2), but does not bind to multipotent stem cells (5). BA-2 also binds to most B lineage ALLs and some T lineage ALLs (3), but does not bind to multipotent stem cells (6). BA-3 is an anti-gp100 (CALLA) antibody, which like other anti-CALLA antibodies, does not bind multipotent stem cells (7). Futhermore, experiments carried out in our laboratories indicate that the cocktail of BA-1, BA-2 and BA-3 does not inhibit multipotent stem cells in the presence of complement (7).

Our studies with BA-1, BA-2, and BA-3 indicate that a great deal of heterogeneity exists relative to the binding of these antibodies to cells from individual cases of ALL, as well as between the various cases (8). Additive killing effects of the antibodies have been demonstrated with regularity; these results have been previously reported using a chromium release assay (7). A more recent analysis using a more sensitive clonogenic assay with ALL cell lines also demonstrated additive killing using more than one antibody (Stepan and LeBien, unpublished). Studies to date in our group have utilized baby rabbit serum as complement source. We have recently initiated a clinical study using the cocktail of BA-1, BA-2 and BA-3 plus one cycle of complement to remove leukemic cells from autologous marrow (15). Patients are eligible

if they are high risk ALL (children who have relapsed or adults in first
remission) and have cells which are BA-1, BA-2, and/or BA-3 positive.
Patients receive cyclophosphamide, 60mg per Kg per day or two days, followed by total body irradiation 165 cG b.i.d. X 4 days followed by
rescue using BA-1, BA-2, BA-3 plus complement treated autologous marrow. Efficacy of marrow cleanup in this study will be determined by (1)
analysis of residual cells in vitro, and (2) by comparison with a group
of patients who receive allogeneic transplantation.

THE USE OF TA1-RICIN, T101-RICIN, AND UCHT1-RICIN TO REMOVE GVHD-PRODUCING LYMPHOCYTES FROM ALLOGENEIC MARROW OR T LEUKEMIC CELLS IN AUTOLOGOUS MARROW.

A second use for monoclonal antibodies is to purge marrow of GVHD-
producing lymphocytes. Abundant evidence has accumulated to indicate
that experimental animals that receive T cell depleted bone marrow can
be successfully transplanted across the major transplantation barriers. Mice that receive untreated marrow inevitably develop severe and
fatal graft versus host disease (9). Marrow may be purged of T lymphocytes using antibody plus complement, and in more recent experiments in
the mouse, T cell antibody conjugated to ricin (10). In these latter
experiments antibody has been conjugated with intact ricin. Ricin is
composed of two chains, the A chain which is responsible for killing and
the B chain which facilitates intracellular movements of the ricin
molecule (16). Ricin is conjugated in these experiments using thioether
linkage (17).

Recently, three human T cell monoclonal antibodies have been produced which bind to >95% of mature lymphocytes (TABLE 1). Each of the
three binds to unique antigenic determinents on cell surfaces (11-13).
These three antibodies have been conjugated to intact ricin using the
same method as was used for the anti-murine antibodies (17). The antibody ricin conjugates have been studied extensively relative to inhibition of T cell function in the phytohemoglulinin (PHA) proliferative
assay, the mixed leucocyte assay, the assay for generation of cytotoxic
T lymphocytes and inhibition of multipotent stem cell function. The
antibody ricin conjugates are extremely effective in elimination of PHA,
MLR, and CTL responses at concentrations which are not inhibitory for

MONOCLONAL ANTIBODIES IN USE AT UNIVERSITY OF MINNESOTA FOR
PURGING BONE MARROW OF LEUKEMIC CELLS IN ALL OR GVHD-PRODUCING T CELLS

Antibody	Reference	Cluster* Designation	Antigen	Rabbit Complement Fixing	Ricin Conjugate Produced	Percentage of Leukemia	Normal Lymphoid Progenitors	Mature Lymphoid Cells	Stem Cell Binding
BA-1	2	NT	?p30	Yes	No	>80% of B-lineage	Yes	Yes (B)	No
BA-2	3	CD 9	p24	Yes	No	>70% of B-lineage some T	Yes	No	No.
BA-3	4	CD 10	gp100 (CALLA)	Yes	No	>70% of B-lineage some T	Yes	No	No
TA-1	11	NT	gp170/95	No	Yes	95% of T	Yes	Yes (T)	No
T101	12	CD 5	p65	Yes	Yes	95% of T	No	Yes (T)	No
UCHT1	13	CD 3	p20	No	Yes	25% of T	No	Yes (T)	No

* First International Leucocyte Differentiation Workshop

multipotent stem cells (14). Additional experiments indicate that these antibodies are more effective when used as a combination (TA-1, UCHT1, and T101) than when used individually (14). This approach using anti- body-ricin has several advantages over other methods of cell lysis: The immunotoxins can be produced using antibodies which are not complement fixing and do not have the problems inherent in the use of complement. The method for antibody-ricin treatment is relatively simple and less labor intensive than other methods of T cell removal, eg. antibody plus complement or the physical removal of T lymphocytes using lectins or sheep erythrocyte rosetting (Filipovich et al, unpublished).

Based on the extensive pre-clinical studies discribed above, we have recently embarked on a Phase I study using the cocktail of TA1-ricin, T101-ricin, and UCHT1 ricin to remove T cells from allogeneic marrow. In initial studies HLA-matched sibling marrow is being used with very high-risk leukemia patients. Analysis of the preliminary data obtained is currently underway (18).

As described in Table 1, the bulk of T cell leukemias bind either TA1, T101, UCHT1 or a combination of these antibodies. We are therefore hopeful that antibody-ricin conjugates using these antibodies may be useful in autologous marrow transplantation for T leukemia. Ex vivo studies using these three immunotoxins are currently under study (Stong et al, unpublished).

CONCLUSION

Extensive characterization of the range of binding of the monoclonal antibodies BA-1, BA-1, BA-3, TA-1, T101 and UCHT1 has previously been reported from this and other laboratories using a wide variety of hemopoietic as well as nonhemopoietic targets. There data clearly indicate that the targets for these antibodies are generally not re- stricted to a single lineage. Furthermore, these antibodies bind to various normal and malignant lymphoid cell targets depending on the particular antibody. The lack of binding of these antibodies to multi- potent stem cells makes these antibodies especially attractive for use in purging either allogeneic or autologous marrow of unwanted cells. These antibodies have been used by us for marrow purging, as either "T" or "B" cocktails. Our experience to date suggests the importance of adequate ex vivo killing of cells without reliance on in vivo killing of

238

antibody coated cells. Effective killing is possible using either complement-mediated cell lysis, or alternatively the use of antibody-ricin (immunotoxin) conjugates. The efficacy of marrow purging for removal of leukemia cells in autologous marrow or GVHD producing T cells in allogeneic marrow transplantation will be determined only after careful clinical trials.

ACKNOWLEDGMENT

The authors gratefully acknowledge Hybritech, Inc., San Diego, who have produced sufficient quantities of antibodies BA-1, BA-2, BA-3, TA-1, and T101 for the preclinical and clinical studies described herein.

REFERENCES

1. Filipovich AH, McGlave P, Ramsay NKC, Goldstein G, Kersey JH. 1982. Pretreatment of donor bone marrow with monoclonal antibodies for prevention of acute Graft vs. Host Disease in allongeneic histocompatible bone marrow transplantation. Lancet 1:1266-1269.
2. Abramson CS, Kersey JH, LeBien TW. 1981. A monoclonal antibody (BA-1) reactive with cells of human B lymphocyte lineage. J Immunol 126:83-88.
3. Kersey JH, LeBien TW, Abramson CS, Newman R, Sutherland R, Greaves M. 1981. p24: A human leukemia-associated and lymphohemopoietic progenitor cell surface structure identified with monoclonal antibody. J Exp Med 153:726-731.
4. LeBien TW, Boue DR, Bradley G, and Kersey JH. 1982. Antibody affinity may influence antigenic modulation of the common acute lymphoblastic leukemia antigen in vitro. J Immunol 129;5:2287-2292.
5. Jansen J, Ash RC, Zanjani ED, LeBien TW, Kersey JH. 1982. Monoclonal antibody BA-1 does not bind to hematopoietic precursor cells. Blood 59:1029-1035.
6. Ash RC, Jansen J, Kersey JH, LeBien TW, Zanjani ED. 1982. Normal human puripotential and committed hematopoietic progenitors do not express the p24 antigen detected by monoclonal antibody BA-2: Implications for immunotherapy of lymphocytic leukemia. Blood 60:1310-1316.
7. LeBien TW, Ash RC, Zanjan ED, Kersey JH. 1983. In vitro cytodestruction of leukemic cells in human bone marrow using a cocktail of monoclonal antibodies. Haematology and Blood Transfusion Vol 28, "Modern Trends in Human Leukemia V", R. Neth, ed., Springer Verlag:112-116.
8. Kersey JH, Goldman A, Abramson C, Nesbit M, Perry G, Gajl-Peczalska K, LeBien TW. 1982. The clinical utility of monoclonal antibody phenotyping in childhood acute lymphoblastic leukemia. Lancet :1419-1423.
9. Vallera DA, Soderling CCB, Carlson GJ, Kersey JH. 1981. Bone marrow transplantation across major histocompatibility barriers in mice: the effect of elimination of T cells from donor grafts by treatment with monoclonal Thy 1.2 plus complement or antibody

alone. Transplantation 31:218-22.

10. Vallera DA, Youle RJ, Neville DM, Kersey JH. 1982. Bone Marrow transplantation across major histocompatibility barriers. V. Protection of mice from lethal GVHD by pretreatment of donor cells with monoclonal anti-thy-1.2 coupled to the toxin lectin ricin. J Exp Med 155:949-954.

11. LeBien TW, Kersey JH. 1980. A monoclonal antibody (TA-1) reactive with human T lymphocytes and monocytes. J Immunol 125:2208-2214.

12. Royston I, Majda JA, Baird SM, Meserve BL, Griffiths JC. 1980. Human T cell antigens defined by monoclonal antibodies: the 65,000-dalton antigen of T cells (T65) is also found on chronic lymphocytic leukemia cells bearing surface immunoglobulin. J Immunol 125:725-731.

13. Beverley PCL, Callard RE. 1981. Distinctive functional characteristics of human T lymphocytes defined by E rosetting or a monoclonal anti-T cell antibody. Eur. J. Immunol 11:329.

14. Vallera DA, Ash RC, Zanjani ED, Kersey JH, LeBien TW, Beverley PCL, Neville DM Jr., Youle RJ. 1983. Anti-T-cell reagents from human bone marrow transplantation: Ricin linked to three monoclonal antibodies. Science In press.

15. Ramsay N, LeBien T, Nesbit M, McGlave P, Weisdorf D, Hurd D, Kenyon P, Goldman A, Kim T, Kersey J. 1983. Autologous bone marrow transplantation for acute lymphoblastic leukemia following marrow treatment BA-1, BA-2, BA-3 and rabbit complement. Blood In press.

16. Neville DM, Youle RJ. 1982. Monoclonal antibody-ricin or ricin-A chain hybrids: Kinetic analysis of cell killing for tumor therapy. Immunol. Rev. 62:75.

17. Youle RJ, Neville DM. 1980. Anti-Thy 1.2 monoclonal antibody linked to ricin is a potent cell-type-specific toxin. Proc. Nat. Acad.Sci. 77:5483.

18. Filipovich AH, Vallera D, Quinones R, Youle RJ, Neville D, Kersey JH. 1983. Bone marrow (BM) pretreatment with anti T-cell immunotoxins (IT) for the prevention of graft versus host disease (GVHD) in human bone marrow transplant (BMT). Blood In press.

TREATMENT OF AUTOLOGOUS BONE MARROW GRAFTS WITH ANTIBODIES AGAINST ALL CELLS.

S. Thierfelder, B. Netzel, G. Hoffmann-Fezer, B. Kranz, J. Haas

1. INTRODUCTION

Protection of the patient against fatal marrow aplasia induced by maximal chemoand radiotherapy is possible by allogeneic bone marrow transplantation. However the majority of patients lack histocompatible donors. Therefore the question was raised whether for such patients remission bone marrow autografts represent an alternative to allogeneic bone marrow transplatation. Autologous bone marrow transplantation circumvents problems of donor selection and histocompatibility. But remission bone marrow has gone through cytoreductive treatment affecting also hemopoietic stem cells. Would a patient in remission have sufficient stem cells to be stored for months or years and still retain the capacity to fully reconstitute his hemopoeisis? The answer is yes and documented in several clinical centers by the collection, preservation and engraftment of the remission marrow in leukemia patients (2). But even if autografting of remission bone marrow is possible in principle the question remains whether it eradicates or reduces the leukemic clone so that cure or at least stable remissions can be obtained. Leukemic relapses must be expected which arise from residual leukemia having resisted the patient's chemotherapy. Even remission bone marrow may contain leukemic cells which would be reimplanted by the autologous transplantation procedure.

We therefore proposed the purging of leukemic bone marrow with antibodies against differentiation antigens expressed on leukemic and normal bone marrow cells but absent from hemopoietic stem cells. In the presence of complement rabbit antimouse T cell globulin could be shown to prevent leukemic bone marrow to kill irradiated syngeneic mice with T cell leukemia (9). These animal studies were encouraging and transplantations of autologous remission bone marrow in patients with common acute lymphoblastic leukemia following treatment with rabbit anti-cALL globulin were performed. (7) Since autologous bone marrow transplantation cannot be proven by genetic markers and also because elimination of leukemic cells can only be assumed after long-term clinical follow-up animal experiments are particularly important. In the following we summarize our experimental and clinical findings.

2. ANIMAL STUDIES

2.1. Material and Methods

2.1.1. Mice (10 to 12 weeks old) skin grafting, absorbed rabbit anti-mouse T cell globulin, absorbed fresh rabbit serum (for complement), thymectomy (at 9 weeks), as described before (9).

2.1.2. Bone marrow transplantation. 2×10^7 bone marrow cells were incubated with anti-T cell globulin (10 mg/ml) in a dilution of 1:4 at $37^\circ C$ for 30 min and transfused to syngeneic mice irradiated with 850 R 24 hr before.

2.1.3. Leukemia. Th-1.1 antigen-bearing lymphocytes from the 7th to 10th passage of a spontaneous AKR/J leukemia was passaged in an ascitic form. Various concentrations of leukemic cells alone or together with bone marrow were incubated with the same volume of antibody or complement or both for 30 min at 37 C before transfer to syngeneic recipients.

2.2. Results and Discussion

2.2.1. Survival after inoculation of leukemic cells treated with anti-T. Groups of six unirradiated AKR/J mice received injections of 10^2, 10^3, 10^4, 10^5,

Group no.	Incubation of donor cells	No. of recipients	Individual survival times (days)
1	Buffer	12	8, 8, 11, 11, 11, 11, 11, 11, 11, 11, 12, 13
2	Complement	12	8, 8, 8, 8, 8, 11, 11, 11, 11, 11, 11, 11
3	Complement + ATCG	12	9, 16, 18, 19, 19, 21, 22, >100, >100, ₊100, >100, >100[a]

No leukemia was detected in group 3 in contrast to the mice of the other groups.

TABLE 1. Survival of irradiated AKR/J mice grafted with syngeneic marrow mixed with 10^5 lymphocytes of an AKR/J T cell leukemia and incubated with anti-T cell globulin

Group no.	Thymectomy[a]	Incubation with ATCG	No. of recipients	Survival of skin grafts[b] (days)
1	+	+	15	84, >100, >100, >100, >100, >100, >100
2	+	-	9	28, 29, 30, 35, 35, 35, 70, 77, 84
3	-	+	9	11, 12, 14, 14, 15, 16, 16, 16, 16

Thymectomy was performed 2 weeks before bone marrow transplantation.

H-2-incompatible C57BL/6 skin was grafted 1 month after bone marrow transplantation.

TABLE 2. Recovery of cellular immunity after transplantation of syngeneic bone marrow incubated with ATCG into normal or thymectomized CBA mice.

10^6 AKR/J T leukemia cells ip. One thousand cells still
killed 100% of the animals. 75% of mice receiving 10^5
leukemic cells incubated with antibody and complement
survived 80 days. When 10^5 leukemic cells were mixed
with $2 \cdot 10^7$ bone marrow cells and transferred to irradiated AKR/J mice the bone marrow recipients died of leukemia within 2 weeks (Table 1). Pretreatment of the leukemic marrow with absorbed anti-T resulted in long term
survival of 40% of the animals. But also mice dying earlier, did not show symptoms of leukemia. They may have
died of a comparatively lower radiation resistance of the
AKR strain. Interestingly complement had to be added to
the antibody treatment (Table 1). The bone marrow recipients' reticulo-endothelial system was apparently not
capable to eliminate enough leukemic cells by opsoni-
zation if the cells were coated by antibody only.

2.2.2. Recovery of cellular immunity after transplantation of bone marrow pretreated with anti-T. CBA recipients of bone marrow whose T cells were lysed by anti-T
and complement did not develop T cell defiency. Their
capacity to reject H-2 incompatible skin grafts recovered
in a normal fashion. Apparently the recipients' thymus
helped the transferred stem cells to quickly build up a
new T cell population. This can be concluded from the
fact that no such recovery occurred in thymectomized mice
(Table 2, Group no 1). Many mice died, but others clearly
survived, whether due to residual T cells having with-
stood the antibody treatment or irradiation is not clear.
Our experimental data indicated that leukemic bone marrow
can be purged of over 99% of leukemic T cells by rabbit
anti-T in the presence of complement. Normal immune reconstitution under the influence of the bone marrow recipient's thymus ensues.

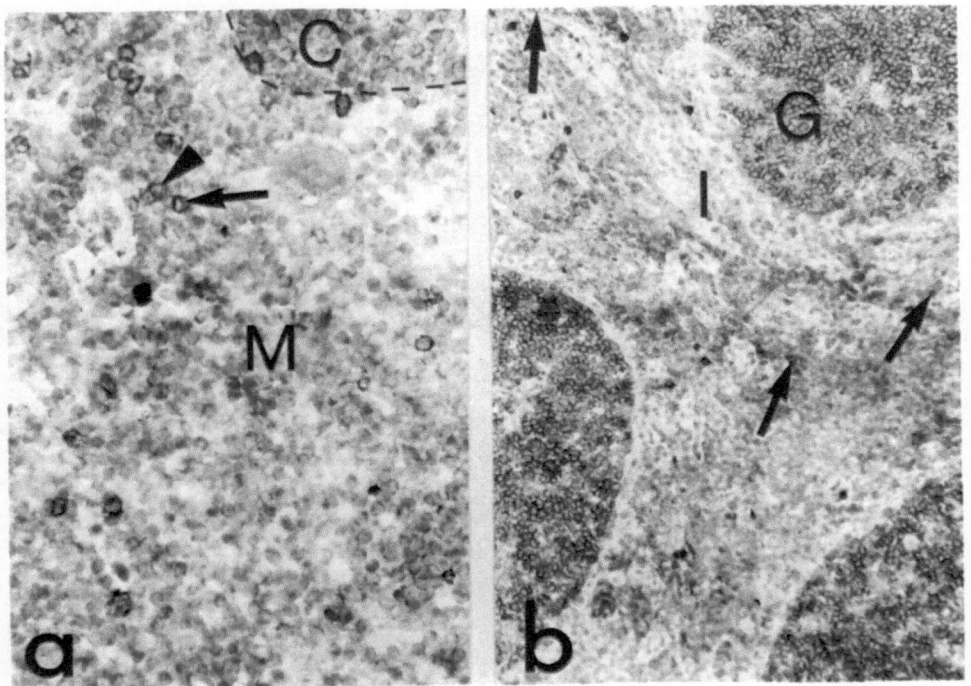

Fig. 1a

Thymic medulla (M) of children with a few strongly
CALL-labeled (↑) and rare faintly labeled cells
(▲), - - - border between thymic cortex (c) and
medulla.

Fig. 1b

Tonsil with many CALL-labeled cells in germinal
centres (G) and singular CALL⁺ cells (↑) in inter-
follicular T-cell zone (I).

246

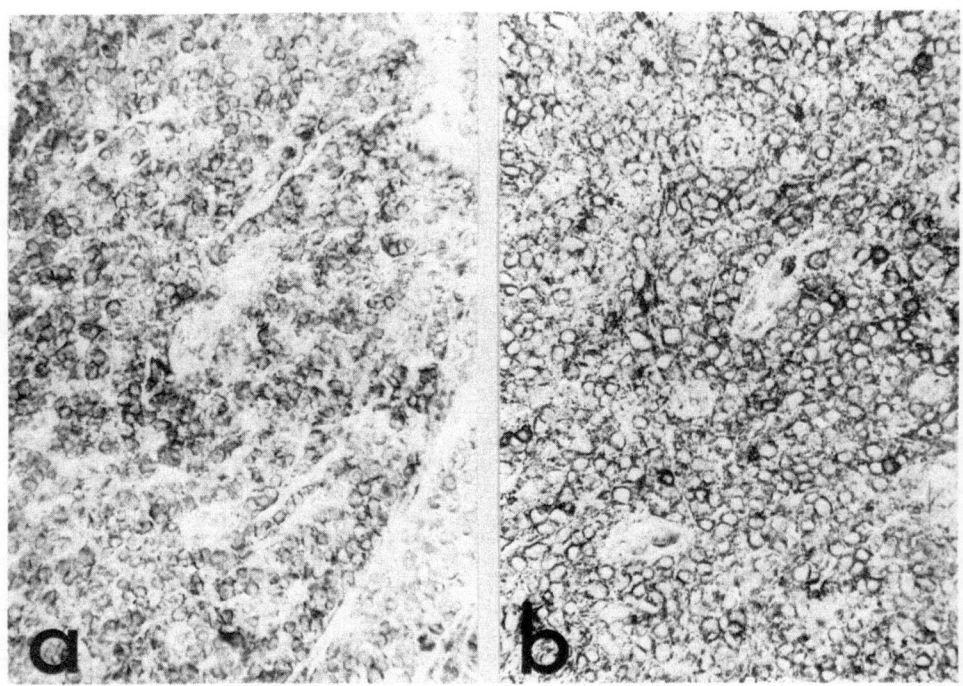

Fig. 2
Lymphoma expressing simultaneously
a) CALLA, b) T-antigens.

3. HUMAN STUDIES

3.1 The CALLA-phenotype

The CALL antigen is a potent antigen originally found on lymphoblasts of common acute lymphoblastic leukemias lacking T and B cell markers (3). Meanwhile poly- as well as monoclonal antibodies were found to react with numerous leukemic and normal hemopoietic and other cells and tissues (5). Using an immunocytochemical slide method we find around 8% of normal bone marrow cells and 30% of its lymphocytes CALLA$^+$. Below 2% peripheral blood lymphocytes are CALLA$^+$. Surprizingly also mature granulocytes are CALLA$^+$ (1). Most of the CALLA$^+$ bone marrow cells are early B cells expressing TDT and Ia antigens. But also thymocytes ($<10\%$) can be CALL$^+$ in thymic cortex as well as medulla (Fig.1a). Up to 20% CALLA$^+$ thymocytes were found on fetal thymus (12th week of gestation). Germinal centers known as peripheral B cell areas contain many CALLA$^+$ lymphocytes but singular or few cells can also be found in interfolicular T cell zones of tonsils (Fig.1b) (4). All these findings explain why CALLA$^+$ lymphomas with B or T markers occur (Figure 2a and b). Although CALLA has been identified in up to 5% of hemopoietic cells in the fetal liver, it does not seem to be expressed on stem cells.

3.2 Anti-CALLA

Polyclonal anti-CALLA antibody was produced in rabbits (8). After thorough absorption on liver and kidney homogenate, B-CLL and transformed LCL the IgG fraction lysed and fixed complement with common acute lymphoblastic leukemia cells but not with granulocytes. The differences between monoand polyclonal anti-CALLA are presently under investigation. So far it has been our experience that cytotoxic monoclonal mouse and polyclonal rabbit IgG antibodies differ by the considerably lower amount of complement fixed by the further. Whether this is due to the configuration of the antibodies or the clustering of polyclonal antibodies around the epitopes of an antigen is open to speculation. The titer of the rabbit anti-CALLA was 1:256 in the microcytotoxicity test.

3.3 Storage and Transplantation of Marrow

Bone marrow from patients in remission was obtained by multiple aspirations from the anterior and posterior iliac crest under general anesthesia and suspended in a preservativefree heparin medium mixture. The bone marrow (800-1700 ml) was filtered through fine screens; after fractionation in a cell separator, the red cell suspension depleted from mononuclear cells was washed and immediately reinfused to the donor. The marrow cell suspension was mixed at $4^{\circ}C$ to a final concentration of 10% DMSO, transferred to polyolefine bags, sandwiched into metal sleeves and frozen to $-30^{\circ}C$ at a rate of $1^{\circ}C/min$ with automatic compensation of the phase transition time, than to $-100^{\circ}C$ at a rate of $5-7^{\circ}C/min$ followed by storage in liquid nitrogen at $-196^{\circ}C$. Thawing was performed in a $45^{\circ}C$ water bath within 2 minutes.

After an ACDA plasma pH correction to a pH of 6.9, the cryopreserved bone marrow is directly infused to the patient without clearing the cryopreservation medium from the marrow.

For the clinical use of incubation with anti-CALLA antisera (final dilution 1:200 of 10 mg/ml antibody preparation) the following requirements had to be satisfied: sterility, pyrogenfree technique, negative hemagglutination titer; no cross-reactions against glomerular beasement membrane, hemopoetic stem cells, plasma proteins and complement.

Cross-reactions of antisera with normal hemopoetic stem
cells were studied in inhibition tests using the CFU-C
assay and the diffusion chamber test (6). Standard methods were applied for microcytotoxicity testing. Remission bone marrow was incubated with the antibody preparation before storage. Patients were conditioned with the
following antileukemic therapeutic regimen: BCNU (200
mg/m^2 on days -13, -12), cytosine arabinoside (200
mg/m^2 on days -12 to -8), cyclophosphamide (1.8 g/m^2
on days -7, -6), and a total body irradiation with 1,000
rad from two opposing ^{60}Co sources at a dosage of 5.5
R/min 24 hours before transplantation. During hospitali-
sation the patients were kept in a laminar flow unit. The
cytotoxic activity of anti-cALL globulin against normal
hemopoietic stem cells was investigated in frozen marrow
cells from patient 1 (Table 3). Short-term incubation of
marrow cells with non-absorbed anti-cALL antiserum and
complement completely inhibited the growth of stem cells
committed to granulocytic-myeloid differentiation
(CFU-C). The absorption of cross-reacting antibodies produced a globulin fraction with no cytotoxic activity
against normal progenitor cells but a high cytotoxic activity against cALL-type leukemic cells.
Figure 3 illustrates the clinical course of patient 1, a
7-year-old girl in her third relapse of cALL. 24 hours
after total body irradiation, 1.9 x 10^8/kg nucleated
marrow cells (86,000 CFU-C/kg) were infused. The marrow
cells had been harvested during her first remission,
cryopreserved in liquid nitrogen for 30 months and prepared with anti-cALL globulin before grafting. The clinical course was uneventful and the patient achieved complete hemopoietic recovery with WBC of 1,000/mm^3 on day
21, a platelet count of 20,000/mm^3 on day 50 and a remission period of 6 months.
The second patient, an 8-year-old boy in his third cALL
relapse, received 3.7 x 10^8/kg nucleated bone marrow

cells cryopreserved at -196°C for 12 months. 7 days after bone marrow transplantation the patient died of cardiac failure. The bone marrow was characterized by an onset of normal myelopoietic and erythropoetic differentiation but no leukemic cells could be detected. Autografting (3.3×10^8/kg marrow cells, preservation at
-196°C for 15 months) was also performed in another
8-year-old girl in her third relapse as well. On day 23
the patient died of septicemia. Histopathology showed the
onset of remission in bone marrow and peripheral blood,
but no leukemic cells.

In spite of the clinical outcome of the 3 patients this
phase-1 study demonstrated that bone marrow cells harvested during the first remission and prepared with antileukemic antisera have the capacity to repopulate the recipient's bone marrow and produce hemopoietic recovery.
The analysis of patient data after allogeneic bone marrow
transplantation showed that leukemic relapse ranked second as mortality cause. There is clear evidence of predominant relapse in those patients with grafting in late
relapse (29,30,33). This was also observed in patient 1
with a relapse 6 months after bone marrow transplantation.
Our present phase-2 study is designed to investigate improvement in survival rates after bone marrow transplantation in the second or latest third remission. Patient
4, an 8 1/2-year-old boy, had a graft of 2.5×10^8/kg
nucleated marrow cells preserved for 51 months at
-196°C in his third remission (Fig.4). The clinical
course after transplantation was uneventful and the
patient is in complete remission 10 months after bone
marrow transplantation.

Patient 5, an 9-year-old girl, had an autograft ($2.2 \times
18^8$/kg nucleated marrow cells preserved for 50 months
at -196°C) in her third remission and is in complete

remission 2 months after bone marrow transplantation.
Whether these observations will translate into an improved cure rate, remains to be determined by long-term
follow-up studies.

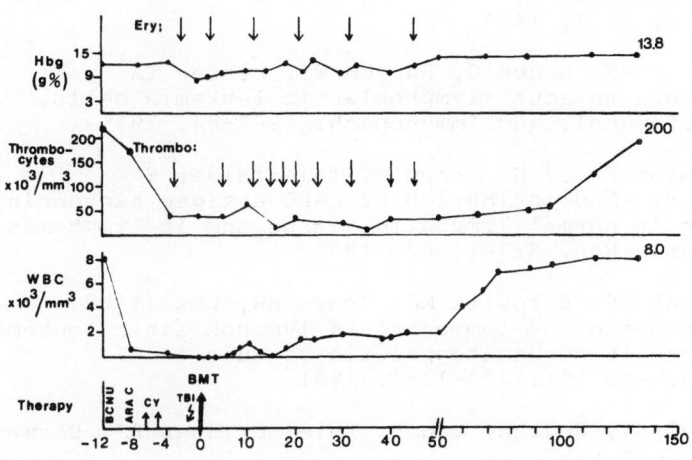

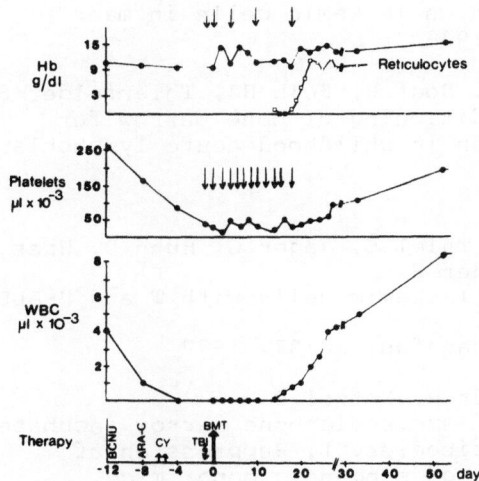

Fig. 3 and 4

Reconstitution after autologous bone marrow
transplantation in patients No. 1 and 4

1. Cossman J, Neckers LM, Leonhard WJ, Greene WC
   Polymorphonuclear neutrophils express the common
   acute lymphoblastic leukemia antigen.
   J. Exp.Med. 157:1064-1069, 1983

2. Deisseroth A, Mangalik A, Robinson W, Weiner R
   Keystone Conference on Autologous Bone Marrow
   Transplantation.
   Exp.Hemat. 7, 1979

3. Greaves MF, Brown G, Rapson NT, Lister TA
   Antisera to acute lymphoblastic leukemia cells.
   Clin.Immunol. and Immunopath. 4:67-84, 1975

4. Hoffmann-Fezer G, Knapp W, Thierfelder S
   Anatomical distribution of CALL antigen expressing
   cells in normal lymphatic tissue and in lymphomas.
   Leukemia Res. 6:761-767, 1982

5. Metzgar RS, Borowitz MJ, Jones NH, Dowell BL
   Distribution of common acute lymphoblastic leukemia
   antigen in nonhematogpoietic tissues.
   J.Exp.Med. 154:1243-1254, 1981

6. Netzel B., Rodt H, Lau B, Thiel E, Haas RJ, Dörmer P,
   Thierfelder S
   Transplantation of syngeneic bone marrow incubated
   with leukocyte antibodies. II. Cytotoxic activity of
   anti-cALL globulin on leukemic cells in man.
   Transpl. 26:157, 1978

7. Netzel B, Haas RJ, Rodt H, Kolb HJ, Thierfelder S
   Immunological conditioning of bone marrow for
   autotransplantation in childhood acute lymphoblastic
   leukemia.
   Lancet I:1332, 1980

8. Rodt H, Netzel B, Thiel E, Jäger G, Huhn D, Haas RJ,
   Götze D, Thierfelder S
   Classification of leukemic cells with T and O-ALL
   specific antisera.
   Haematol. Blood Transfus. 20:87, 1977

9. Thierfelder S, Rodt H, Netzel B
   Transplantation of syngeneic bone marrow incubated
   with leucocyte antibodies. I. Suppression of
   lymphatic leukemia of syngeneic donor mice.
   Transpl. 26:460, 1977

10. Thomas ED, Buckner CD, Clift RA, Fefer A, Johnson FL,
    Neiman PE, Sale GE, Sanders JE, Singer JW, Shulman H,
    Storb R, Weiden PL
    Marrow transplantation for acute non-lymphoblastic
    leukemia in first remission.
    N. Engl. J. Med. 302:597, 1979

11. Thomas ED, Sanders JE, Johnson FL, Buckner CD, Clift
    RA, Fefer A, Goodell BW, Storb R, Weiden PL
    Marrow transplantation for patients with acute
    lymphoblastic leukemia in remission.
    Blood 54:468, 1979

12. Weiden PL, Flurnoy N, Thomas ED, Prentice R, Fefer A,
    Buckner CD, Storb R
    Antileukemic effect of graft-versus-host disease in
    human recipients of allogeneic-marrow graft.
    N. Engl. J. Med. 300:1068, 1979

AUTOLOGOUS BONE MARROW TRANSPLANTATION IN CALLA POSITIVE ACUTE LYMPHOBLASTIC LEUKEMIA

S.E. SALLAN, R.C. BAST, JR, J.M. LIPTON, J. RITZ

INTRODUCTION

Chemotherapy is the primary treatment for childhood and adult acute lymphoblastic leukemia. The disease-free survival for children is 50% (1) and for adults approximately 40% (2). However, for patients who relapse while receiving drugs, or shortly after the elective cessation of chemotherapy, subsequent treatment has been unsatisfactory (3,4). Although second complete remissions can usually be attained, the median duration of such remissions has usually been less than six months (3,4).

Bone marrow transplantation offers an alternative form of therapy for patients with acute lymphoblastic leukemia who have failed initial chemotherapy. Between 25 and 50% of patients with relapsed acute lymphoblastic leukemia who receive allogeneic bone marrow transplantation have prolonged, leukemia-free survival (5-7). However, less than 40% of patients have an allogenic donor, and in the transplanted population an additional 30-50% endure graft-versus-host disease (6,7).

Autologous bone marrow transplantation offers an opportunity to expand the pool of transplant recipients and to avoid graft-versus-host disease (6,7). Our initial experience with autologous bone marrow transplantation and elimination of leukemic cells from human bone marrow has been previously published (8,9). In this report we provide an update of our clinical experience, as well as the rationale for protocol changes that have been instituted since our previous reports. These changes were intended to deal more effectively with two major problems: removal of leukemic cells from the marrow in vitro and removal of leukemic cells from the patient in vivo.

METHODS

Elimination of leukemic cells from human bone marrow in
vitro:

The method for generating, characterizing, and utilizing
murine monoclonal antibodies to eliminate leukemic cells
from human bone marrow have been described previously (9,10).
The J5 antibody reacts with the common acute lymphoblastic
leukemia antigen (CALLA), and the J2 monoclonal antibody react:
with a glycoprotein of molecular weight 26,000 daltons (10,11)

Three changes have been made in this methodology based
upon work with a model system that permits measurement of up t
5 logs of malignant cells (12). Two monoclonal antibodies, J5
and J2, are now used in combination. The rationale for the tw
antibody treatment was based upon experimental observation in
artificial, in vitro system utilizing a Burkitt cell line unde:
conditions comparable to the use of antibody in the presence o
bone marrow excess. We found that the addition of two antibod.
resulted in a 4-5 log cell kill compared to a 1-3 log cell kil
when one antibody was used (12). In addition, we found that
rabbit complement works more effectively if human serum compon
are excluded from the system. Moreover, repeated washing of
marrow is not required between the three cycles of treatment w.
antibody and complement.

Cytoreductive chemoradiotherapy in vivo:

Patients with acute lymphoblastic leukemia who relapsed
after receiving standard chemotherapy and whose leukemic cells
expressed CALLA were eligible for this protocol. Patients wit
normal identical twins or histocompatible siblings, and patien
in whom a complete remission could not be induced with chemotherapy alone, were excluded. One patient, #10, had Philadelp:
chromosome positive acute lymphoblastic leukemia and initiall:
failed remission induction. He was transplanted as soon as hi
bone marrow had fewer than 5% lymphoblasts and normal cytogene
tics.

After induction of a second or subsequent remission
(usually with vincristine, prednisone and asparaginase),

patients were subjected to an intensive course of chemotherapy. All patients received VM 26, cytosine arabinoside, and asparaginase. Intrathecal central nervous system reprophylaxis was performed with hydrocortisone and cytosine arabinoside. Those who had not previously received intensive treatment with an anthracycline were also given a single dose of doxorubicin during this intensive course of chemotherapy. After recovery from intensification, patients underwent a bone marrow harvest under general anesthesia. Initially, patients had bone marrow harvested after their reinduction therapy and prior to intensification therapy. This marrow was not antibody treated, but instead was used as a "backup". The practice of two harvests was abandoned after the first five patients had demonstrated engraftment of their antibody-treated marrows. Presently, a single large bone marrow harvest is performed after intensification. Approximately 2×10^7 cells/kg of marrow is cryopreserved immediately without antibody treatment to be used as a backup should the need arise. The remainder of the marrow is treated and cryopreserved as previously described (8,9). After completion of the harvest, patients receive ablative chemotherapy. In general, the treatment has consisted of total body irradiation and a standardized chemotherapy regimen, the details of which follow.

All patients received total body irradiation: 850 rad were delivered as a single dose in five rad per minute fractions for the first 13 patients, whereas 1200 rad were delivered in six, 200 rad fractions at 5 rad per minute administered every 12 hours for the last six patients. All patients received cyclophosphamide 60 mg/kg/dose intravenously on the two days preceeding the initiation of total body irradiation. They also received a continuous infusion of subcutaneous cytosine arabinoside (500 mg/m^2/day) ending on the day preceeding the administration of cyclophosphamide. The first 13 patients received five-day infusions and the last six patients received seven-day infusions. All patients also received VM26 (200 mg/m^2/dose) intravenously on the first and last day of the cytosine arabinoside infusion. Additionally, the last six patients received a single dose of

asparaginase (25,000 IU/m²) intramuscularly on the first day o
ablative therapy.

Approximately 12 hours after the completion of total body
irradiation, the cryopreserved, antibody-treated marrow was
rapidly thawed at 37°C and reinfused through a central venous
catheter. The number of cells infused per kilogram body weight
varied between 2.1 x 10^7 and 1.8 x 10^8 (median 5.2 x 10^7). Th
time to engraftment did not appear to be a function of the num]
of cells infused.

RESULTS

Tables 1 and 2 show the clinical characteristics and post
transplantation status as of October 1st, 1983 for all 19
patients.

Of the 19, one was too recently treated to be evaluated.
remain in continuous remission from 2 to 35 months (median 20.
months), seven relapsed (six of them within 100 days and one a
eight months), and there were five remission deaths (all withi
100 days). Of the latter, two were the result of hemorrhage i
patients #4 and #8, both of whom did not have sufficient plate
recovery at the time of death. Their antemortem bone marrow
aspirations did, however, show megakaryocyte recovery and ther
was no evidence of peripheral platelet destruction. The other
remission deaths occurred as the result of central nervous sys
toxoplasmosis (diagnosed at autopsy), fungal sepsis, and presu
gram negative sepsis.

Of the seven patients who remain in remission, three have
been followed for less than one year, two from one to two year
and two from two to three years. Of the four who have been in
remission for over one year, three were transplanted in second
remission and one in third remission. All four had had previo
remissions of greater than two years duration. The sites of
relapse prior to transplant varied in the four longterm surviv
bone marrow only in one patient, testes only in one patient; b
marrow, testes and central nervous system in one patient; and
testes only in the patient transplanted in third remission (wh

TABLE 1

CLINICAL CHARACTERISTICS

PATIENT	SEX	INITIAL WBC/MM^3	AGE AT DIAGNOSIS (YRS)
1	M	2,000	5
2	M	150,000	1 1/2
3	M	22,000	1 1/2
4	M	31,000	3
5	M	90,000	7
6	M	5,900	3
7	M	5,000	2
8	M	7,000	9
9	M	16,000	1 1/2
10	M	37,000	8
11	F	2,100	18
12	M	4,000	7
13	M	4,000	6
14	F	13,400	3
15	M	1,800	16
16	M	5,100	5
17	F	9,400	13
18	F	85,000	2
19	M	42,000	41

TABLE 2

DURATION OF 1st REMISSION AND POST-TRANSPLANTATION STATUS

PATIENT	DURATION 1st CR (mos)	RELAPSE SITE FIRST (SECOND)	POST-TRANSPLANT STATUS
1	50	BM	CCR 35 months
2	32	Testes	CCR 33 months
3	15	CNS (BM)	Relapse 2 mos
4	2	BM	RD 3 months
5	29	BM (Testes)	CCR 21 months
6	24	BM/CNS/Testes	CCR 20 months
7	16	BM	Relapse 8 mos
8	11	CNS/Testes	RD 3 months
9	11	BM (BM)	Relapse 3 mos
10	-	Ind Failure	RD 2 months
11	9	BM (BM)	RD 2 months
12	10	BM	Relapse 3 mos
13	3	BM	Relapse 3 mos
14	39	BM	CCR 7 months
15	16	BM (BM)	Relapse 3 mos
16	47	BM (BM/Testes)	RD 2 months
17	24	BM	Relapse 2 mos
18	30	BM	CCR 2 months
19	12	BM	CCR <1 month

CCR = continuous complete remission
RD = remission death

had previously had a bone marrow relapse). Of the patients who relapsed, four had been transplanted in their second remission and three others in their third remission.

None of the patients had manifestations of graft-versus-host disease. With the exception of the five patients who died from complications of transplant, none of the others had major, life-threatening complications during the post-transplantation period.

This autologous transplantation program was begun in November 1980. During a similar period of time, beginning in 1978, 17 children from our institution who had relapsed acute lymphoblastic leukemia, an HLA compatible donor and clinical characteristics similar to the 19 patients reported here, were referred for allogeneic bone marrow transplantation in one of the two major transplant centers in the United States. The Figure shows a Kaplan-Meier analysis of the length of transplant induced remission in the two patient populations as of August 1983. It can be seen that there is no statistically significant difference in leukemia-free survival between the autologous and allogeneic transplant groups.

DISCUSSION

The purpose of this clinical investigation was to assess whether antibody-treated bone marrow that had been cryopreserved and subsequently thawed would engraft, and whether in vitro anti-leukemic therapy, coupled with intensive chemotherapy and total body irradiation, could eradicate leukemia in relapsed, CALLA positive patients. We have established that engraftment of antibody treated marrow can be routinely observed.

Whether autologous bone marrow transplantation can be curative for patients with relapsed leukemia remains uncertain. We have been concerned by the high incidence of leukemic recurrence following the procedure. It has been especially difficult to eradicate leukemic cells in patients who had previously relapsed while receiving chemotherapy. However, our experience has not differed markedly from that of centers performing allogeneic transplantation (5). It is of interest that nearly identical results have been observed in 17 of our patients who underwent allogeneic transplantation during the same time period during which this trial of autologous transplantation was conducted (Figure).

We have also noted that the duration of initial complete remission has been important in predicting the post-transplantation duration of remission. A similar observation was apparent in an allogeneic transplant population (7). Of the four patients for whom post-transplantation remissions have exceede one year, all had an initial duration of remission of at least two years on chemotherapy. We found that the longterm survivo of allogeneic transplantation had a median duration of first, chemotherapy-maintained remission of 34 months. Other investi gators have suggested that children who relapse more than one year after the elective cessation of drugs can be successfully retreated by chemotherapy (13). With the exception of patient #1, we have only transplanted patients whose pre-transplantion relapse occurred while they were receiving chemotherapy or within one year of the elective cessation of chemotherapy. Patients who relapse one or more years after the elective cess tion of drugs are treated with further chemotherapy and not transplanted.

On the other hand, of the seven patients who relapsed, th duration of first remission was relatively short, ranging from three to twenty-four months, with a median time to relapse of 10.5 months. Thus, none of the patients who remained in conti uous remission have had a post-transplantation duration of remission that exceeds their initial chemotherapy-maintained remission. It is possible that this small group of successful treated patients has a more treatable disease characterized by a slower proliferative capacity of their leukemic cells; wheth they are cured remains uncertain. The results of allogeneic transplantation at other centers should be similarly scrutiniz

After evaluation of the first thirteen patients, we re- assessed our program to explore possibilities to improve resul It was impossible to determine whether the leukemic relapses occurred as a result of failure to eradicate leukemic cells _in_

vivo, in vitro or both. We knew from the allogeneic experience
of the Seattle Transplantation Team that most failures in acute
lymphoblastic leukemia were the result of failure of the chemotherapy and radiation therapy used in pre-transplantation conditioning (5,7). Therefore, we chose to further intensify our
in vivo therapy. The last six patients received a longer duration of cytosine arabinoside infusion (from five to seven days),
a higher dose of total body irradiation (from 850 to 1200 rad),
and a single dose of pre-transplantation asparaginase was added.
In addition, we intensified in vitro therapy for the last four
patients treated, by the use of the combination of J5 and J2
antibodies. These changes were begun within the last six
months, too soon to evaluate the impact of such adjustments on
longterm results.

Treatment of additional patients and longer follow-up will
be necessary to determine if this regimen is a clinically effective modality for the majority of patients with CALLA positive,
relapsed acute lymphoblastic leukemia.

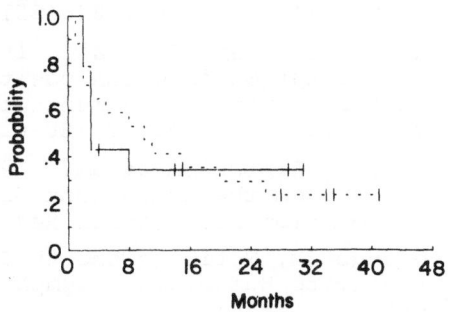

TYPE	BMT	CCR	FAIL	TOTAL
——	AUTO	5	9	14
· · ·	ALLO	4	13	17

August 1983

Probability of leukemia-free survival from
the time of transplantation for 31 patients
with relapsed acute lymphoblastic leukemia.
Allogeneic transplantation (allo) (N = 17)
was begun in 1978. Autologous transplantation (auto) (N = 14) began in 1980.
CCR = continuous complete remission

REFERENCES

1. Inati A, Sallan SE, Cassady JR et al. 1983. Efficacy and morbidity of central nervous system "prophylaxis" in childhood acute lymphoblastic leukemia: Eight years' experience with cranial irradiation and intrathecal methotrexate. Blood 61, 297-303.

2. Schauer P, Arlin ZA, Mertelsmann R et al. 1983. Treatment of acute lymphoblastic leukemia in adults: Results of the L10 and L10M protocols. J Clin Oncol 1, 462-470.

3. Poplack DG, Reaman GH, Wesley R. 1981. Treatment of acute lymphoblastic leukemia in relapse: Efficacy of a four-drug reinduction regimen. Can Treat Rep 65, 93-96.

4. Sallan SE, Hitchcock-Bryan S. 1981. Relapse in childhood acute lymphoblastic leukemia after elective cessation of initial treatment: Failure of subsequent treatment. Med Pe Oncol 9, 455-462.

5. nomas ED. 1983. Bone marrow transplantation: A lifesavir applied art. J Amer Med Assn 249, 2528-2536.

6. Dinsmore R, Kirkpatrick D, Flomenberg N et al. 1983. Allc geneic bone marrow transplantation for patients with acute lymphoblastic leukemia. Blood 62, 381-388.

7. Johnson FL, Thomas ED, Clark BS et al. 1981. A comparisor of bone marrow transplantation with chemotherapy for childr with acute lymphoblastic leukemia in second or subsequent remission. N Engl J Med 305, 846-851.

8. Ritz J, Sallan SE, Bast RC et al. 1982. Autologous bone marrow transplantation in CALLA positive acute lymphoblasti leukaemia after in vitro treatment with J5 monoclonal antibody and complement. Lancet 2, 60-62.

9. Bast RC, Ritz J, Lipton JM et al. 1983. Elimination of leukemic cells from the human bone marrow using monoclonal antibody and complement. Cancer Res 43, 1389-1394.

10. Ritz J, Pesando JM, Notis-McConarty J et al. 1980. A monc clonal antibody to human acute lymphoblastic leukaemic anti gen. Nature 283, 583-585.

11. Herchend T, Nadler LM, Pesando JM, Reinherz EL, Schlossman SF, Ritz J. 1981. Expression of a 26,000 dalton glycoprotein on activated human T-cells. Cell Immunol 64, 192.

12. Bast RC Jr, DeFabritiis P, Maver C et al. 1983. Elimination of malignant clonogenic cells from human bone marrow using multiple monoclonal antibodies and complement (C'). Amer Assn Can Res 24, 223.

13. Rivera G, George SL, Bowman WP et al. 1983. Second centra nervous system prophylaxis in children with acute lymphobla tic leukemia who relapse after elective cessation of therap J Clin Oncol 1, 471-476.

AUTOLOGOUS BONE MARROW TRANSPLANTATION IN ACUTE MYELOID LEUKAEMIA IN FIRST REMISSION

A.K. BURNETT, P. TANSEY, M. ALCORN, C.R.J. SINGER,
G.A. McDONALD and A.G. ROBERTSON

SUMMARY

Allogeneic Bone Marrow Transplantation currently offers the best chance of prolonged remission in Acute Myeloid Leukaemia, with a leukaemia relapse rate of 10-15%. It is, however, only available to less than 10% of those with the disease. There is also associated morbidity and mortality due to the transplant related complications of immunosuppression, graft-versus-host disease and pneumonitis. Autologous remission bone marrow is potentially available to all patients as a source of stem cells. We report our preliminary experience in nine patients who received supralethal chemoradiotherapy with cyclophosphamide and total body irradiation in first remission. The toxicity of the protocol was acceptable. Eight of nine patients remain in remission 15-103 weeks post graft. One patient died at 20 weeks due to adenovirus pneumonitis, but also in early relapse. Similar defects of immune recovery, and pulmonary function and patterns of viral infection were seen in this series, as are familiar in allogeneic BMT. For this study bone marrow was stored at 4°C for 54 hours, and resulted in acceptable haematological reconstitution.

INTRODUCTION

With aggressive chemotherapy, improved initial remission rates can be achieved in acute myeloid leukaemia (AML) (1,2). Therapeutic modalities designed to prolong remission and achieve cure for the majority of patients remain however elusive.

Currently, allogeneic bone marrow transplantation (Allo-BMT) offers the best chance of long term survival but is severely restricted by criteria of remission status, age and availability of an HLA-identical donor(3,4,5,6). These criteria restrict this procedure to less than 10% of all patients with AML. Even for HLA-identical patients the transplant related complications of immunosuppression, graft-versus-host disease (GVHD) and pneumonitis contribute to significant morbidity and mortality. Although a major advance and contribution, allogeneic BMT currently plays a minor role in the overall treatment of acute myeloid leukaemia. However, experience of this technique in a number of centres indicates that relapse of leukaemia only occurs in 10-15% of patients at risk. This suggests that the chemoradiotherapy protocol generally employed, Cyclophosphamide and Total Body Irradiation (TBI), is extremely effective maintenance therapy. There is therefore considerable incentive to administer this treatment to a wider group of patients for whom a fully matched donor is not available. The use of donors who are not fully HLA compatible is currently under evaluation but initial experience(7) has highlighted the considerable problems which beset this approach.

Autologous remission bone marrow represents an alternative source of marrow stem cells. This has the additional benefit of avoiding graft-versus-host disease with its associated immunosuppression.

We report our preliminary experience of the elective use of cyclophosphamide and TBI with autologous bone marrow transplantation in first remission of acute myeloid leukaemia. This protocol was carried out storing bone marrow at 4°C for 54 hours. The effects on pulmonary function, immune reconstitution, and patterns of viral infection are described.

PATIENTS AND METHODS

Nine patients with acute myeloid leukaemia who attained complete remission with 2-3 pulses of "DAT" chemotherapy (Daunorubicin 50mgs/m^2 I.V. Day 1, Cytosine-arabinoside 100mgs/m^2 I.V. 12-hourly Days 1-5, and Thioguanine 100mgs/m^2 orally 12-hourly Days 1-5) received further 5-13 pulses of consolidation/maintenance chemotherapy. Patients were aged 28-53 years. Patients under the age of 40 years with an HLA-identical donor were excluded and received allogeneic BMT. Reserve bone marrow was cryopreserved at least 6 weeks before embarking on the final autograft protocol which is shown in Figure 1. Informed consent was obtained from each patient.

Bone marrow was collected under general anaesthetic into blood collection bags (Tuta) containing 70mls citrate phosphate dextrose (CPD) per 500mls. The final volumes were pooled in larger dry bags and sealed in sterile conditions. The autograft was stored at 4°C for administration at the conclusion of irradiation therapy. Sufficient marrow was aspirated to ensure a minimum "dose" of 1×10^8 nucleated cells/kg. Patients were nursed in laminar flow beds with reverse barrier nursing. They received gut decontamination regime FRACON (Framycetin, Colistin and Nystatin) and sterile food. Isolation was discontinued as the patients' neutrophil count returned to 0.5×10^9/l. All patients received irradiated blood products. Where appropriate these products were obtained from CMV negative community donors. Patients received no further chemotherapy post-autograft.

Bone marrow precursor studies.

CFU-GM and BFU-E survival studies in 4°C storage conditions were measured by minor modifications of standard techniques(8,9).

Immune reconstitution

Serial phenotypic analysis of circulating T-lymphocytes was carried out in four patients periodically for several weeks, by fluorescent microscopy using monoclonal antibodies

OKT3, OKT 4 and OKT 8. Humoral immunity was assessed by
serial measurement of IgG, IgA and IgM.

Pulmonary function testing

This was performed using standard spirometric techniques
with diffusion capacity (D_LCO) measured by the single
breath technique. Taking patient age and weight into
account, all pulmonary function tests were performed when
the haemoglobin was within normal limits and were repeated
at four week intervals.

FIGURE 1. AUTOLOGOUS BMT PROTOCOL

-54 hours	B.M. Harvest	
-52 hours	Cyclophosphamide 60mg/kg	
-32 hours	Cyclophosphamide 60mgs/kg	Storage at 4°C
-8 hours	TBI 9.5Gy (5.5 cGy/min)	
0 hours	Marrow reinfusion	

RESULTS

The characteristics of the nine patients are shown in
Table 1. All patients entered complete remission of
disease promptly with 2 or 3 courses of induction
chemotherapy. They then received 5-13 pulses of consolidation,
maintenance chemotherapy. Bone marrow was cryopreserved
prior to autograft for each patient in the event of graft
failure but no patient required this reserve marrow.

Before the clinical introduction of this protocol
marrow stem cell assays (CFU-GM and BFU-E) were used to
assess marrow viability after 24, 48 and 72 hours storage at
4°C. The results are shown in Table 2. Since about one
third to one half of these precursor cells remained viable,
as large a number of marrow cells was harvested as possible.
The nucleated cell dose was $1.27 - 3.80 \times 10^8$ cells/kg.
Peripheral blood regeneration has been satisfactory.
Neutrophil counts of greater than 1×10^9/l were achieved

at 35 $\pm$ 4.1 (mean $\pm$ SEM) days. Platelet counts recovery was variable but no patient had a haemorrhagic episode. In patients numbers 2-5 (Table 3) prompt platelet recovery was noted. Counts of greater than 100 x 10^9/l were achieved in 4-10 weeks. In more recent patients, numbers 1 and 6-9, the platelet count was still below 100 x 10^9/l but above 30 x 10^9/l 7-15 weeks post-graft.

All patients tolerated the procedure without difficulty and were discharged from hospital within four weeks of autograft. As soon as adequate haematological reconstitution had taken place each patient received prophylactic low dose Septrin orally. Non-life-threatening viral infections were frequent in the first 4-6 months but one 53 year old patient died 20 weeks post autograft. He was admitted with progressive dyspnoea. There was substantial deterioration of his pulmonary function resulting in death despite assisted ventilation. Adenovirus was cultured from the lungs and was assumed to be the causative agent. At the time of death leukaemia relapse was also detected. A second patient developed pneumonitis 18 weeks post graft which was of unknown aetiology despite extensive investigation including lung biopsy, but recovery has taken place. The remaining seven patients are well in continuing complete remission between 15 and 103 weeks post graft (Table 3).

Table 1. Elective autograft in remission: patient details

Patient No	Sex	Age	FAB	Marrow Blasts	Induction Pulses	Consolidation/ Maintenance Pulses
1	M	41	M2	80%	2	12
2	M	33	M2	50%	3	13
3	M	34	M1	80%	3	8
4	M	53	M1	95%	3	9
5	M	53	M1	45%	2	8
6	F	28	M2	60%	3	5
7	M	33	M2	50%	2	6
8	F	44	M1	80%	3	11
9	F	27	M2	75%	3	5

Table 2: <u>Survival of Marrow Stem Cells at $4^{\circ}C$ (%)</u>

	0 hrs	24 hrs	48 hrs	72 hrs
CFU-GM	100	84 $\pm$ 10.3* (n=22)	81.5 $\pm$ 14.5 (n=14)	37 $\pm$ 8.5 (n=9)
BFU-E	100	83 $\pm$ 9.3 (n=6)	45 $\pm$ 12.3 (n=6)	28 $\pm$ 7.5 (n=11)

*Mean $\pm$ sem.

Table 3: <u>Elective Autograft in Remission: Present Status</u>

Patient No.	Cell Dose ($\times 10^8$/kg)	Remission (weeks) Pre	Post-ABMT	Total	Status
1	1.33	48	103+	151+	A and W
2	1.50	55	88+	143+	A and W
3	3.80	90	76+	166+	A and W
4	2.30	42	20	62	Died Adeno Pneum. Relapse
5	1.90	31	35+	66	A and W
6	2.2	18	27+	45+	A and W
7	2.0	20	22+	42+	A and W
8	1.54	48	21+	69+	A and W
9	1.27	19	15+	34+	A and W

Pulmonary Function Tests:

When serial pulmonary function was commenced shortly
prior to chemoradiotherapy, minor lung dysfunction was found
in all patients. Following autologous grafting(Fig 2) there
was a significant fall in vital capacity (v.c.) and diffusion
capacity ($D_L CO$), with significant increase in residual
volume. This restrictive defect was observed in all patients
but was variable in severity from one to another. It was
maximal between days 90-140 with static lung volumes tending
to return towards normal thereafter. Diffusion capacity
($D_L CO$), however, remains sub-normal in two out of three
patients surviving more than 52 weeks with no radiological
evidence of chronic radiation lung disease. There was no
difference in degree or progression of abnormalities in the
two patients who developed pneumonitis.

Figure 2: Serial Pulmonary Functions Post Cyclo/TBI +
Autologous Marrow

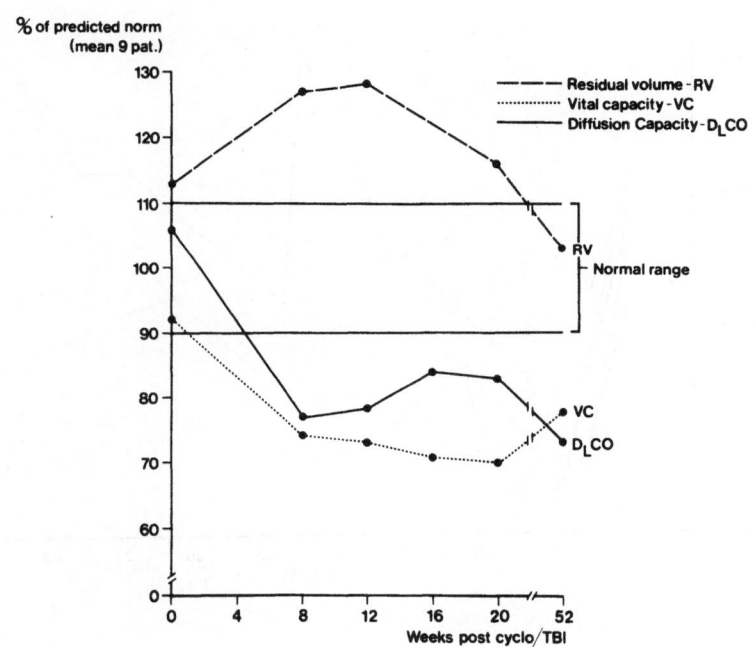

Immune recovery:

     Immunoglobulin levels have remained within normal limits
in all but 2 patients; one with a minor, isolated drop in
IgM; the other with severe reductions in both IgG and IgM.

     Serial measurement of T4:T8 peripheral blood
T lymphocyte ratios showed a normal ratio (2.0 - 2.5) pre-
chemoradiotherapy. As marrow function recovered, marked
inversion of this ratio (Fig 3) was seen (between 0.2 - 0.5)
with an absolute reduction in helper and absolute increase
in suppressor subsets. With time this ratio reverted to
normal. These T-lymphocyte abnormalities and the high
incidence of viral infections indicate that cellular
immunity is considerably influenced by this protocol in the
absence of graft-versus-host disease.

Figure 3: T Cell Subset regeneration following ABMT
(T4:T8 ratio)

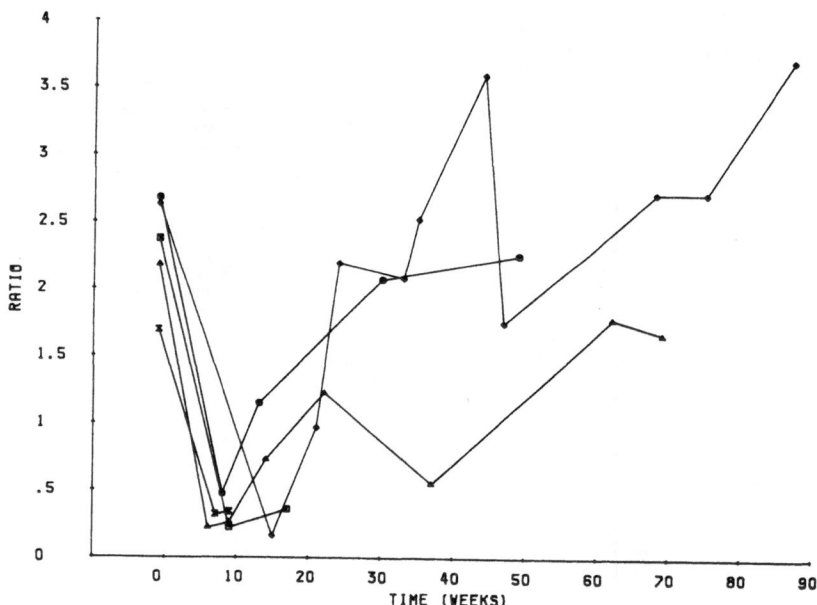

The range of viral infections with time is shown in
Fig 4. The majority of patients experienced Herpes Simplex
infections of the lip/oropharynx in the first 14 days. Two
CMV reactivations occurred but no primary cases were seen.
Adenovirus and Herpes Simplex infections were contracted
after the 100th day; in addition, there was a high incidence
of upper respiratory tract pathogens of the influenza group
in the first 100 days.

Figure 4: Infections - Viral   Post Cyclo/TBI + Autologous
                                                    Marrow

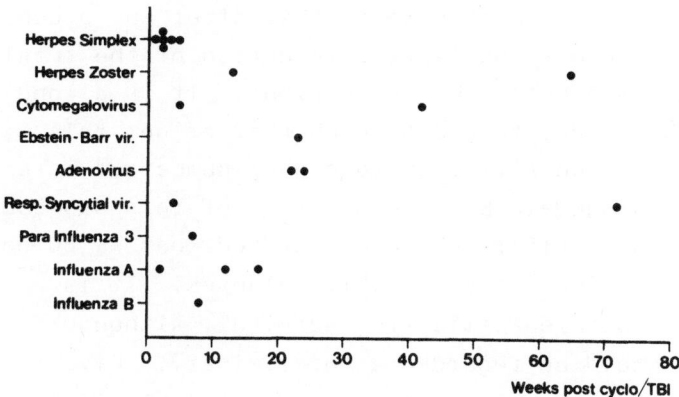

DISCUSSION

The supralethal combination of Cyclophosphamide and TBI
is highly effective therapy for acute myeloid leukaemia if
given in first remission. Other anti-leukaemia effects may
be operative however. For example, most initial studies
used methotrexate as graft-versus-host-disease prophylaxis.

In more recent experience the non-cytotoxic drug Cyclosporin A has been substituted. There has been no significant increase in leukaemia relapse rate(10,11). Similarly, a graft-versus-leukaemia effect has been demonstrated in experimental allografts(12) and statistical evidence of its effect has been suggested in humans when transplanted in relapse(13,14), but an antileukaemic effect in acute myeloid leukaemia allografted in remission has not been shown. We did not feel therefore that elimination of these two effects should make a substantial difference to the leukaemia free survival. Of greater concern is the possibility that the autograft contains residual clonogenic leukaemia cells. We expect however that after the procedure there will have been a substantial reduction of the total number of leukaemia cells in each patient. It is a long term aim of this study to evaluate whether or not this postulated reinfusion will lead to higher number of late relapses. In allogeneic BMT the majority of relapses occur within twelve months(15); we are encouraged that we do not yet have a higher incidence of early relapses. It is emphasised that our leukaemia free survival, although encouraging, should be regarded as preliminary. Five patients were more than 9 months into first remission before undergoing autograft and could be considered a selected group. Subsequent patients have been autografted earlier in remission.

The toxicity of the protocol has been acceptable in this wide age range of patients. Serial measurement of pulmonary function revealed a restrictive defect in all patients maximal between 90 and 140 days with subsequent improvement in lung function. These defects are similar to those demonstrated in allogeneic transplantation where subclinical GVHD could be present(16). One patient in this series died primarily due to pneumonitis due to adenovirus. This patient was also noted to have leukaemic relapse during the few days before death at 20 weeks post-graft.

immune deficiency as measured by serial immunoglobulins and
T-cell subset analysis also parallels that seen in allogeneic
BMT. Depression of humoral immunity in this series was less
severe than in allogeneic transplantation but apparently
more severe than in ABMT protocols involving high dose
chemotherapy without irradiation for solid tumours.(17,18).
The T-cell subset disturbances are similar to those
reported after allograft and previously associated by some
with the pathogenesis of GVHD.(19,20) We believe these
changes are non-specific. We, and others, have reported
similar findings following high-dose cyclophosphamide(21,22).
The pattern of opportunistic viral infection in these patients
was similar to that which we have experienced in allogeneic
grafts and to that found in large series, but we found a
higher incidence of infection with influenza group viruses
in the first 100 days.(23) In this study bone marrow was stored
at 4°C for 54 hours prior to reinfusion. Marrow precursor
assays (CFU-GM and BFU-E) suggested reduced viability at
48 and 72 hours storage in these conditions, but all patients
achieved acceptable haematological reconstitution, confirming
our recent report(24), and are independent of all blood
product support. Platelet reconstitution has been variable;
possible reasons for this are currently under investigation.
In no patient did thrombocytopenia cause a clinical problem.

Our experience of this protocol suggests that it has
acceptable toxicity in patients of an age range which will
encompass about 50-60% of patients with the disease. These
preliminary results provide encouragement that significant
leukaemia free survival may be achieved.

ACKNOWLEDGEMENTS:
    This work is supported by The Leukaemia Research Fund
of Great Britain.

REFERENCES
1. Gale R.P., Cline M.J. (1977) High remission-induction
    rate in acute myeloid leukemia. Lancet, 1:497-9
2. Rees J.K.H., Sandler R.M., Challener J., Hayhoe F.,(1977)
    Treatment of acute myeloid leukaemia with a triple
    cytotoxic regime:DAT. Brit J Cancer 36:770-6
3. Thomas E.D., Buckner D.C., Clift R.A. et al. Marrow
    Transplantation for acute non-lymphoblastic leukaemia in
    first remission . N. Engl.J.Med. 1979:301:597-9.
4. Blume K.G., Beutler E., Bross K.J. et al. Bone-marrow
    ablation and allogeneic marrow transplantation in acute
    leukaemia . N. Engl. J. Med. 1980:302:1041-6.
5. Powles R.L., Morgenstern G., Clink H.M. et al.   The place
    of bone-marrow transplantation in acute myelogenous
    leukaemia   Lancet 1980; 1:1047-50.
6. Gale R.P., Kay H.E.M., Rimm A.A., Bartin M.M.   Bone
    Marrow Transplantation for Acute Leukaemia in First
    Remission . Lancet 1982: ii, 1006-1009.
7. Powles R.L., Kay H.E.M., Clink H.M., et al (1983)
    Mismatched Family donors for bone marrow transplantation
    as treatment for acute leukaemia. Lancet 1; 612-615.
8. Pike B.L., Robinson W.A. (1970) Human bone marrow
    colony growth in agar gel. J. Cell Physiol. 76:77-84.
9. Iscove N.N., Sieber F. (1975). Erythroid progenitors
    in mouse bone marrow detected by macroscopic colony
    formation in culture. Exp. Hemat. 3:32.
10. Powles R.L., Clink H.M., Spence D. et al (1980).
    Cyclosporin A to prevent graft-versus-host disease in
    man after allogeneic bone marrow transplantation.
    Lancet 1: 327-329.
11. Zwaan F.E., Hermans J. (1983). Bone marrow trans-
    plantation for leukemia: European results of 487 cases.
    Exp. Hemat. 11: Suppl. 14:180.
12. Boranic M (1968). Transient graft-versus-host reaction
    in the treatment of leukemia in mice. J. Natl. Cancer
    Inst. 41: 421-437.
13. Weiden P.L., Flournoy N., Thomas E.D., et al. Anti-
    leukemic effect of graft-versus-host disease in human
    recipients of allogeneic marrow grafts. (1979)
    N. Eng. J. Med. 300: 1068-1073.
14. Weiden P.L., Sullivan K.M., Flournoy N. et al.(1981)
    Anti-leukaemia effect of chronic graft-versus-host
    disease . N. Eng. J. Med 304: 1529-32.
15. Zwaan F.E., Hermans J. (1983). Bone marrow trans-
    plantation for leukemia - European results in 264 cases.
    Exp. Hemat. 10 Suppl. 10: 64-69.
16. Depledge M.H., Barrett A., Powles R.L. (1983). Lung
    Function after Bone Marrow Grafting. Int. J. Radiation
    Oncol. Biol. Phys. 9: 145-151.
17. Atkinson K., Hansen J.A., Storb R. et al. (1982)
    T-cell subpopulations identified by monoclonal anti-
    bodies after human marrow transplantation. I Helper-
    inducer and cytotoxic-suppressor subsets. Blood 59:
    1292-1298.

18. Gorin N.C., Muller J.Y., Salmon C, Duhamel G (1980)
     Immunological studies in Patients submitted to
     Autologous Bone Marrow Transplantation. Immunobiology
     of Bone Marrow Transplantation, 263-273. Editor -
     Thierfelder S, Rodt H and Kolb H.J. Springer and
     Verlag, N.Y.
19. Reinherz E.L., Parkman R., Rappeport J et al (1979)
     Aberrations of suppressor T-cells in human graft-versus-
     host disease. N. Engl. J. Mec. 300: 1061-1068.
20. Bacigalupo A., Mingari M.C., Moretta L et al (1981)
     Imbalance of T-cell subpopulations and defective pokeweed
     mitogen-induced B-cell differentiation after bone-marrow
     transplantation in man. Clin. Imm. Immunopath 20:137-145
21. Singer C.R.J., Tansey P.J., Burnett A.K. (1983)
     T-lymphocyte reconstitution following autologous bone
     marrow transplantation. Clin. Exp. Immunol. 51:455-460.
22. Linch D.C., Knott L.J., Thomas R.M., et al (1983)
     T-cell regeneration after allogeneic and autologous
     bone marrow transplantation. Brit. J. Haematol.
     53: 451-458.
23. Watson J.G. (1983) Problems of infection after bone
     marrow transplantation. J. Clin. Pathol. 36: 683-692.
24. Burnett A.K., Tansey P.J., Hills C et al. (1983)
     Haematological reconstitution following high dose and
     supralethal chemo-radiotherapy using stored, non-
     cryopreserved autologous bone marrow.
     Brit. J. Haemat. 54: 309-316.

AUTOLOGOUS BONE MARROW TRANSPLANTATION IN PATIENTS WITH AML
WITHOUT TUMOR CELL PURGING AND POST TRANSPLANT CHEMOTHERAPY.

Bob Löwenberg , Johan Abels , Dirk W. van Bekkum , Gorda Dzoljic ,
Anton Hagenbeek , Willem D.H. Hendriks , Johan van de Poel ,
Willemijn Sizoo , Krijn Sintnicolaas , Gerard Wagemaker .

1. SUMMARY

Four consecutive patients with AML who did not have an HLA
matched bone marrow donor in the family, were subjected to
autologous bone marrow transplantation. The marrow had been
aspirated in remission, was cryopreserved and then reinfused
following antileukemic chemo-/radiotherapy. All patients had good
hemopoietic recoveries and continued in a new phase of stable
remission. One patient had a relapse at 13 month post transplant
and died. The other three patients continue in first remission at
45+, 18+ and 3+ months without any further therapy.

2. INTRODUCTION

Allogeneic bone marrow transplantation following high dose
chemotherapy and total body irradiation, when applied during
complete remission, has given promising disease free survival
rates (1-4). Major limitations of the wide employment of this
therapeutic modality, unfortunately, apply to: the restriction of
fully HLA compatible family donors, the high rate of
immunobiologic complication (GvHD; interstitial pneumonia; viral
infections; etc.), and the poor results in patients of age beyond
40 years of age.
These problems can be avoided to a large extent with autologous
BMT, and this explains the interest in autologous BMT, even though

the marrow may be contaminated with subclinical tumor.

One of the aims of developing autologous BMT towards general clinical applicability is to establish the advantages of the approach relative to the risks (higher rate of relapse). We ha suggested that the reinfusion of autologous marrow per se, ev contaminated with a small tumor cell burden, may lead to a significant tumor reduction and prevent recurrences as a resu tumor cell loss due to ineffective seeding in the host tissue (5). Only when baseline values of autologous BMT are availabl can be seen whether purging of the grafts from tumor cells do further improve the results.

Here we present the results of transplantation of non-modifie autologous bone marrow in four patients with AML.

3. METHODS

Bone marrow was collected from the iliac crest and pelvic in 2-4 ml aspirates and collected in bottles containing heparinised Hanks Balanced Salt Solution. The buffy coat (pre by centrifugation at 2000 g) was filtered through a nylon gau and then through a glass filter. Nucleated cells were counted Türck solution. Samples from the graft were sent for bacterio logical and GM-CFU cultures. Cells were frozen in 10% DMSO an calf serum using a controlled rate freezer (Cryoson, Beemster Holland) at $1^{\circ}C$/min and stored in liquid nitrogen (6).

Cyclophosphamide (60 mg/kg) was administered in saline during hr infusion on two subsequent days under conditions of forced diuresis (>125 ml/hr) and alkalinization of the urine (pH >6.(In patients No. 2, 3 and 4, Mesna was given in divided portior -10 min, +4 hr, +8 hr and +12 hr following the start of the cyclophosphamide infusion up to a total dose of 48 mg/kg on e of two days.

Total body irradiation (25 MV photon-beam, average treatment distance, 420 cm) was administered on day -1 with two horizont beams (AP and PA; with patient on either side) and delivered one session at an average dose rate of 15.0 cGy/min (pts. No. and No. 2) or 5.5 cGy/min (pts. No. 3 and No. 4). The total d

vas 8.0 Gy to the midline of the body with partial lung shielding
resulting in a dose of 7.0 Gy to the lungs.

The marrow graft was thawed on day 0 and step-wise diluted with
IBSS according to previously described methods (6) and then
reinfused during 30-45 min.

GM-CFU cultures were done by a double agar layer technique with a
leukocyte feeder as previously described (7).

Blood products for transfusion were irradiated (15 Gy);
leukocyte-poor cotton-wool filtrated red cells were given;
platelet and granulocyte transfusions were always prepared from
single donors using an Aminco continuous flow cell separator.

All patients were nursed in reverse isolation in a room (pts. No.
1 and No. 4) or a laminar air flow unit (pts. No. 2 and No. 3)
from about day -10 until the granulocyte count had reached a value
of $0.5 \times 10^9/1$.

No autologous BMT in patients with AML performed in our
institution were excluded from the analysis.

Clinical data were evaluated as of October 1, 1983.

4. RESULTS

Four consecutive patients were treated with high dose cyclophosphamide and total body irradiation and autologous BMT. All
patients had AML and were in first complete remission. The
clinical features of the disease, the seize of the graft and post
transplant events are all summarized in the Table.

5. DISCUSSION

From the experiences it is evident that bone marrow which had
previously been exposed to heavy remission induction therapy and
is likely to contain occult AML cells, permits excellent
hemopoietic repopulation and results in stable remissions. One
patient had a relapse, which was progressive in spite a trial of
new chemotherapy. The other three patients now experience a total
remission duration of 52+, 28+ and 7+ months if the transplant
intermission is included. Probably the most important implication

Clinical characteristics of 4 patients with AML; outcome of autologous BMT during first remission.

	patient no	1	2	3	4
Pre-transplant	age (yrs)	30	48	15	35
	sex	F	F	M	F
	diagnosis (FAB subtype of AML)	M4	M4	M3	M2
	duration of CR until transplant (mo)	7	7	10	4
Transplant	cell dosis (frozen) per kg b.w.	2.5×10^8	1.5×10^8	1.9×10^8	3.8×10^8
	CFU-c per kg body weight	3.1×10^4	2.1×10^4	1.0×10^4	8.2×10^4
Post transplant	hemopoietic recovery (day)				
	granulocytes above 500/mm^3	day 36	day 23	day 27	day 24
	platelets above 50.000/mm^3	day 67	day 39	day 39	day 40
	complications	pneumonia	-	- herpes simplex infection, - staph.epid. septicemia, - hydradenitis	-
	cause of death	-	relapse AML at 13 mo	-	-
	survival post transplant (mo)	45+	14	18+	3+

All data are expressed relative to the time of transplantation (time 0).
Evaluated as of October 1, 1983.

of these observations is that investigators developing tumor
separation methods for autologous BMT require baseline controls,
since non-modified grafts per se may give satisfying results.
The probability of the successful establishment of the neoplasm in
the host following i.v. transfer of cells is thought to be based
on: a) the number of clonogenic cells in the tumor and b) the
efficiency of the cells to reach a suitable tissue environment for
re-initiating cell proliferation. It is conceivable that the i.v.
infusion of small numbers of AML cells is associated with a
significant tumor reduction as a consequence of seeding at
inappropriate sites in the body. In fact autologous BMT in canines
with lymphoma with a high rate of marrow involvement has resulted
in high cure rates (8). The phenomenon of cell loss due to
ineffective seeding has been well recognized in animal models and
may, although it is difficult to prove at this stage, also hold
for clinical transplantation biology. We propose that a systematic
development of autologous BMT should be pursued with unfractionated grafts first because a) tumor cleaning may not be required
at all in a certain proportion of instances, b) tumor cell
cleaning at present is usually a blind procedure without
evaluating for the specific removal of the tumor clonogenic cells
and may be an ineffective cell manipulation (9,10), c) the effect
of tumor cleaning of autologous grafts can only be assessed in the
presence of data without separation.

ACKNOWLEDGEMENTS
This work was supported by the Netherlands Cancer Society "The
Queen Wilhelmina Fund".

6. REFERENCES

1. Thomas E.D., Buckner C.D., Clift R.A. et al.
   Marrow transplantation for acute non lymphoblastic leukemia in
   first remission.
   NEJM, 1979, 301, 597-599.

2. Blume K.G., Beutler E., Bross K.J. et al.
   Bone marrow ablation and allogeneic marrow transplantation
   acute leukemia.
   NEJM, 1980, 302, 1041-1046.

3. Powles R.L., Clink H.M., Bandini G., et al.
   The place of bone marrow transplantation in acute myelogenc
   leukemia.
   The Lancet, 1980, i, 1047-1050.

4. Thomas E.D., Clift R.A. and Buckner C.D.
   Marrow transplantation for patients with acute non
   lymphoblastic leukemia who achieve a first remission.
   Cancer Treat.Rep., 1982, 66, 1463-1466.

5. B. Löwenberg et al.
   Transplantation of non-purified autologous bone marrow in
   patients with AML in first remission.
   Cancer, 1984, in press.

6. Schaefer U.W., Dicke K.A. and Van Bekkum D.W.
   Recovery of haemopoiesis in lethally irradiated monkeys by
   frozen allogeneic bone marrow grafts.
   Rev.Europ.Etudes Clin. et Biol., 1972, 17, 483-488.

7. Löwenberg B. and de Zeeuw M.H.C.
   A method for cloning T lymphocytic precursors in agar.
   Am.J.Hematol., 1979, 6, 35-43.

8. Weiden P.L., Storb R., Deeg R.J. and Graham T.C.
   Total body irradiation and autologous bone marrow
   transplantation as consolidation therapy for spontaneous
   canine lymphoma in remission.
   Exp.Hemat., 1979, 7 (suppl. 5), 160-164.

9. Touw I.P. and Löwenberg B.
   Differentiation of human acute myeloid leukemias following

colony formation in vitro.
Submitted.

10. Wouters R. and Löwenberg B.
On the maturation order of AML cells: a distinction on the basis of self-renewal properties and immunologic phenotypes. Blood, 1984, in press.

DOUBLE ABLATIVE CHEMOTHERAPY WITH AUTOLOGOUS MARROW RESCUE
IN THE TREATMENT OF ACUTE LEUKAEMIA

A.H. GOLDSTONE, D.C. LINCH, C.C. ANDERSON, M. JONES,
S.P. CLOSS, J.C. CAWLEY & J.D.M. RICHARDS

SUMMARY

Seventeen patients with acute leukaemia (8 AML and 9 ALL) have entered a trial protocol involving two courses of ablative chemotherapy followed by rescue with autologous bone marrow transplantation (ABMT). The treatment was generally well tolerated and only one patient died during the period of marrow aplasia. Only one of the 10 patients receiving ablative chemotherapy with ABMT after first remission has survived for a prolonged period. This patient completed the double ABMT procedure and is well at 538 days. Among first remission patients, there has been only one early relapse (Thy-ALL), and the others are well at 60-960 days. Double ablative chemotherapy with ABMT may be useful in reducing minimal residual disease, thereby prolonging first remission in adult acute leukaemia.

1. Introduction

One of the major current therapeutic problems in adult acute leukaemia is the achievement of prolonged remission in patients for whom allogenic transplantation is not an option.

The main approaches to this problem have been intensive consolidation maintenance chemotherapy (for example 3), or ablative chemotherapy (± total body irradiation) with rescue by autologous bone marrow transplantation (ABMT) (reviewed in 2). Since the autologous marrow is likely to contain residual leukaemic cells, there has been considerable interest in methods to remove such cells before reinfusion (Experimental Haematology, 1983, Vol 11 Suppl 14 p 7-13). However, because no ideal purging procedures are yet available, especially for acute myeloid leukaemea, and because those in current use are of unproven value, we have used

very high dose chemotherapy with rescue by unpurged autologous
marrow. In an attempt to reduce the number of presumed residu
leukaemic cells, we adopted a double ABMT technique. The seco
ABMT is performed on the hypothesis that normal marrow will ha
regenerated more rapidly than leukaemic cells, so that leukaem
contamination will be at its nadir at the time of the second A
In this paper we report early results with our first 18 patien

2   Patients and Protocol
2.1   Patients.

A total of 17 patients (8 AML and 9 ALL) (10 male, 7 fema
1 child with Thy-ALL aged 6 years, others 16-57 years) have
received the first ABMT. 6 of these patients have undergone t
second ABMT. of the 11 remaining patients, 4 are awaiting seco
marrow harvest (all > 60 days post ABMT), 3 relapsed before th
second ABMT, 2 patients refused, one died of intracranial haem
rhage while thrombocytopenic and one had vomiting which persis
until she relapsed 225 days after ABMT. Seven of the patients
in first remission, while the remaining 10 patients received
ablative chemotherapy and ABMT after first remission (5 in sec
remission and 5 in relapse — these patients were induced with
protocol chemotherapy and ABMT). The first marrow harvest and
cryopreservation was performed in first remission in 14 patien
(time from diagnosis to harvest 262±130 days, range 106-548 da

2.2   Protocol

All patients with AML or poor risk ALL (T-cell or age > 1
years), aged less than 60 years and, when aged less than 45 ye
without an HLA-identical sibling, were considered eligible.
Identical chemotherapy was given before both ABMT reinfusions
consisted of cyclophosphamide 1.5 g/m² IV on days 1, 2 & 3,
adriamycin 50 mg/m² IV on day 1, BCNU 300 mg/m² IV on day 1 an
cytosine arabinoside 100 mg/m² IV and 6-thioguanine 100 mg/m²
orally 12 hourly on days 1,2,3 & 4. The autologous bone marro
was returned on day 6. The first harvest and subsequent chemo
therapy was performed as early as possible after induction/
consolidation, but for a variety of reasons was often delayed.
The second ABMT was performed as soon as possible after the

peripheral count had returned to normal providing the marrow aspirate was cellular and still in remission (50-105 days; mean 75 days). AML patients received no further chemotherapy while ALL patients were given maintenance with mercaptopurine, methotrexate, vincristine and prednisolone. Harvested bone marrow was concentrated by centrifugation on a Haemonetics 30 and frozen and stored as previously described and $0.6-4 \times 10^8$ nucleated cells/kg frozen, in all instances, an aliquot of frozen marrow was shown to contain viable CFUc ($5-30 \times 10^4$ CFUc/kg).

3 Results
3.1 Haematological recovery after first and second ABMT
3.1.1 First ABMT.

The time taken for the peripheral neutrophil count to reach 0.5×10^9 was 20 ± 5 days (range 14-31), for $1 \times 10^9/1$, 24 ± 7 days (range 17-36 days). The time taken for the platelet count to reach $50 \times 10^9/1$ was 29 ± 20 days (13 to 99 days) for $100 \times 10^9/1$, 38 ± 31 days (range 15-145 days).

3.1.2 Second ABMT

Peripheral neutrophils reached $0.5 \times 10^9/1$ in 26 ± 5 days (range 16-30 days), for $1 \times 10^9/1$, 31 ± 8 days (range 20-43 days). The platelet count reached $50 \times 10^9/1$ in 37 ± 8 days (range 26-45 days) and $100 \times 10^9/1$ in 48 ± 12 days (range 31-61 days). The differences in haematological recovery after the first and second ABMT were not statistically significant. Haematological recovery, especially of platelets, after the first ABMT was longer in AML than ALL pateints taken as groups but none of the differences were statistically significant (Neutrophils $0.5 \times 10^9/1$, AML 21 ± 5 days (range 15-30 days), ALL 19 ± 5 (range 14-31 days), neutrophils to $1.0 \times 10^9/1$, AML 26 ± 5 (range 15-34 days), ALL 25 ± 8 (range 16-36 days), platelets to $50 \times 10^9/1$, AML 37 ± 28 days (range 17-99 days), ALL 23 ± 7 days, (range 13-33 days), platelets to $100 \times 10^9/1$, AML 52 ± 46 days (range 18-145 days), ALL 27 ± 9 (range 15-42 days)).

3.2 Patients successfully completing the second ABMT

All patients survived the second ABMT without unexpected complications (one patient had an aspergilloma which responded amphotericin, 2 of the patients have relapsed (both ALL at 109 169 days), while the other 4 (2 ALL and 2 AML) remain in good remission at 108, 466, 538 and 960 days). Both the patients w relapsed were transplanted after first remission as were 2 of surviving patients (now 108 and 538 days post ABMT).

3.3 Patients completing only the first ABMT

Four patients will receive their second ABMT in the near future. Of the remaining 7 patients, one died on day 12, 5 ha relapsed (3 ALL at 67, 69 and 220 days; 2 AML at 59 and 225 da and one (AML) is well 763 days post ABMT.

The long survivor was treated in first remission. Four o the relapsed patients were treated after first remission, and other patient had T-ALL.

DISCUSSION

The present study clearly shows that our double ablative chemotherapy regime, together with ABMT, is well tolerated in patients.

Only one of the patients submitted to the protocol after first remission has survived for a prolonged period, and we co clude that the procedure is unlikely to be of significant bene to such patients.

Of the seven patients treated in first remission, all hav done well except one with Thy-ALL. Although only three have s far completed the second ABMT, the other four will do so in th near future. The relatively small number of our patients who so far completed the second ABMT is likely to be a consequence the high proportion of the initial patients treated beyond fir remission who relapsed before the second ABMT could be perform

In conclusion, double ablative chemotherapy with ABMT seel to be a possible approach to prolonging first remission, but m experience is necessary to compare the technique with the othe therapeutic options currently available.

REFERENCES

1. Linch DC, Knott LJ, Patterson KG, Cowan DA & Harper PG.
    (1982) Bone marrow processing and cryopreservation. J. Clin.
    Pathol. 35, 186-190.

2. Spitzer G, Vellekoop L, Zander A, Tannir NM, Verma D, Kanojia
    M, Jagganath S & Dicke K. (1983) Autologous bone marrow
    transplantation in leukaemia and lymphoma. Personal communica-
    tion.

3. Weinstein HJ, Mayer RJ, Rosenthal DS, Lamitta BM, Coral PS,
    Nathan DG & Frei E. (1980) Treatment of acute meyologenous
    leukaemia in children and adults. New Eng. J. Med. 303,
    473-478.

FACTORS ASSOCIATED WITH RELAPSE FOLLOWING ALLOGENEIC BONE MARROW TRANSPLANTATION FOR ACUTE LEUKEMIA IN REMISSION

F.E. ZWAAN   and J. HERMANS
(for the E.B.M.T.-Leukaemia Working Party)

A. INTRODUCTION

Although the advances in the treatment of patients with acute nonlymphoblastic leukemia (ANL) obtained with combination chemotherapy and supportive care are promising, the overall long-term leukemia-free survival and possible cure rates of the majority of these patients is poor (1).
The median duration of the first remission is approximately one year and only 15%-35% of the patients are alive after 3 years (2).
Various centers have reported the improvements made in the chemotherapy of acute lymphoblastic leukemia (ALL) with better survivals in poor prognostic categories (3-5). Once a marrow relapse occurs, however, the prognosis is poor. Over 70% of children will enter a second remission, but the median duration of the second remission is usually in the range of 2 to 8 months (6,7).
For adolescent and adult ALL the mean survival and relapse-free survival was 17 and 16 months, respectively, with a 5-year leukemia-free survival of 25%. After first relapse, the median survival is 8 months, with a median duration of the second remission of 5.5 months (8).
Attempts to carry out bone marrow transplants in man in the treatment of acute leukemia were reported in the late Fifties (9,10), but, with the exception of a few identical twin transplants (11), these grafts were unsuccessful. The development of better supportive care techniques and particularly, of the techniques for and knowledge of human histocompatibility typing set the stage for renewed efforts of bone marrow trans-

plantation (BMT) in man.
The use of BMT provides two potential therapeutic advantages
over more conventional approaches. First, it enables one to
extend the intensity of cytoreductive therapy without regard
to hematopoietic toxicity since the infusion of marrow is able
to "rescue" the patient from otherwise lethal therapy.
Secondly, posttransplant changes in immunoregulatory processes
particularly graft-versus-host disease (GVHD) may provide im-
munotherapeutic effects against residual tumor cells (12).

Initially, transplants were only carried out in patients
with acute leukemia, who had relapsed after failure to respond
to the best available chemotherapy.
Total body irradiation (TBI) alone, TBI in combination with
cyclophosphamide (CY) (13), CY alone or in combination with
busulfan (BU) (14), and TBI in combination with piperazinedione
(15) were most commonly used as preparative treatments in these
early studies.
Long-term leukemia-free survival were between 0-15%, depending
on the series, and estimates of leukemic relapse rates were
in the order of 70-100%.
Bone marrow transplantation following CY and TBI can also
eradicate leukemia in a small proportion of patients with refractory ALL (13).

About 1975, allogeneic BMT was undertaken earlier in the
course of leukemia, i.e., during a period of complete remission

Marrow transplantation for ANL in first remission was
initiated by the Seattle bone marrow transplant team using CY
and single dosis of TBI as their preparative regimens (16).
Nineteen patients were prepared with CY and 920 Rads TBI and
given marrow from HLA-identical siblings. Ten of these 19
patients are alive now and in remission 5.0-7.0 years after
grafting. Only two patients relapsed. Three additional patients
were transplanted on this regimen, and two of them are alive
and in remission. Thus, the median remission duration for these
patients now is longer than 5 years. Various marrow transplant
centers have now described the results of marrow grafting for
patients with ANL in first remission with long-term survival

in the order of 50-60%, and a probability of leukemia-free
survival in the order of 80-90%. The actuarial survival (17-26)
of patients with ANL grafted in second remission was 20%, while
the probability of being in remission was 50% (27,28).
Also in 1976, a programme was initiated in Seattle to transplant patients with ALL in second or subsequent remission -
the first 22 patients were reported in 1979 (29). Most of
these patients were children; 18 were younger than 16 years
of age. An actuarial survival of 50% at 2 years was obtained,
with a probability of leukemia-free survival of 50% at the
same point of time. A total of 10 relapses occurred (all within
281 days posttransplant), 4 of them extramedullary. Relapses
occurred predominantly between 2 months to one year, but later
relapses have been described by others (30). Although most recurrent leukemias occur in cells of host origin, relapses in
donor cells have been observed in both <u>ANL</u> (31,32) and <u>ALL</u>
(33-37). The incidence of recurrence of the leukemia in donor
cells after allogeneic BMT was studied in a group of 243 patients
with acute leukemia (transplanted in relapse and in remission),
who received a marrow graft from a donor of the opposite sex
(38). Seventy-five patients subsequently relapsed. Three relapses were in donor-type cells, while all these 3 patients
were grafted for ALL. Therefore, recurrence of the leukemia
in donor cells in patients grafted for ANL is extremely rare.
    Since a large number of leukemia patients have been trans-
planted in Europe (39), factors of possible importance in predicting subsequent leukemia relapse after BMT for ANL and ALL
(transplanted in remission) have been evaluated and will be
reported in this paper.

3. PATIENTS AND METHODS
    In the E.G.B.M.T. (European Cooperative Group for Bone
Marrow Transplantation)-computer files in Leiden, data on a
total of 229 ANL-BMT patients and on 192 ALL-BMT patients are
currently stored. These patients have been transplanted by 32
BMT teams throughout Europe during the past 5 years. An update
of the current European transplantation results for leukemia

have recently been published (39). For this study only patient
transplanted in complete remission with donors who were HLA
identical, and mutually unresponsive in mixed leucocyte cultur
tests were analyzed; syngeneic or histo-incompatible grafts
were also excluded from this study.
Each center was advised to report all transplant experience.
The status of the leukemia was determined just before pretrans
plant chemo-radiotherapy. GVHD was classified as absent, mild,
moderate, or severe, according to criteria proposed by the
International Bone Marrow Transplant Registry (40). A GVHD sco
was given, based on severity and duration of dermatitis, liver
function abnormalities, diarrhoea, and other clinical variable
Measures to prevent GVHD consisted of methotrexate (MTX), cycl
sporin-A (CyA), bone marrow incubation with OKT3, or antilymph
cyte globulin (ALG).
Factors studied for prognostic value with respect to relapse
were: 1) age (recipient/donor), 2) sex (recipient/donor), 3)
time interval remission - BMT, 4) time interval diagnosis - BM
5) cytogenetic abnormalities at diagnosis, 6) extramedullary
disease at diagnosis, 7) year of transplant, 8) number of remission before BMT, 9) total TBI dose, 10) TBI dose-rate/min,
11) total lung dose, 12) method of GVHD-prevention, 13) occurr
of acute GVHD, 14) severity of acute GVHD, 15) time interval B
acute GVHD, 16) method of GVHD-treatment, 17) occurrence of
chronic GVHD, 18) interstitial pneumonitis, 19) leukemia subtypes.

C. STATISTICAL METHODS

Time from transplantation to treatment failure has been
studied in ANL and ALL-BMT patients. Standard statistical
techniques available in the computer programme package SPSS (4]
and BMDP (42) were used.
The analysis concentrated on the comparison of actuarial incidence rates of relapse, using univariate analysis (LEE-DESU
statistics) as well as multivariate analysis (Cox-regression).
A stepwise linear discriminant analysis was performed to compare the variables in different subcategories of patients.

D. RESULTS

1) Relapse in ANL after BMT:

Two hundred and seventeen patients who underwent marrow transplantation for ANL were studied. The sex of the patients was male in 128, and female in 89. The median age was 24 years (range 1-44), while 77 were < 20 years and 140 > 21 years. Grafted in 1st remission were 173 patients, while 41 were grafted in 2nd remission and 3 in 3rd remission (i.e., 44 in ≥ 2nd remission).

In 18 patients a relapse after BMT was observed: 10/173 in the 1st remission group, 8/41 in the 2nd remission group and 0/3 in the 3rd remission group of patients.

The actuarial relapse incidence (i.e., the probability of leukemia-free survival) in the various remission groups is demonstrated in Fig. 1. The actuarial probability of relapse for the various ANL subgroups is presented in Fig. 2. Fifteen pre- and posttransplant factors (see Patients and Methods) were studied with both univariate and multivariate analysis. Those factors that were associated with a significant higher actuarial probability of relapse after BMT for ANL are presented in Table 1. It is obvious, that ANL subtypes with a monocytic component (M5, M4, respectively) and Cy-A prophylaxis for acute GVHD, is associated with a significantly higher probability of relapse.

2) Relapse in ALL after BMT:

For 168 patients with ALL the same procedure was followed. The sex of the patients was male in 115, and female in 53. The median age was 16 (range 0-42). Grafted in 1st remission were 48 patients, while 84 were grafted in 2nd remission and 36 in ≥ 3rd remission. The distribution of ALL subtypes was as follows: T-ALL: 43 (mainly grafted in 1st remission); B-ALL: 11, non-B non-T-ALL: 105 and in 9 patients the subtype was unknown (i.e., non-typed). A total of 30 relapses were observed; 2/48 in the 1st remission group, 16/84 in the 2nd remission group and 12/36 in the ≥ 3rd remission group. Specified to the ALL subtype, the number of relapses were: 5/43 in T-ALL, 1/11 in B-ALL, 17/105 in non-B non-T-ALL, and

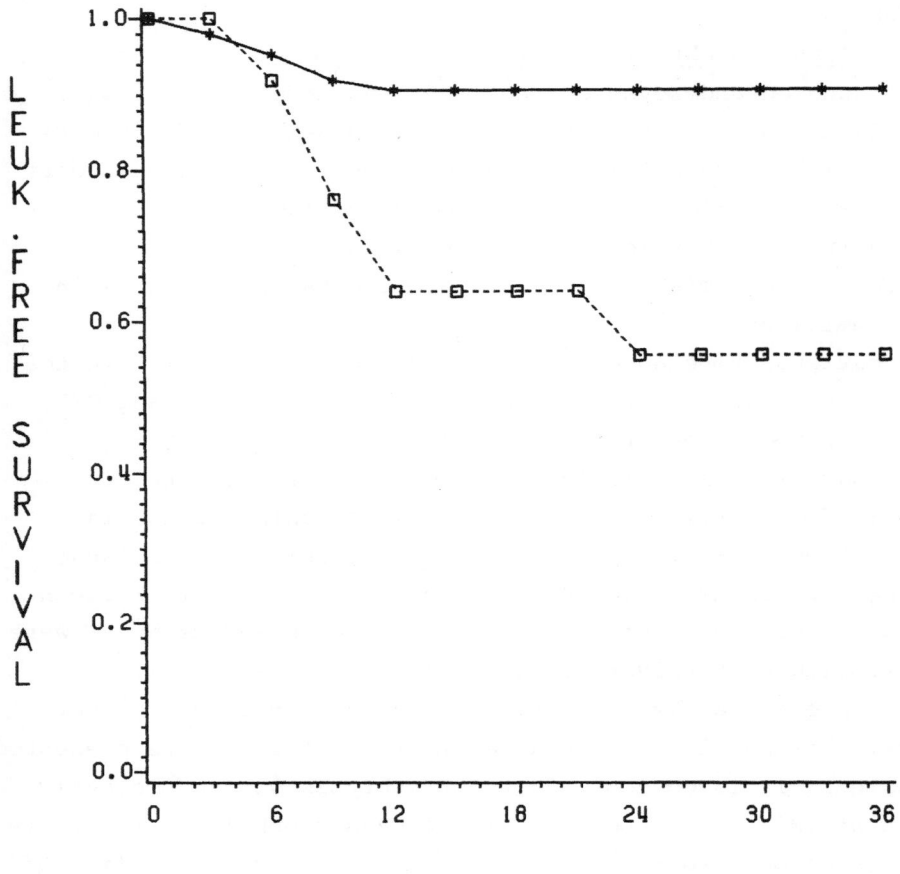

Fig. 1: The probability of leukemia-free survival after bone
marrow transplantation for ANL in first remission (✱)
and second or subsequent remission (▢).

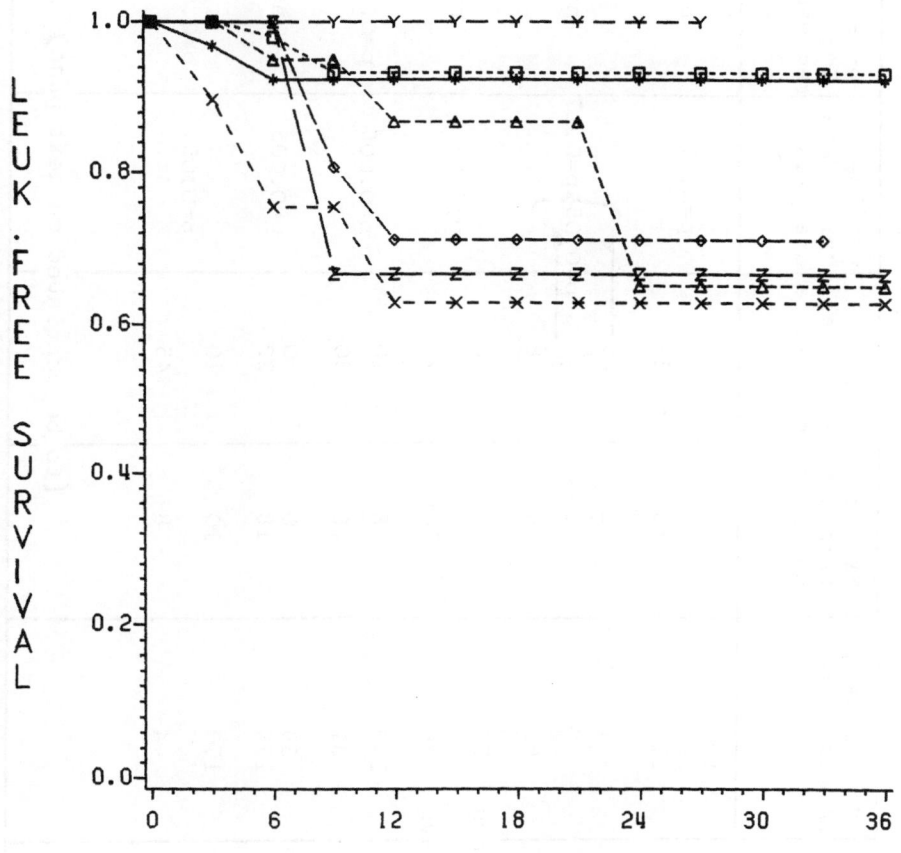

Fig. 2: The probability of leukemia-free survival after bone marrow transplantation for ANL subtypes: M1: ✱ , M2: ☐ , M3: △ , M4: ◇ , M5: ✗ ,M6: Y , and acute undifferentiated: Z .

Table 1: Factors associated with leukemic relapse after BMT for ANL

Variable		Nr. of pat. in each group	Nr. of relapses observed	2-year actuarial relapse rate(%)	p-value univariate analysis	p-value Cox regression analysis
sex recipient	male	106	5	12	p=0.07	ns
	female	111	13	22		
sex combined	RMDF	41	1	5	p=0.05 p=0.27	ns
	RMDM	65	4	8		
	RFDE	48	7	30		
	RFDM	63	6	8		
interval (days) between remission and BMT	≥ 150 days	53	1	0	p=0.03	ns
	≤ 60 days	76	10	25		
GVHD-prophylaxis	MTX	157	8	10	p=0.006	p=0.002
	Cyclosporin-A	31	6	30		
chronic GVHD	yes	39	0	0	p=0.005	ns
	no	175	18	22		
remission nr.	first	173	10	10	p=0.05	p=0.05
	≥ second	44	8	45		

(to be continued on next page)

Variable	Nr. of pat. in each group	Nr. of relapses observed	2-year actuarial relapse rate(%)	p-value univariate analysis	p-value Cox regression analysis
ANL subtypes M1	38	2	7		
M2	79	3	7		
M3	24	3	30		$p=0.04$
M4	39	4	36	$p=0.01$	$p=0.017$
M5	22	5	49		$p=0.0009$
M6	5	0	0		
acute undifferentiated	10	1	34		

6/9 in the non-typed group.

The actuarial probability of relapse in the various remission groups is demonstrated in Fig. 3. The actuarial probability of relapse for the various ALL subtypes is presented in Fig. 4. Those factors that were associated with a significant higher actuarial probability of relapse after BMT for ALL are presente in Table 2. In this analysis the remission number in which the patient is transplanted appears to be the most important factor (p=0.002), while the ALL subtypes and sex of the recipient/dono are of borderline significance.

3) Early versus late relapse:

In analyzing these 18 ANL and 30 ALL relapse patients, we were also interested to see if factors were associated with early relapse (≤ 6 months after BMT, group 1) or late relapse (> 6 months after BMT, group 2). Therefore, the ANL- (8 in group 1, 10 in group 2) and ALL- (14 in group 1, 16 in group 2) relapse patients were further studied, using linear stepwise discrimina analysis.

For both groups of leukemia, only the ages of the patient (AML, p=0.006; ALL, p=0.02) and donor (AML, p=0.006; ALL, p=0.04) wer of significant value in discriminating between an early or late relapse probability; e.g. older patients (and donors) had a higher probability of early relapse compared to younger patient donor combinations. This correlation was especially significant (p=0.006) in ANL-BMT patients, for while the median age of "ear relapse" patients was 29.8 years, the median age for "late rela patients was 17.5 years.

E. DISCUSSION

Intensive antileukemic therapy followed by marrow transplant-ation has resulted in prolonged disease-free survival and cure in some patients with refractory leukemia (13). Despite rigorou chemotherapy and TBI, persistence or subsequent relapse of leukemia following marrow grafting remains a problem in end-sta leukemia patients.

Factors of possible importance in predicting subsequent leukemia relapse have been evaluated by Harrison et al. (43) in a grou

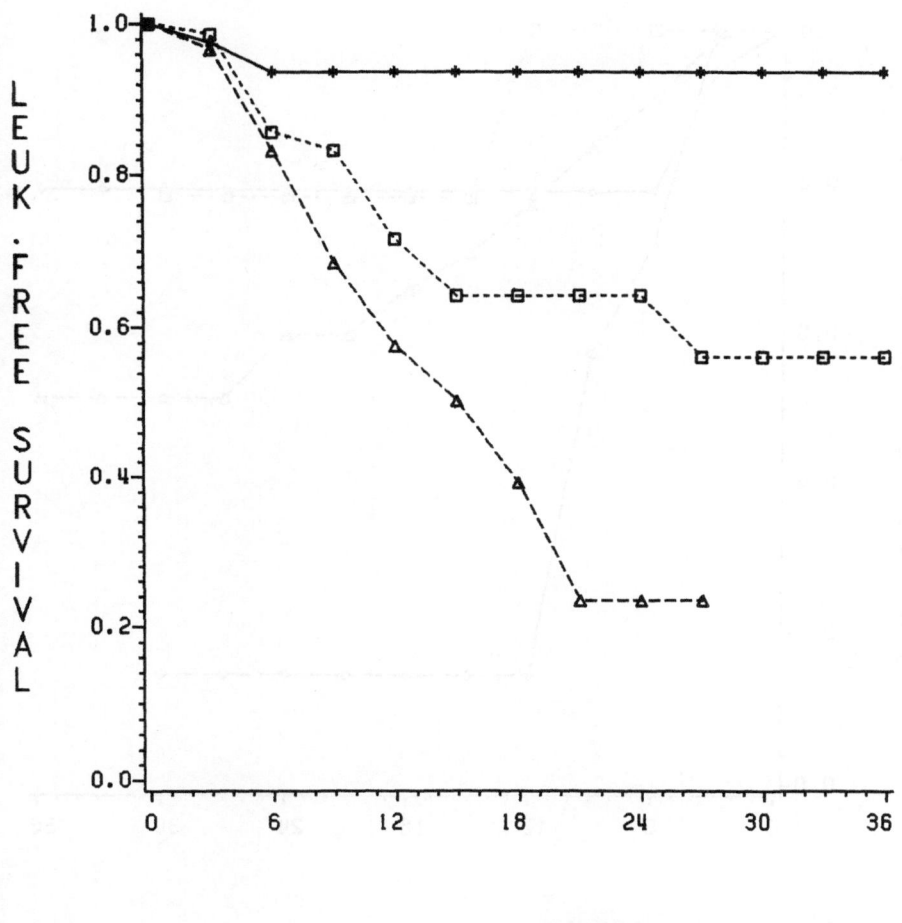

MONTHS AFTER BMT

Fig. 3: The probability of leukemia-free survival after bone
marrow transplantation for ALL in first (✽), second
(◘), and third or subsequent remission (△).

304

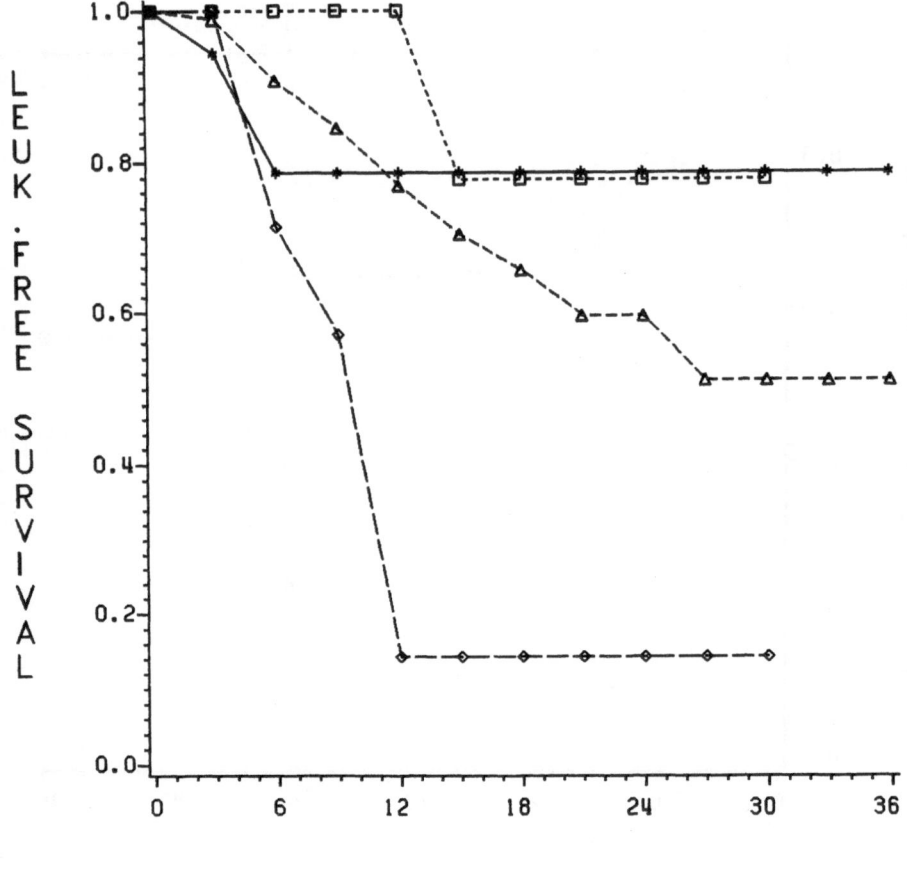

MONTHS AFTER BMT

Fig. 4: The probability of leukemia-free survival after bon
marrow transplantation for ALL subtypes: T-ALL (✦
B-ALL (◘), non-B non-T-ALL (▲), and non-typed
ALL (◆).

Table 2: Factors associated with leukemic relapse after BMT for ALL

Variable		Nr. of pat. in each group	Nr. of relapses observed	2-year actuarial relapse rate(%)	p-value univariate analysis	p-value Cox regression analysis
sex donor	female	76	9	30	p=0.03	ns
	male	92	21	55		
sex combined	RMDF	50	5	25	p=0.04	p=0.06
	RMDM	65	15	60	p=0.17	
	RFDF	26	4	35		
	RFDM	27	6	45		
ALL subtypes	T-ALL	43	6	20	p=0.03	p=0.07
	B-ALL	11	1	27		
	non-B non-T-ALL	105	17	40		
	ALL non-typed	9	6	75		
Remission	first	48	2	7	p=0.04	p=0.002
	second	84	16	35	p=0.13	
	third	36	12	76		

of 136 patients, who underwent a marrow transplantation in Sea
They found that the presence of an enlarged spleen, either at
diagnosis or at transplantation, was associated with an increa
probability of relapse (p<0.006) among patients with ANL. In
patients with ALL, active central nervous system (CNS) disease
the time of transplantation significantly increased the risk o
relapse in the CNS (p<0.01). Patients with a white blood-cell
count greater than 20,000/mm^3 at admission for transplantation
had an increased rate of relapse (p<0.003). Patients whose leu
ic cells showed a karyotypic abnormality on cytogenetic analys
had an increased probability of relapse as compared to those w
karyotypically normal leukemic cells (p=0.04). Following trans
plantation, the persistence of leukemic cells in the marrow on
week after transplantation indicated an increased likelihood o
failure to achieve remission and an increased likelihood of su
sequent relapse in those who achieved a remission (p<0.001).
From that study, it is obvious that in end-stage leukemia pati
the tumor load at diagnosis, or failure to eradicate leukemic
cells by the preparative regimen was the major factor correlat
with relapse after transplantation. For patients transplanted
remission, such a single center study is not yet available.
The analysis described in this study identifies factors that
appear to be related to recurrence of leukemia following marro
transplantation during remission. For ANL, the monocytic component (especially M-5 ANL) appears to predict a high probabil
of relapse. Therefore, for this category of patients, addition
chemotherapy before or after transplantation must be considere
The use of CyA in ANL transplant patients also appears to be
related with a higher probability of relapse, although it has
be mentioned that this phenomenon was not found in a prospecti
randomized trial performed by the Seattle bone marrow transpla
team (44). On the other hand, the abrogation of the antileukem
potential of acute GVHD by CyA has been confirmed in animal
studies (45). More patients, with longer follow-up, need to be
studied before this particular question can be answered. For Al
the only significant factor found is the remission state in wh
the patient is grafted. Therefore, to diminish the relapse pro

bability, bone marrow transplantation for ALL should be performed
during first remission.
From this study it is clear that the number of patients with a
relapse after marrow grafting during remission is rather limited.
Therefore, the statistical significance of various factors can
be changing in time when more patients are entered in this study.
It is also important that the data mentioned were not based on a
prospective single center study. Thus, factors that appeared to
have significant association with relapse may have been influenced
by the difference between centers. Therefore, the findings reported here represent conservative estimates of the associations that
will be found where controlled studies are employed.

. ACKNOWLEDGEMENTS
   We would like to thank the medical staff of the following
institutions that have contributed data on their patients for
this report: University of Vienna, Austria; Cliniques universi-
taires St.-Luc, Brussels, Belgium; St.-Raphael Hospital, Louvain,
Belgium; The Finsen Institute, Copenhagen, Denmark; Royal Free
Hospital, London, England; University College Hospital, London,
England; Westminster Hospital, London, England; Meilahti Hospital,
Helsinki, Finland; University of Helsinki, Finland; University of
Turku, Finland; Blood Transfusion Center, Besançon, France;
Ôpital Henri Mondor, Créteil, France; Hôpital E. Herriot, Lyon,
France; Institut J. Paoli I Calmettes, Marseille, France; Hôpital
St.-Louis, Paris, France; Hôpital Bellevue, St. Etienne, France;
University of Tübingen, West Germany; University of Ulm, West
Germany; San Martino Hospital, Genova, Italy; Bone Marrow Trans-
plantation Centre, Hospital of Pesaro, Italy; Isolation Ward,
University of Leiden, The Netherlands; Department of Pediatrics,
University of Leiden, The Netherlands; Radboud Hospital, Univer-
sity of Nijmegen, The Netherlands, Dijkzigt Hospital, Rotterdam,
The Netherlands; University of Utrecht, The Netherlands; University of Oslo, Norway; University of Barcelona, Spain; University Hospital, Huddinge, Sweden; Kantonsspital, Basle, Switzerland; University Hospital, Zürich, Switzerland.
The data analysis by Ms A.W. Lyklema and the secretarial assistance
from Ms J. Kooreman in preparing this paper are acknowledged.

308

REFERENCES

1. Lister TA, Rohatiner AZS. 1982. The treatment of acute myelogenous leukemia in adults. Seminars in Hematology 19: 172-192.
2. Preisler HD. 1982. Therapy for patients with acute myelocytic leukemia who enter remission: bone marrow transplantation or chemotherapy? Cancer Treatment Reports 66: 1467-1473.
3. Miller DR, Leikin S, Albo V. 1981. Intensive therapy and prognostic factors in acute lymphoblastic leukaemia in childhood CCG 141. Modern Trends in Human Leukaemia IV. (ed. by R. Neth, R.C. Gallo, T. Graf, K. Mannweiler and K. Winkler), pp. 76-88, Springer Verlag, Berlin.
4. Henze G, Langermann HG, Ritter J, et al. 1981. Treatment strategy for different risk groups in childhood acute lymphoblastic leukaemia. A report from the BFM Study Group. Modern Trends in Human Leukaemia IV. (ed. by R. Neth, R.C. Gallo, T. Graf, K. Mannweiler and K. Winkler), pp. 87-93, Springer Verlag, Berlin.
5. Haghbin M, Murphy ML, Tan CTC, et al.1981.Intensive chemo therapy in children with acute lymphoblastic leukaemia (protocol). Cancer 33: 1491-1498.
6. Chessells JM, Cornbleet M. 1979. Combination chemotherapy for bone marrow relapse in childhood lymphoblastic leukaemia. Medical and Pediatric Oncology 6: 359-365.
7. Reaman GH, Ladisch S, Echelberger C, et al. 1980. Improved treatment results in the management of single and multiple relapses of acute lymphoblastic leukemia. Cancer 45: 3090-3094.
8. Baccarani M, Corbelli G, Amadori S, et al. 1982. Adolescent and adult acute lymphoblastic leukemia: prognostic features and outcome of therapy. A study of 293 patients. Blood 60: 677-684.
9. Mathé G, Jammet H, Pendic B, et al. 1959. Transfusions et greffes de moelle osseuse homologue chez des humains irradiés a haute dose accidentellement. Rev Franc Etudes Clin Biol 4: 226-238.
10. Thomas ED, Lochte HL Jr, Lu WC, et al. 1957. Intravenous infusion of bone marrow in patients receiving radiation and chemotherapy. New England Journal of Medicine 257: 491-496.
11. Thomas ED, Lochte HL Jr, Cannon JH, et al. 1959. Supralethal whole body irradiation and isologous marrow transplantation in man. Journal of Clinical Investigation 38: 1709-1716.
12. Weiden PL, Sullivan KM, Flournoy N, et al. 1981. Antileukemic effect of chronic graft-versus-host disease: contribution to improved survival after allogeneic bone marrow transplantation. New England Journal of Medicine 304: 1529-1533.
13. Thomas ED, Buckner CD, Banaji M, et al. 1977. One hundred patients with acute leukemia treated by chemotherapy, total body irradiation, and allogeneic marrow transplantation. Blood 49: 511-533.

14. Tutschka PJ, Elfenbein GJ, Sensenbrenner LL, et al. 1980.
    Preparative regimens for marrow transplantation in acute
    leukemia and aplastic anemia - Baltimore experience.
    American Journal of Pediatric Hematology/Oncology 2: 363-
    370.
15. Dicke KA, Kanojia MD, Zander AR. 1983. Allogeneic bone
    marrow transplantation in hematologic disorders. Cancer
    Bulletin 35: 23-29.
16. Thomas ED, Buckner CD, Clift RA, et al. 1979. Marrow
    transplantation for acute nonlymphoblastic leukemia in
    first remission. New England Journal of Medicine 301:
    597-599.
17. Blume KG, Beutler E, Bross KJ, et al. 1980. Bone-marrow
    ablation and allogeneic marrow transplantation in acute
    leukemia. New England Journal of Medicine 302: 1041-1046.
18. Forman SJ, Spruce WE, Farbstein MJ, et al. 1983. Bone
    marrow ablation followed by allogeneic marrow grafting
    during first complete remission of acute nonlymphoblastic
    leukemia. Blood 61: 439-442.
19. Gale RP: Clinical trials of bone marrow transplantation
    in leukemia. In: Gale RP, Fox CF (eds.). Biology of bone
    marrow transplantation. Academic Press, New York, 1980,
    pp. 11-27.
20. Kersey JH, Ramsay NKC, Kim T, et al. 1982. Allogeneic
    bone marrow transplantation in acute nonlymphoblastic
    leukemia: a pilot study. Blood 60: 400-403.
21. Mannoni P, Vernant JP, Rodet M, et al. 1980. Marrow
    transplantation for acute nonlymphoblastic leukemia in
    first remission. Blut 41: 220-225.
22. Morgenstern GR, Powles RL. 1981. Allogeneic bone marrow
    transplantation for acute myeloid leukemia in first re-
    mission. Haematology and Blood Transfusion 26: 139-142.
23. Powles RL, Clink HM, Bandini G, et al. 1980. The place
    of bone marrow transplantation in acute myelogenous
    leukemia. Lancet i: 1047-1050.
24. Speck B, Gratwohl A, Nissen C, et al. 1981. Further ex-
    perience with cyclosporin A in allogeneic bone marrow
    transplantation. Experimental Hematology 9 (suppl. 9):
    124 (Abstract).
25. Thomas ED, Clift RA, Buckner CD. 1982. Marrow transplantation
    for patients with acute nonlymphoblastic leukemia who achieve
    a first remission. Cancer Treatment Reports 66: 1463-1466.
26. Zwaan FE, Jansen J, Colpin GGD, Simonis RFA. 1982. Marrow
    grafting for acute leukemia during remission - results in
    23 patients. Experimental Hematology 10 (suppl. 10): 87.
27. Appelbaum FR, Clift RA, Buckner CD, et al. 1983. Allo-
    geneic bone marrow transplantation for acute nonlympho-
    blastic leukemia after first relapse. Blood 61: 949-953.
28. Buckner CD, Clift RA, Thomas ED, et al. 1982. Allogeneic
    marrow transplantation for patients with acute non-lympho-
    blastic leukemia in second remission. Leukemia Research
    6: 395-399.

310

29. Thomas ED, Sanders JE, Flournoy N, et al. 1979. Marrow transplantation for patients with acute lymphoblastic leukemia in remission. Blood 54: 468-476.
30. Barrett AJ, Kendra JR, Lucas CF, et al. 1982. Bone marrow transplantation for acute lymphoblastic leukaemia. British Journal of Haematology 52: 181-188.
31. Elfenbein GJ, Brogaonkar DS, Bias WB, et al. 1978. Cytogenetic evidence for recurrence of acute myelogenous leuke after allogeneic bone marrow transplantation in donor hema poietic cells. Blood 52: 627-636.
32. Gossett TC, Gale RP, Fleischman H, et al. 1979. Immunoblas sarcoma in donor cells after bone-marrow transplantation. New England Journal of Medicine 300: 904-907.
33. Fialkow PJ, Thomas ED, Bryant JI, et al. 1971. Leukaemic transformation of engrafted human marrow cells in vivo. Lancet i: 251.
34. Goh K, Klemperer MR. 1977. In vivo leukemic transformation cytogenetic evidence of in vivo leukemic transformation of engrafted marrow cells. American Journal of Hematology 2: 283-290.
35. Newburger PE, Latt SA, Pesando JM, et al. 1981. Leukemia relapse in donor cells after allogeneic bone-marrow transplantation. New England Journal of Medicine 304: 712-714.
36. Schubach WH, Hackman R, Neiman PE, et al. 1982. A monoclon immunoblastic sarcoma in donor cells bearing Epstein-Barr virus genomes following allogeneic marrow grafting for acu lymphoblastic leukemia. Blood 60: 180-187.
37. Thomas ED, Bryant JI, Buckner CD, et al. 1972. Leukaemic transformation of engrafted human marrow cells in vivo. Lancet i: 1310-1313.
38. Boyd CN, Ramberg RC, Thomas ED. 1982. The incidence of recurrence of leukemia in donor cells after allogeneic bone marrow transplantation. Leukemia Research 6: 833-837.
39. Zwaan FE, Hermans J. 1983. Report of the E.B.M.T.- Leukaem Working Party. Experimental Hematology 11 (suppl. 13): 3-6
40. ACS/NIH Bone Marrow Transplantation Report. 1975. Experime Hematology 3: 149-155.
41. Hull CH, Nie NH. 1981. SPSS - update 7-9. Mac Graw Hill, New York.
42. Dixon WJ, Brown MB, Engelman L, et al. 1981. BMDP - statistical software 1981. University of California Press, Berkeley.
43. Harrison DT, Flournoy N, Ramberg R, et al. 1978. Relapse following marrow transplantation for acute leukemia. Ameri Journal of Hematology 5: 191-202.
44. Deeg HJ, Storb R, Thomas ED, et al. 1983. Marrow transplan ation for acute nonlymphoblastic leukemia in first remissi preliminary results of a randomized trial comparing cyclo- sporine and methotrexate for the prophylaxis of graft-vers host disease. Transplantation Proceedings 15: 1385-1388.
45. Denham S, Attridge S, Barfoot RK, Alexander P.1983. Effect of cyclosporin A on the anti-leukaemia action associated with graft-versus-host disease. British Journal of Cancer 47: 791-795.

BONE MARROW TRANSPLANTATION FOR MINIMAL RESIDUAL DISEASE IN ALL IN CHILDREN: AN OVERVIEW

J.M. VOSSEN

1. INTRODUCTION

Acute lymphoblastic leukemia (ALL) is the commonest malignancy in children and adolescents. It comprises about 83% of all leukemias in that age-group (Van Steensel-Moll, 1983). In the last decade the progress with the management of ALL has been slow, the most important innovations in the conventional cytoreductive regimens occurred in the intensification of the treatment protocols for the groups of patients discerned as having a poor prognosis (Chessels, 1982; Henze et al., 1982). Despite the overall rate of about 95% of complete remissions following "standard" remission-induction therapy, and the use of more intensive maintenance programs for bad-risk patients, a longlasting complete continuous remission (CCR) was only attained in 43% of the patients with poor prognostic factors in the study of the Children's Cancer Study Group (CCSG), comprising 880 patients (Miller et al., 1983). The overall cure rate of children with ALL, i.e. a disease-free survival at 4 years and later after stopping chemotherapy is about 50% with the current treatment protocols.

Leukemic relapse during treatment occurs in 20 to 60% of the patients (Miller et al., 1983). The relapse rate after elective cessation of therapy is about 25% (George et al., 1979). Although a second marrow remission can be achieved in 80 to 90% of these children, their long-term prognosis is poor: second remissions lasting 2 years or more can only be achieved in up to 25% of those patients who relapsed 12 months or later after cessation of maintenance therapy (Cornbleet and Chessels, 1978; Reaman et al., 1980; Chessels and Breatnach, 1981; Rivera, 1981); the duration of a second remission is mostly shorter than 1 year in the patients who relapsed during chemotherapy or early after its cessation.

312

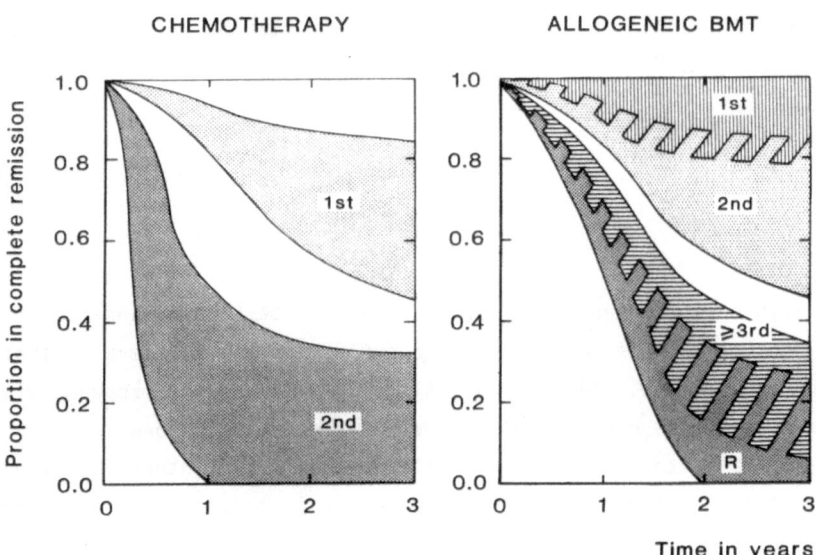

CHEMOTHERAPY   ALLOGENEIC BMT

FIGURE. Schematic representation of the probability of being in remission
following either chemotherapy or allogeneic bone marrow transplantation
for ALL (1st: first remission, 2nd: second remission, ⩾3rd: third and
subsequent remission, R: relapse).

In the figure the probability for children suffering from ALL to
remain in complete first c.q. second remission with the currently used
remission-induction and maintenance chemotherapy is drawn schematically,
taking together the data from several large studies comprising the results
of patients with good and poor prognosis (Cornbleet and Chessels, 1978;
Miller, 1980; Palmer et al., 1980; Chessels and Breatnach, 1981; Rivera,
1981; Feldges et al., 1982; Henze et al., 1982; Miller et al., 1983). In
view of the low cure rate with chemotherapy for patients with ALL after
relapse, and after it was proven that long-term disease-free survival
could be obtained after ablative chemoradiotherapy followed by bone marrow
transplantation (BMT) in patients with end-stage leukemia, the Seattle
group initiated BMT for ALL in second and subsequent remission (Thomas
et al., 1979).

2. RESULTS OF ALLOGENEIC BONE MARROW TRANSPLANTATION FOR CHILDREN AND ADOLESCENTS WITH ALL IN REMISSION: THE PROBLEM OF LEUKEMIC RELAPSE

Almost all centres employ cyclophosphamide (60 mg/kg/day x 2) and either single-dose or fractionated total-body irradiation (TBI) as preparative regimen for BMT. The results from the International Bone Marrow Transplant Registry (IBMTR) (Gale et al., 1983) and the European Group for Bone Marrow Transplantation (EGBMT) (Zwaan et al., 1984) as reported recently, are summarized in Table 1.

Table 1. Probability of long-term remission after allogeneic BMT for ALL

BMT centres/ cooperative groups	ALL remission state	No of patients	Probability of CCR at 3 years		References
IBMTR	1st	20	68%	72%[1]	Gale et al., 1983
	2nd	86		69% 72%	
	≥3rd	30	33%		
	relapse	68			
EGBMT	1st	57	94%	100%[2] 90%	Zwaan et al., 1984
	2nd	96	55%	51%[3] 52%	
	≥3rd	39	27%		
London, Westminster Hosp.	1st	5	35%		Barrett et al., 1982
	2nd	11			
	3rd	4			
Minneapolis, Univ. of Minnesota	2nd	11	43%		Woods et al., 1983
	3rd	4			
New York, Memorial Sloan-Kettering CC	2nd	22	86%		Dinsmore et al., 1983
	3rd	15	40%		
	relapse	15			
Seattle, Fred Hutchinson CC	2nd	14	40%		Johnson et al., 1981
	3rd	5			
	4th	5			
	relapse	63	13%		Sanders et al., 1983

[1] At 2 years after BMT 72% of 20 high-risk patients grafted in 1st remission, 69% of 46 high-risk patients grafted in 2nd remission, and 72% of 40 standard-risk patients grafted in 2nd remission in CCR.
[2] 100% of 25 patients with non B-non T-ALL and 90% of 20 patients with T-ALL in CCR.
[3] 51% of 63 patients with non B-non T-ALL and 52% of 17 patients with T-ALL in CCR.

The majority of patients included in these evaluations was younger than 40 years of age. Also data from several BMT centres treating a majority of children and adolescents are included in Table 1. From these data it can be seen that the proportion of patients with ALL, who will remain in CCR for 3 years and more, and who may be cured is more than 50% for those grafted in first and second remission, and less than 40% for those grafted in third and subsequent remission or in relapse. The probability for patients with ALL to remain in CCR after allogeneic BMT is also schematical ly depicted in the Figure. Comparison of the results from chemotherapy and allogeneic BMT for ALL in the different remission states suggests that one may get a second chance of cure with allogeneic BMT for patients with ALL, who relapsed on chemotherapy.

The results of BMT in first and second remission are clearly superior to those achieved in a subsequent remission state or in relapse. The major obstacle to cure in the latter cases was recurrence of the leukemia. The reasons for relapse of the ALL after ablative chemoradiotherapy in the usually unmaintained remission period after BMT may of course be several: either the quantity or the quality or both of the residual leukemia in intra- and extramedullary sites may break through the (allogeneic) tumor surveillance barriers and proliferate again until a relapse is diagnosed when a number of 10^9 tumor cells is passed.

In two recently reported cooperative studies on BMT in ALL patients (Gale et al., 1983; Zwaan et al., 1984) relapse rates for patients transplanted in second complete remission were comparable for those considered to belong to the high-risk category under conventional chemo- therapy, and those with standard-risk qualifications (see Table 1). Prognostic factors such as a high leukocyte count of > 50 x 10^9/l and an extramedullary localisation at diagnosis - parameters of leukemic burden - which are known to affect adversely the duration of the CCR after chemo- therapy (Miller et al., 1983) did not seem to have the same effect on the relapse rate after BMT.

We evaluated the effect of prior CNS relapse on the relapse rate of children, adolescents and young adult patients, transplanted in second and subsequent complete remission of ALL. Data from four centres, collected by questionnaire, were combined and are presented in Table 2.

Table 2. Effect of prior CNS relapse on relapse rate after allogeneic BMT of young patients with ALL

ALL remission state	n⁰ of patients relapsing after BMT/ n⁰ of patients grafted			site of relapse after BMT		
	with prior CNS relapse	without prior CNS relapse	total	CNS	BM	testic.
2nd remission	6/13 (46%)	14/58[1](24%)	20/71 (28%)	4	16[4]	1
≥ 3rd remission	8/14[2](57%)	18/40[3](45%)	26/54 (48%)	4	24[5]	1

[1] 1 with prior skin relapse, 1 with prior testicular relapse
[2] 1 with prior testicular relapse
[3] 2 with prior testicular relapse
[4] 1 with CNS plus BM relapse
[5] 3 with CNS plus BM relapse

The data for this table were kindly provided by R. Joshi, Dep. of Haematology, Westminster Hospital, London; J.H. Kersey, Dep. of Pediatrics, Univ. of Minnesota, Minneapolis; R.J. O'Reilly, Memorial Sloan-Kettering Cancer Center, New York and Jean E. Sanders, Univ. of Washington and Fred Hutchinson Cancer Research Center, Seattle.

Except for some patients of the Westminster BMT team, detailed data on all patients included in the Table have been published (Barrett et al., 1982; Dinsmore et al., 1983; Sanders et al., 1983; Woods et al., 1983). All patients included in the Table were more than 1 year post-transplant, the majority being more than 18 months post-transplant. The results from this retrospective evaluation indicate a lower relapse rate in the group of patients grafted in second complete remission, who had no prior CNS relapse. In two separate studies, from which data are included in Table 2, no significantly different relapse rates were seen in patients with or without prior extramedullary disease (Dinsmore et al., 1983; Sanders et al., 1983). However, the number of patients transplanted in second complete remission with prior extramedullary relapse, was small in the separate studies; no distinction was made between different sites of prior extramedullary relapse, and in the study of Sanders c.s. more than half of the patients enroled were grafted in marrow relapse. From the data in Table 2 it may be concluded that leukemic relapse in the CNS, a pharmacological sanctuary, results in a focus of residual leukemic cells, hardly to eradicate by the intensive cytoreductive treatment before BMT, and giving rise to recurrent of the leukemia mostly in the bone marrow (i.e. in 4 out of 6, and 7 out of 8 relapses in the patients of Table 2, who were grafted in second and ≥ third remission respectively, after previous CNS relapse). Comparable results, i.e. an increased actuarial relapse rate of 62% in 11 ALL patients with previous extramedullary involvement as compared to an over-all actuarial relapse rate of 30% in the 33 patients with ALL transplanted in ≥ second remission was reported by Champlin et al. (1982).

Not only the quantity of residual leukemic cells, but also the "resistance" of the clonogenic leukemic cells remaining after BMT is a possible origin for relapse. Although an increased proliferative rate, as seen in blasts with T and B cell markers (Scarffe et al., 1980) may predispose to an early regrowth of drug-resistant clones, the phenotype of the pre-BMT lymphoblasts may have little prognostic value. First, leukemic cells are often phenotypically heterogeneous, and second, data suggest that the malignant transformation in ALL occurs in a cell more primitive than the leukemic blast predominating in the blood and bone marrow (Foon et al., 1982). A phenotype shift in a few children relapsing from ALL after conventional chemotherapy has been described by Borella et al. (1979). Also studies of the DNA content of the blasts by flow cytometry (Look et al., 1982) and chromosome analysis of leukemic cells (Williams et al., 1982) point to some heterogeneity in the genotype of the leukemic cells in a small number of patients with ALL. These studies moreover indicate that the leukemic cell lines with the lower ploidy are more likely to become drug-resistant and may recur, a finding which needs further confirmation. For the moment being, however, it is not feasible to trace the relevant target cell for malignant transformation and to determine in vitro its sensitivity and growth potential, because no clonogenic assay is available for ALL.

3. EFFORTS TO PREVENT LEUKEMIC RELAPSE AFTER ALLOGENEIC BMT FOR ALL IN REMISSION

A first approach to this problem could be to try and improve the detection methods of residual leukemia. It is well known that when a complete remission is reached, i.e. when ≤ 5% lymphoblasts are found in the bone marrow with the conventional cytochemical and immunological methods available, and no extramedullary lymphoblasts are demonstrable, the total number of residual leukemic cells may still be as high as 10^9. With the use of e.g. a combined membrane-immunofluorescence and intra-cellular cytochemical staining technique (Janossy et al., 1980) on cryostat sections from bone marrow (Pizzolo et al., 1982; Wood and Warnke, 1982) the detection limit might probably be lowered ten times; however, not for all types of ALL. The combination of membrane-staining with a monoclonal antibody against thymocytes and a nuclear terminal transferase (TdT) staining will be highly effective in tracing residual Thy-ALL blasts, because such cells, normally present in the thymus, are virtually absent in the normal and regenerating bone marrow. However, the combination of membrane anti-common ALL-antigen (CALLA) and nuclear TdT staining is not useful because $\geqslant 10\%$ of normal blasts in the bone marrow of normal children (Greaves et al., 1983) and in regenerating marrow (Janossy et al., 1980; Greaves et al., 1983) are stained with this combination. Also ALL blasts with a pre-B ($CALLA^+$, TdT^+, Ia^+, $cIgM^+$) or a B ($CALLA^{+/-}$, Ia^+, sIg^+) phenotype have their normal counterparts in the bone marrow. One obstacle in lowering the detection limit is obviously the apparent failing of tumor-specific antigens on leukemic cells, and only the finding of cells with a distinct phenotype in tissues where such cells do not home normally is useful for monitoring residual leukemic blasts. Another problem with the finding of low numbers of residual cells with a possibly malignant phenotype in the bone marrow of patients after treatment with chemotherapy is that the biological meaning of such finding is not known so far. As was already said before, the relevant clonogenic cells in ALL cannot yet be discerned and investigated in vitro.

Although the preparative treatment for BMT reduces the number of leukemic blasts with several decades, a relapse rate of more than 60% at 3 years after allogeneic BMT for patients with ALL in $\geqslant$ third remission, and even a relapse rate of 25 to 50% at 3 years for patients with ALL grafted in second remission demonstrate an inadequate suppression of residual leukemia by the usual regimen of high-dose cyclophosphamide and TBI. The search for more efficacious pretreatment regimens is warranted. The use of hyper-fractionated TBI followed by high-dose cyclophosphamide by the Sloan-Kettering group resulted in an actual relapse at $\geqslant 1$ year after BMT in only 1 out of 16 patients (Dinsmore et al., 1983). Although the use of fractionated TBI, given in a different way than the former hyperfractionated TBI, and preceded by high-dose cyclophosphamide, gave no improvement of disease-free survival of ALL patients grafted by the Seattle group, in comparison with historical controls (Clift et al., 1982), the relapse rate of < 10% reported by the Sloan-Kettering group is strikingly low and demands confirmation. Another approach to the improvement of disease-free survival after BMT is the use of more appropriate pretreatment prior to TBI, e.g. with VM26 and cytosine-arabinoside, known to be effective against refractory ALL (Rivera et al., 1980). Such a proposal has been made by the Westminster group (Barrett, 1983) to apply on a multi-centre basis as a cooperative EGBMT study, in order to obtain information at short notice. It should, however, be kept in mind that a more aggressive preparative regimen implies an increased toxicity, and may result in a decreased survival rate, as was found in the past in end-stage leukemia BMT with the regimens known as BACT (Graw et al., 1974) and SCARI (UCLA BMT group, 1977). From the data on an increased relapse rate after previous extramedullary involvement (Champlin et al., 1982; Table 2) some CNS and testicular intensification therapy should also be considered in an appropriate pretreatment regimen.

Apart from the possible anti-leukemic effect of methotrexate, given until day +102 post-transplant to prevent graft-versus-host disease (GvHD), and the additional administration after day +102 post-transplant of eight doses of methotrexate intrathecally, given every other month to recipients with a history of prior CNS disease (Sanders, 1983), the remission following BMT is unmaintained. The preliminary results of a pilot study of Woods et al. (1983) suggest that maintenance chemotherapy with 6-MP and methotrexate after BMT for ALL may decrease the relapse rate. However, more than half of the patients eligible for maintenance chemotherapy either never received it or had to cease from taking it because of several reasons, such as (repeated) viral reactivations, infections and poor general condition. Studies should be undertaken to find out more appropriate individual maintenance c.q. consolidation treatment schedules, based on kinetic parameters of the leukemic blasts.

Although a graft-versus-leukemia reaction has been shown to be brought about by acute and chronic GvHD (Weiden et al., 1979, 1981), the potential short-term and long-term adverse reactions of GvHD and its unpredictable course do not allow for a provocation of this disease. In the studies of Weiden et al. (1979, 1981) the lesser probability of recurrent leukemia was offset by a greater probability of non-leukemic causes of death.

Aspecific immunomodulation, e.g. with BCG, has no proven effect on the relapse rate in childhood ALL. After the initial study of Mathé et al. (1969) showed a beneficial effect attributed to BCG, later trials with immunotherapy conducted either after a short course of chemotherapy (Medical Research Council, 1971; Heyn et al., 1975) or after a prolonged course of 1 year of chemotherapy (Stryckmans et al., 1983) could not confirm the decreased relapse rate in children given immunotherapy. On the contrary, in the EORTC study (Stryckmans et al., 1983) a significant superiority for disease-free survival was seen in the chemotherapy-maintenance group. Even after a complete course of 3 years of chemo-therapy, no effect of oral BCG was seen on the post-therapy 20 to 25% recurrence rate of the disease by Haghbin et al. (1980). Because it has recently been shown that cell-mediated cytotoxicity against leukemic blasts can be generated in vitro in the autologous (Zarlin and Bach, 1979) and allogeneic (HLA identical sibling) combinations (Taylor and Bradley, 1979), such an approach should be elaborated, because it may provide a specific and potent antileukemic reaction, without GvHD.

4. CONCLUSION

Ablative chemoradiotherapy followed by allogeneic BMT of patients suffering from ALL is superior for the eradication of residual leukemia than chemotherapy alone. The cure rate after allogeneic BMT, however, is adversely affected by transplantation-associated complications as GvHD, infections and interstitial pneumonitis. Nevertheless, for children with diagnostic characteristics of a poor prognosis, the strongest predictors of outcome being a high leukocyte count and pseudodiploidy at chromosomal analysis, the probability of failure with conventional cytostatic therapy is so great that allogeneic BMT is indicated in the first remission.

After relapse of the leukemia the probability of disease-free long-term survival after BMT is still $\geqslant 50\%$, but it is obvious that recurrence of the disease is a major obstacle to cure. With the use of modern sensitive labelling techniques the detection limit of residual leukemia can be lowered, but as long as the biological significance of the remaining of a low number of leukemic cells is not clear, such finding will have no therapeutical consequences. Studies of the kinetics of

clonogenic lymphatic leukemia cells and of the tumor surveillance
mechanisms are badly needed to understand the problem of recurrence of
the disease. At this time trials with more appropriate cytoreductive
regimens may improve the results. Various modifications of the preparative
and/or maintenance treatment of grafted patients have been tried by
individual centres, as described before, in order to prevent leukemic
relapse. Extension of such studies e.g. by cooperative multi-centre
trials is needed to improve the cure rate after allogeneic BMT for ALL.

ACKNOWLEDGEMENTS

I am indebted to A.J. Barrett and R. Joshi, Dep. of Haematology,
Westminster Hospital, London; J.H. Kersey, Dep. of Pediatrics, Univ. of
Minnesota, Minneapolis; R.J. O'Reilly, Memorial Sloan-Kettering Cancer
Center, New York and Jean E. Sanders, Univ. of Washington and Fred
Hutchinson Cancer Research Center, Seattle, for their contribution to
this report.

REFERENCES
1. Barrett A.J., Kendra J.R., Lucas C.F. et al.: Bone marrow transplantation for acute lymphoblastic leukaemia. Brit. J. Haemat. 52: 181,
   1982.
2. Barrett A.J., personal communication, 1983.
3. Borella L., Casper J.T. and Lauer S.J.: Shifts in expression of cell
   membrane phenotypes in childhood lymphoid malignancies at relapse.
   Blood 54: 64, 1979.
4. Champlin R.E., Feig S.A., Ho W.G. et al.: Bone marrow transplantation
   (BMT) for acute lymphoblastic leukemia in remission: importance of
   extramedullary involvement. Blood 60: 165a, 1982.
5. Chessels J.M. and Breatnach F.: Late marrow recurrences in childhood
   acute lymphoblastic leukaemia. Brit. med. J. 283: 749, 1981.
6. Chessels J.M.: Acute lymphoblastic leukaemia. Seminars in Hematology
   19: 155, 1982.
7. Clift R.A., Buckner C.D., Thomas E.D. et al.: Allogeneic marrow
   transplantation for acute lymphoblastic leukemia in remission using
   fractionated total body irradiation. Leukemia Research 6: 409, 1982.
8. Cornbleet M.A. and Chessels J.M.: Bone-marrow relapse in acute lymphoblastic leukaemia in childhood. Brit. med. J. 2: 104, 1978.
9. Dinsmore R., Kirkpatrick D., Flomenberg N. et al.: Allogeneic bone
   marrow transplantation for patients with acute lymphoblastic leukemia.
   Blood 62: 381, 1983.
10. Feldges A., Imbach P. Lüthy A. et al.: Chance einer Zweitremission
    bei prognostisch günstiger kindlicher akuter lymphoblastischer
    Leukämie. Sweiz. med. Wschr. 112: 1070, 1982.
11. Foon K.A., Schroff R.W. and Gale R.P.: Surface markers on leukemia
    and lymphoma cells: recent advances. Blood 60: 1, 1982.

12. Gale R.P., Kersey J.H., Bortin M.M. et al.: Bone-marrow transplantation for acute lymphoblastic leukaemia. Lancet ii: 663, 1983.
13. George S.L., Aur R.J.A., Mauer A.M. et al.: A reappraisal of the results of stopping therapy in childhood leukemia. NEJM 300: 269, 1979.
14. Graw R.G., Lohrmann H.-P., Bull M.I. et al.: Bone-marrow transplantation following combination chemotherapy immunosuppression (B.A.C.T.) in patients with acute leukemia. Transplantation Proceedings 6: 349, 1974.
15. Greaves M.F., Hariri G., Newman R.A. et al.: Selective expression of the common acute lymphoblastic leukemia (gp100) antigen on immature lymphoid cells and their malignant counterparts. Blood 61: 628, 1983.
16. Haghbin M., Cunningham-Rundles S., Tzvi Thaler H. et al.: Immunotherapy with oral BCG and serial immune evaluation in childhood lymphoblastic leukemia following three years of chemotherapy. Cancer 46: 2577, 1980.
17. Henze G., Langermann H.-J., Fengler R. et al.: Therapiestudie BFM 79/81 zur Behandlung der akuten lymphoblastischen Leukämie bei Kindern und Jugendlichen: intensivierte Reinduktionstherapie für Patientengruppen mit unterschiedlichem Rezidivrisiko. Klin. Pädiat. 194: 195, 1982.
18. Heyn R.M., Joo P., Karon M. et al.: BCG in the treatment of acute lymphoblastic leukemia. Blood 46: 431, 1975.
19. Janossy G., Bollum F.J., Bradstock K.F. et al.: Cellular phenotypes of normal and leukemic hemopoietic cells determined by analysis with selected antibody combinations. Blood 56: 430, 1980.
20. Johnson F.L., Thomas E.D., Clark B.S. et al.: A comparison of marrow transplantation with chemotherapy for children with acute lymphoblastic leukemia in second or subsequent remission. NEJM 305, 846, 1981.
21. Look A.Th., Melvin S.L., Williams D.L. et al.: Aneuploidy and percentages of S-phase cells determined by flow cytometry correlate with cell phenotype in childhood acute leukemia. Blood 60: 959, 1982.
22. Mathé G., Amiel J.L., Schwartzenberg L. et al.: Active immunotherapy for acute lymphoblastic leukemia. Lancet i: 697, 1969.
23. Medical Research Council's Working Party for Leukemia in Childhood Treatment of Acute Lymphoblastic Leukemia: Comparison of immunotherapy (BCG), intermittent methotrexate, and no therapy after a five month intensive cytotoxic regimen (Concord Trial). Brit. med. J. 4: 189, 1971.
24. Miller D.R.: Acute lymphoblastic leukemia. Pediatric Clinics of North America 27: 269, 1980.
25. Miller D.R., Leikin S., Albo V. et al.: Prognostic factors and therapy in acute lymphoblastic leukemia of childhood: CCG-141. Cancer 51: 1041, 1983.
6. Palmer M.K., Hann I.M., Jones P.M. et al.: A score at diagnosis for predicting length of remission in childhood acute lymphoblastic leukaemia. Br. J. Cancer 42: 841, 1980.
7. Pizzolo G., Chilosi M., Cetto G.L. et al.: Immuno-histological analysis of bone marrow involvement in lymphoproliferative disorders. Brit. J. Haemat. 50: 95, 1982.
8. Reaman G.H., Ladisch S., Echelberger C. et al.: Improved treatment results in the management of single and multiple relapses of acute lymphoblastic leukemia. Cancer 45: 3090, 1980.

322

29. Rivera G., Aur R.J., Dahl G.V. et al.: Combined VM-26 and cytosine arabinoside in treatment of refractory childhood lymphocytic leukemia. Cancer 45: 1284, 1980.
30. Rivera G.: Recurrent childhood lymphocytic leukemia: outcome of marrow relapses after cessation of therapy. Haematology and Blood Transfusion 26: 94, 1981.
31. Sanders J., Flournoy N., and the Seattle Marrow Transplant Group: Allogeneic marrow transplantation for acute lymphoblastic leukemia (ALL) in children. Experimental Haematology 11, suppl. 14: 131, 1983.
32. Sanders J., personal communication, 1983.
33. Scarffe J.H., Hann I.M., Evans D.I.K. et al.: Relationship between the pretreatment proliferative activity of marrow blast cells and prognosis of acute lymphoblastic leukaemia of childhood. Br. J. Cancer 41: 764, 1980.
34. Steensel-Moll H.A. van: Childhood leukaemia in The Netherlands. A register based epidemiologic study. Thesis, Rotterdam, 1983.
35. Stryckmans P.A., Otten J., Delbeke M.J. et al.: Comparison of chemotherapy with immunotherapy for maintenance of acute lymphoblastic leukemia in children and adults. Blood 62: 606, 1983.
36. Taylor G.M. and Bradley B.A.: Graft-versus-leukaemia without graft-versus-host? Lancet ii: 959, 1979.
37. Thomas E.D., Sanders J.E., Flournoy N. et al.: Marrow transplantation for patients with acute lymphoblastic leukemia in remission. Blood 54: 468, 1979.
38. UCLA Bone Marrow Transplantation Group: Bone marrow transplantation with intensive combination chemotherapy/radiation therapy (SCARI) in acute leukemia. Ann. intern. Med. 86: 155, 1977.
39. Weiden P.L., Flournoy N., Thomas E.D. et al.: Antileukemic effect of graft-versus-host disease in human recipients of allogeneic-marrow grafts. NEJM 300: 1068, 1979.
40. Weiden P.L., Sullivan K.M., Flournoy N. et al.: Antileukemic effect of chronic graft-versus-host disease. NEJM 304: 1529, 1981.
41. Williams D.L., Tsiatis A., Brodeur G.M. et al.: Prognostic importance of chromosome number in 136 untreated children with acute lymphoblastic leukemia. Blood 60: 864, 1982.
42. Wood G.S. and Warnke R.A.: The immunolgic phenotyping of bone marrow biopsies and aspirates: frozen section techniques. Blood 59: 913, 1982.
43. Woods W.G., Nesbit M.E., Ramsay N.K.C. et al.: Intensive therapy followed by bone marrow transplantation for patients with acute lymphocytic leukemia in second or subsequent remission: determination of prognostic factors (A report from the University of Minnesota Bone Marrow Transplantation Team). Blood 61: 1182, 1983.
44. Zarling J.M. and Bach F.H.: Continuous culture of T cells cytotoxic for autologous human leukaemia cells. Nature 280: 685, 1979.
45. Zwaan F.E., Hermans J., Barrett A.J. et al.: Bone marrow transplantation for acute lymphoblastic leukaemia: a survey of the European Group for Bone Marrow Transplantation (E.G.B.M.T.). 1984, Brit. J. Haemat. (in press).

ALLOGENEIC AND SYNGENEIC MARROW TRANSPLANTATION IN ACUTE LEUKEMIA WITH MINIMAL RESIDUAL DISEASE

GEORGE W. SANTOS

Bone marrow transplantation (BMT) offers two potential therapeutic advantages over that of more conventional therapy in leukemia. The use of this procedure allows one to give very intensive cytoreductive therapy without regard to marrow toxicities since the marrow infusion is able to "rescue" the patient from this otherwise lethal toxicity. In addition, allogeneic marrow appears to have an additional antileukemic effect by way of graft-versus-host disease (GVHD). GVHD is, of course, a two-edged sword since its antileukemic effects are balanced by the morbidity and mortality it may produce. Marrow transplantation was initially confined to end-stage leukemic patients. The long-term survivals and cures were only about 10-15%. It was estimated that the actuarial relapse rate was somewhere near 70%, it should be noted, however, that at least 50% of the patients died of non-leukemic causes. In the mid-1970's marrow transplantation was performed in patients in remission. It was surmised that such patients would be in better general clinical condition (i.e., no infections, adequate nutrition, normal peripheral counts, etc.) and would because of remission status have minimal residual disease. Thus, it was hoped that deaths from non-leukemic causes might be decreased and that leukemic relapse rate would be lower. The present communication deals only with patients transplanted with minimal residual disease and considers only those patients having genotypical HLA identical allogeneic or syngeneic donors.

Supported by PHS Grants CA-15396 and CAO-6973 awarded by the National Cancer Institute, DHHS

ALLOGENEIC TRANSPLANTATION FOR ACUTE LYMPHOCYTIC LEUKEMIA (ALL)

Thomas et al. (1) reported a series of patients transplanted for ALL either in second or subsequent remission or
at relapse. In this series, transplantation in remission was
shown to be associated with a significantly improved survival
due to decrease in deaths from both leukemic and non-leukemic
causes. Nevertheless at the time of the report, 10/22 patients in the remission group had relapsed by one year post-
transplant and the actuarial probability of relapse was
greater than 50%. In this small series there was no survival
advantage to BMT in second remission as opposed to later remission. In a recent follow-up of the remission patients,
27% were alive in unmaintained remission at 3.5-5 years
post-BMT (2). In a pediatric series from the same group containing seven patients reported previously (1) 9/24 patients
were alive in complete remission at 17-55 months following
BMT for ALL in second or subsequent remission (3). Again
relapse rate was high as 12/24 had relapsed at the time of
the report and eight had done so within the first year. A
survival advantage was not shown for early transplantation
when results were compared for transplantation performed in
second versus subsequent remission. In these Seattle studies
the preparative regimen consisted generally of cyclophosphamide (CY) 60 mg/kg given on two successive days followed in
one or two days by 1000 rad of mid-line total body irradiation (TBI).

Scott et al. (4) used a preparative regimen slightly
modified from that of one used by the Seattle group. In
addition to the CY they added cytosine arabinoside and gave
TBI in a single setting from a linear accelerator with a mean
dose of 986 rad. Eight out of 14 such patients transplanted
in first complete remission were alive in continuous complete
remission from 7-30 months with a median survival of 19
months. Eight out of 20 patients transplanted in second or
third remission were in continuous complete remission 8-41
months after transplantation with a median survival of 22
months. There were no relapses in the first remission

patients but 7/20 relapsed when they were transplanted in the second or third remission. The actuarial two-year survival was 57% for first remission patients versus 34% for those transplanted in subsequent remissions. Kendra et al. (5) reported a similar advantage of transplanting patients in first remission as opposed to second remission. In a subsequent follow-up report Kendra et al. (6) reported on 12 patients transplanted in first remission, 21 in second remission and 13 in third or fourth remission. Patients transplanted in first remission had a two-year disease-free survival of 80% compared with a two-year disease-free survival varying between 33-38% for all other groups. Their preparative regimen consisted of a protocol called, "V-RAPID". It included VM26, intrathecal methotrexate, cytosine arabinoside, methyl prednisolone, daunorubicin, and 950 rad of TBI. No relapses were seen in first remission but a relatively high relapse rate was seen in second and subsequent remissions.

Woods et al. (7) employed a preparative regimen quite similar to that employed in Seattle except they used the linear accelerator to deliver 750 rad TBI. Fifteen patients with acute lymphocytic leukemia in second or subsequent remission were transplanted, twelve in the second remission and three in third remission. Five patients survive in continuous complete remission from 24^+-48^+ months. There were seven relapses in this group, all within 14 months after transplantation.

Dinsmore et al. (8) reported a series of patients who were prepared with hyperfractionated TBI for a total dose of 1320 rad delivered in four days. This was followed by two days of CY (60 mg/kg) on each of two successive days. Of those transplanted in second remission 15/22 survive, 14 in complete remission with a median follow-up of 24 months. The two-year actuarial projected survival was 67% with 62% projected being free of relapse. There were two observed relapses in this group at 9 and 15 months. Of third remission patients 6/15 survive, five in complete remission for 15-20

months, (median 16 months). The projected two-year survival
and disease-free survial were 33% and 27% respectively. Six
of 15 were observed to relapse 1-9 months after transplantation.

The Baltimore group recently reported their preliminary
findings in transplantation in acute lymphocytic leukemia in
remission (9). Their preparative regimen consists of CY 50
mg/kg given on each of four successive days for a total dose
of 200 mg/kg followed immediately by TBI delivered at the
rate of 300 rad a day for four consecutive days with the
lungs completely shielded for the third dose. Fourteen
patients were transplanted in second remission, and 13 in
third remission. These two groups taken together showed an
actuarial two-year disease-free survival of 40% and actuarial
two-year relapse rate of 30%. Leukemic relapses were only
seen in third remission and these occurred at 2-3 months in
the marrow, the CNS at eight months and one testicular relapse at eight months. The patients transplanted in the
second remission have a 50% projected two-year disease-free
survival. Patients transplanted in the third remission have
a projected 37% two-year disease-free survival. There were
no statistical differences between the two disease-free survival curves, however, it was evident that there were more
relapses in patients transplanted in third remission. Thus,
there are two reports cited above where transplantation
appears to be better in the earlier remissions as opposed to
subsequent remissions. However, there are two reports that
are unique in that the relapse rate is quite low in second
remission. Both of these protocols are somewhat different
from that originally proposed by the Seattle group. The
Memorial Sloan-Kettering group uses hyperfractionated radiation followed by CY and the Baltimore group uses more CY
than the Seattle group but in addition gives fractionated
radiation on a daily basis for four days. It is conceivable
that if these series are followed long enough that these two
latter treatments may prove to be better preparative regimens
as far as the incidence of relapse is concerned.

ALLOGENEIC MARROW TRANSPLANTATION FOR ACUTE NON-LYMPHOCYTIC LEUKEMIA (ANL)

In early 1976 the Seattle group using CY plus single or fractionated doses of TBI (10) began allogeneic transplantation in ANL in first remission. Twelve of the first 22 patients are alive in unmaintained remission for 4 1/4 to 6 1/4 years later (11). An actuarial analysis of the likelihood of remaining in remission shows a plateau at 80% attesting to the efficacy of the CY and TBI regimen. These exciting results continue to be seen with larger numbers of patients transplanted in Seattle (12) and also in other centers using the Seattle protocol as is or with slight modification (13-18).

Therapeutic results in patients with ANL transplanted in second remission were less favorable in the Seattle experience. Their projected actuarial relapse rate was 45% and actuarial survival was 25% (19), a result not better than patients transplanted in first relapse (20). An exception to this finding is the experience of the Memorial Sloan-Kettering group (21). This group employs hyperfractionated TBI for a total dose of 1320 rad followed by CY (60 mg/kg) given on two consecutive days. Thirty patients were transplanted in first remission with an actuarial survival and disease-free survival of 57% and 55% respectively. Only three patients relapsed and the three-year actuarial probability of being in remission was 83%. Seven of 11 patients transplanted in second remission showed a projected disease-free survival of 64% which was not different from patients transplanted in first remission. There were no relapses in this group.

The Baltimore group is the only one that does not employ TBI in patients with ANL. Instead, they employ busulfan (BU) combined with CY. Eighteen patients were transplanted in first remission and 17 transplanted in the second or third remission or early relapse. Actuarial two-year survivals were 44% and 29% respectively. Survivors range from 14 to 52 months with a median of survivors of 31 months. Only one relapse was seen at 12 months and that was in a patient age 36 who was transplanted in his third remission (22).

Except for one report to the contrary (18) the general findings indicate that survival is better in the younger patient. Similarly, except for the findings from the Memorial Sloan-Kettering group, most reports indicate that survival in first remission patients is better than that of subsequent remissions.

SYNGENEIC MARROW TRANSPLANTATION

Marrow transplantation with monozygotic twin donors offers a unique opportunity to study transplantation without the problems associated with GVHD. A series of 34 such patients with refractory leukemia in relapse (18 ALL, 16 ANL) have been transplanted following treatment with CY and single-dose TBI (23). Recurrence of leukemia (13 ALL and 10 ANL) was the principle cause of death. Three patients with ALL and five with ANL at the time of the report remained in complete unmaintained remission from 24 to 103 months.

Subsequently, the same group has transplanted a number of patients in complete remission. Four patients with ALL were transplanted in first remission. Three survive free of leukemia for 11, 36 and 120 months while one relapsed at three months. Seven patients with ALL were transplanted in their second and third remission. Three survive for 31, 48, and 56 months free of leukemia and four relapsed 4-7 months following transplantation. Eight patients with ANL were transplanted in their first remission and two in their second remission. Three patients transplanted in first remission survive free of leukemia for 4, 24, and 53 months, and five relapsed from 4-12 months following transplantation. Two patients transplanted in their second remission survive free of leukemia for 22 and 74 months (24).

The Baltimore group (unpublished observations) have transplanted two patients in their first remission for ALL and one in third complete remission. One patient in first remission and one in the third remission each survive for 23 months free of leukemia. The remaining patient transplanted in first remission relapsed in the mediastinum at ten months, and after remission induction, died of complications related to chemotherapy maintenance 23 months after transplantation. Four patients were transplanted for AML in first remission, two survive continuously free of leukemia for 22 and 52 months.

The European group (25) reported that marrow transplantation was performed in ten cases of ALL and eight cases of ANL. Their report does not give their survival nor in which remission they were transplanted. One can surmise, however, that the therapeutic results were at least as good as reported above, since an identical twin transplant was a strong favorable prognostic factor in their entire series of allogeneic and syngeneic transplants.

It appears, therefore, that the relapse rate in ALL and ANL following syngeneic marrow transplantation will be close to 50%. With small numbers, however, one cannot determine a difference in therapeutic outcome when patients are compared as to which remission existed when they were transplanted. These data provide an important yardstick for autologous transplants performed in acute leukemia in remission.

COMPLICATIONS OF MARROW TRANSPLANTATION

More than 80% of the deaths following allogeneic transplantation in the Baltimore and other centers' experience is related to acute and chronic GVHD or viral infections in the form of gastroenteritis and interstitial pneumonitis. Leukemic relapse following allogeneic transplantation does not appear to be a problem for patients in first remission and remains a problem in second remission patients only with the use of certain preparative regimens. A high rate of relapse, however, is the major problem associated with syngeneic transplantation.

Approaches to preventing or lessening the mortality due to GVHD and viral infections are being actively pursued in a number of centers and have been discussed previously at some length (26-29). Patients over 20 or 30 years of age given allogeneic transplants have a decreased survival as compared to younger patients. The reasons for this have been speculated upon, but in truth no one has yet given evidence for the real biological basis of this observation. Solutions or at least partial solutions to the problems noted at the beginning of this paragraph should improve this situation.

Problems of high leukemic relapse rates seen in the syngeneic transplants are probably best approached by chemotherapeutic maintenance therapy or immunologic (i.e., systemic monoclonal antibody, biological response modifiers, etc.) maneuvers applied following the transplant. Increasing the intensity of the cytoreductive preparative regimens does not at this juncture appear to be an attractive approach since the protocols already in current use produce tolerable but considerable toxicity.

REFERENCES

1. Thomas ED, Sanders JE, Flournoy N et al. 1979. Marrow transplantation for patients with acute lymphoblastic leukemia in remission. Blood 54: 468.
2. Storb R. 1982. Bone marrow transplantation. Cancer Clin. Trials 5: 146.
3. Johnson FL, Thomas ED, Clark BS et al. 1981. A comparison of marrow transplantation with chemotherapy for children with acute lymphoblastic leukemia in second or subsequent remission. N. Engl. J. Med. 305: 846.
4. Scott EP, Forman SJ, Spruce WE et al. 1983. Bone marrow ablation followed by allogeneic bone marrow transplantation for patients with high-risk acute lymphoblastic leukemia during complete remission. Transplant. Proc. 15: 1395.
5. Kendra JR, Barrett AJ, Lucas C et al. 1982. Bone marrow transplantation for acute lymphoblastic leukemia. Exp. Hematol. 10 (Suppl. 10) (abstr.): 72.
6. Kendra JR, Joshi R, Desai M et al. 1983. Bone marrow transplantation for acute lymphoblastic leukemia with matched allogeneic donors. Exp. Hematol. 11 (Suppl. 13) (abstr.): 9.
7. Woods WG, Nesbitt NE, Ramsey NKC et al. 1983. Intensive therapy followed by bone marrow transplantation for patients with acute lymphocytic leukemia in second or subsequent remission: Determination of prognostic factors (A report from the University of Minnesota Bone Marrow Transplantation Team). Blood 61: 1182.
8. Dinsmore R, Kirkpatrick D, Flomenberg N et al. 1983. Allogeneic bone marrow transplantation for patients with acute lymphoblastic leukemia. Blood 62: 381.

9. Santos GW, Bias WB, Beschorner WE et al. 1983. Allogeneic and syngeneic marrow transplantation for acute lymphocytic leukemia (ALL) in remission - Baltimore experience. Exp. Hematol. 11 (Suppl. 14) (abstr.): 132.

10. Thomas ED, Buckner CD, Clift RA et al. 1979. Marrow transplantation for acute nonlymphoblastic leukemia in first remission. New Engl. J. Med. 301: 597.

11. Storb R and Santos GW. 1983, in press. Application of marrow transplantation in leukemia and aplastic anemia. Clin. Haematol.

12. Grouse LD and Young RK. 1983. Clinical perspectives in bone marrow transplantation. A lifesaving applied art. An interview with E. Donnal Thomas, M.D. JAMA 249: 2528.

13. Forman SJ, Spruce WE, Farbstein MJ et al. 1983. Bone marrow ablation followed by allogeneic marrow grafting during first complete remission of acute nonlymphocytic leukemia. Blood 61: 439.

14. Powles RL, Morgenstern G, Clink HM et al. 1980. The place of bone-marrow transplantation in acute myelogenous leukaemia. Lancet 1: 1047.

15. Kersey JH, Ramsey NKC, Kim T et al. 1982. Allogeneic bone-marrow transplantation in acute non-lymphocytic leukemia: A pilot study. Blood 60: 400.

16. Zwaan FE and Hermans J for the E.B.M.T-leukaemia working party. 1982. Bone-marrow transplantation for leukaemia. European results in 264 cases. Exp. Hematol. 10 (suppl. 10): 64.

17. Mannon P, Vernant JP, Roden M et al. 1980. Marrow transplantation for acute nonlymphoblastic leukemia in first remission. BLUT 41: 220.

18. Gale RP, Kay HEM, Rimm AA et al. 1982. Bone-marrow transplantation for acute leukaemia in first remission. Lancet 2: 1006.

19. Buckner CD, Clift RA, Thomas ED et al. 1982. Allogeneic marrow transplantation for patients with acute nonlymphoblastic leukemia in second remission. Leuk. Res. 6: 395.

20. Appelbaum FR, Clift RA, Buckner CD et al. 1983. Allogeneic marrow transplantation for acute non-lymphoblastic leukemia after first relapse. Blood 61: 949.

21. Dinsmore R. Personal communication.

22. Santos GW, Tutschka PJ, Brookmeyer R et al. 1983, in press. Marrow transplantation for acute non-lymphocytic leukemia following treatment with busulfan and cyclophosphamide. N. Engl. J. Med.

23. Fefer A, Cheever MA, Thomas ED et al. 1981. Bone marrow transplantation for refractory acute leukemia in 34 patients with identical twins. Blood 57: 421.

24. Fefer A, Cheever MA, Greenberg PD et al. 1983. Bone marrow transplantation (BMT) with identical twins: Improved results with BMT in complete remission (CR). Proc. Am. Soc. Clin. Oncol. 2 (abstr.): 182.

25. Zwaan FE and Hermans J. 1983. Report of the E.B.M.T. - Leukaemia Working Party. Exp. Hematol. 11 (Suppl. 13) (abstr.): 3.

26. Santos GW and Kaizer H. 1982. Bone marrow transplantation in acute leukemia. Sem. Hematol. 19: 227.
27. O'Reilly RJ, Reisner Y, Kapoor N. 1981. The use of separated allogeneic hematopoietic precursors to circumvent graft vs. host disease following marrow transplantation. In JH Burchenal, HF Oettgen (Eds.): Cancer, Achievements, Challenges, and Prospects for the 1980s, pp. 649.
28. Storb R, Atkinson K, Lum LG et al. 1981. Graft-versus-host disease, immunologic reconstitution and graft-host tolerance in marrow graft recipients. In JH Burchenal, HF Oettgen (Eds.): Cancer, Achievements, Challenges, and Prospects for the 1980s, pp. 639.
29. Thomas ED. 1981. Bone marrow transplantation. In JH Burchenal, HF Oettgen (Eds.): Cancer, Achievements, Challenges, and Prospects for the 1980s, pp. 625.

BONE MARROW TRANSPLANTATION FOR MINIMAL RESIDUAL DISEASE IN
LEUKEMIA *

B. SPECK, A. GRATWOHL FOR THE BASLE BONE MARROW TRANSPLANT
TEAM

1. INTRODUCTION

Between 1974 and March 1979 we transplanted 18 patients
with terminal drug-resistant acute leukemia. 17 patients
died. 14 of them died without evidence of disease due to
transplant related complications e.g. Graft-versus-Host-Disease and interstitial pneumonia. Three died of leukemic relapse. One patient survived and is today eight years after
transplantation leading a normal life (1). These results confirmed those obtained by others (2): Marrow transplantation
could cure leukemia resistant to chemotherapy, complications
however were too frequent in terminally ill patients. In sum-
mer 1979 we initiated a new program. We tried to transplant
patients under optimal conditions: patients with acute leukemia in first remission. Such patients are clinically healthy
and have a minimal tumor load. In this new series of patients
Cyclosporine (CyA) was used for prophylaxis of Graft-versus-
Host-Disease (GvHD) (3). We continued to transplant patients
in later stages of their disease or patients who never gained remission. The aim of this study was to test if earlier
transplantation could indeed reduce both, transplant related
and disease related mortality. Incidently we began to transplant patients with chronic myelogenous leukemia in chronic
phase in 1979 (4).

* Supported by Grants of the Swiss Science Foundation 3.846.
  0.79 and the Swiss Cancer League 4141.LR79 and the Swiss Pu-
  blic Health Service.

2. PROCEDURE

2.1.1. Patients and methods

From July 1979 to August 1983 59 HLA-identical bone marrow grafts were performed. The median age of the patients was 29 years (18 - 42 y). The median observation period is 20 months (3 - 48 m). Four additional patients were transplanted from HLA-one-haplotype identical family member. All patients were conditioned with 2x60 mg/kg Cyclophosphamide (Cy) and 10 Gy total body irradiation (TBI) midline tissue dose from a linear accelerator at a dose rate of 7.5 cGy per minute. In the initial 15 patients the lungs were shielded to receive 8 Gy. Lung shielding was discontinued in the subsequent patients.

2.1.2. HLA-identical sibling transplants in leukemia (N=59)

22 had acute myelogenous leukemia (AML). 16 were in first complete remission, 6 in other stages of the disease. 20 patients had acute lymphoblastic leukemia (ALL). Seven were in first complete remission, 13 in other stages of the disease. 17 had CML. 15 were in chronic - two in accelerated phase of the disease. All CML patients were splenectomized before BMT.

2.1.3. HLA-one-haplotype identical transplants from family members (N=4)

Three patients had ALL. Two were in first complete remission, one in second relapse. One patient had AML. He never reached remission on chemotherapy.

All patients were nursed in sterile laminar air flow rooms with gastrointestinal decontamination, skin cleansing and sterile food. The patients remained for 21 to 45 days (median 28 days) in the sterile rooms after transplantation.

CyA was given intramuscularly 20 mg/kg per day in a single daily dose, starting 24 hours before the infusion of the marrow and continued for seven days in the initial 15 patients.

The next 11 patients were given the same dose of CyA as a continuous i.v. infusion, starting 24 hours before marrow transplantation and continued for five days. All the other patients had CyA as a continuous i.v. infusion, 20 mg/kg on the day before marrow transplantation, then 10 mg/kg for five days and afterwards for 5 more days 5 mg/kg per day as a continuous i.v. infusion. All patients then received the drug orally in a single daily dose of 12.5 mg/kg. This dose was maintained for six months, then slowly reduced and stopped at 12 months (5, 6).

2.2. Results
2.2.1. HLA-identical sibling transplants in leukemia (N=59)

Of the 16 patients with AML in first remission 10 (63 %) survive without evidence of leukemia and without chronic problems. Six patients died: 4 of relapse, 2 of GvHD, in one instance associated with interstitial pneumonia. Of the six patients with AML in later stages, three survive in complete remission. All three deaths were due to leukemic relapse. Of the seven patients with ALL in first remission four survive without evidence of leukemia. One is alive with relapse and is back on chemotherapy. Two patients died: one from GvHD and one from aspergillosis. Of the 13 patients with ALL transplanted in disease stages other than first remission, three survive without evidence of leukemia, one survives with relapse and is back on chemotherapy. There were nine deaths. Eight were caused by leukemic relapse and one by cytomegalovirus-infection (CMV). Of 15 patients with CML in chronic phase, ten survive without evidence of leukemia. Of the five deaths, four were due to GvHD and one to acute sepsis at six months after transplantation. Both transplants in accelerated phase were failures: one never went into remission after transplantation and finally died from the leukemia, the other died of GvHD.

2.2.2. <u>HLA-one-haplotype identical transplants from family members (N=4)</u>

One patient is alive and well with mild chronic cutaneous GvHD at over 20 months after BMT. Three had severe acute GvHD which was fatal in two. One patient recovered from acute GvHD, but died of recurrent disease (T-ALL).

2.3. <u>Discussion</u>

These results confirm that best results can be achieved by transplanting acute leukemia in first remission and chronic myelogenous leukemia in chronic phase (figure 1).

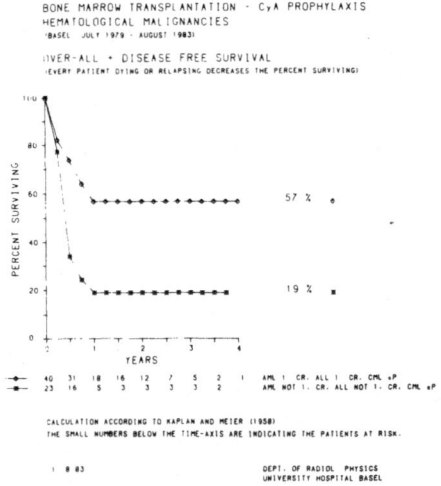

Relapse however remains a problem. It occurs in one of 16 patients with AML in 1. CR and in one of seven with ALL in 1. CR. Relapse could be due to insufficient Graft-versus-Tumor-Activity in patients given Cyclosporine (7), due to resistant leukemia or due to the fact that the state of minimal residual disease was not reached before transplantation. The latter point might be supported by the results of transplantation in patients with ALL other than first remission. In these patients relapse rate is extremely high.

There is one major aspect to contradict the importance
of tumor load at the time of transplantation. The fact that
we did not see any relapse in patients transplanted for CML
in chronic phase is surprising. None of these patients was
in cytogenetic remission before transplantation. All had the
Philadelphia-chromosome in all cells tested and the peripheral white cell count at the time of transplantation was between 10 and $40x10^9/1$. Indeed, a transplantation against an
enormous tumor load. So far all patients went into complete
remission and no relapse has been seen.

In view of these results we could conclude that minimal
residual disease is mandatory for successfull bone marrow
in the majority of patients. Minimal however, might relate
much less to the quantity of tumor rather than to a minimal
resistance of tumor cells against cytotoxic drugs and/or
radiation.

REFERENCES

1. Speck B, Cornu P, Sartorius J, Nissen C, Gratwohl A,
   Burri P, Jeannet M. 1979. Fortschritte in der Knochenmarktransplantation bei akuter Leukämie und aplastischer
   Anämie. Schweiz Med Wschr 109, 1883-1885.
2. Thomas ED, Buckner CD, Banaji M, Clift RA, Fefer A, Fluornoy N, Goodell BW, Hickman RD, Lerner KG, Neimann PE,
   Sale GE, Sanders JE, Singer J, Stevens M, Storb R, Weiden
   PL. 1977. One hundred patients with acute leukemia treated
   with chemotherapy, total body irradiation and allogeneic
   marrow transplantation. Blood 49, 511-533.
3. Speck B, Gratwohl A, Nissen C, et al. 1981. Cyclosporin-A
   for prophylaxis of GvHD in clinical bone marrow transplantation. Exp Hemat today 3, 117-120.
4. Speck B, Gratwohl A, Nissen C, Osterwalder B, Müller M,
   Bannert P, Müller Hj, Jeannet M. 1982. Allogeneic marrow
   transplantation for chronic granulocytic leukemia. Blut
   45, 237-242.
5. Speck B, Gratwohl A, Nissen C, Osterwalder B, Signer E,
   Jeannet M. 1983. Knochenmarktransplantation bei Leukämie
   und aplastischer Anämie. Schweiz Med Wschr 113, 622-629.

6. Gratwohl A, Speck B, Wenk M, Forster I, Müller M, Osterwalder B, Nissen C, Follath F. 1983. Cyclosporin-A in human Bone Marrow Transplantation, Serum concentration,
   Graft-versus-Host-Disease and Nephrotoxicity. Transplantation 36, 40-44.
7. Weiden PL, Sullivan KM, Fluornoy N, Storb R, Thomas ED.
   1981. Antileukemic effect of chronic graft versus host
   disease. Contribution to improved survival after allogeneic marrow transplantation. New Engl J Med 304, 1529-
   1534.

COMPARISON OF HLA MATCHED AND MISMATCHED BONE MARROW TRANSPLANTATION IN ACUTE LEUKEMIA

E. DONNALL THOMAS, M.D.

The majority of bone marrow transplants have utilized HLA-identical siblings as donor. However, the majority of patients who are candidates for bone marrow transplantation do not have HLA-identical siblings. More than six years ago the Seattle Marrow Transplant Team began a cautious exploration of the use of family-member donors other than HLA-identical siblings for patients with acute leukemia (1-3). These donor recipient pairs were haploidentical, that is, genetically identical for one of the HLA haplotypes. The other haplotype was partially matched, that is, phenotypically identical for one or more of the major HLA loci (HLA-A, -B, and -D/DR). These patients were prepared for transplantation with the same regimens of cyclophosphamide and total body irradiation as those employed for patients who received HLA-identical marrow grafts. They also received the same posttransplant prophylaxis for acute graft-versus-host disease in the form of intermittent methotrexate through day 100 after transplantation.

An overview of this experience for patients with acute leukemia in relapse is shown in Figure 1 which presents an analysis of 62 recipients of syngeneic marrow, 297 recipients of HLA-identical marrow, and 50 recipients of partially matched marrow. Although there is a trend

This investigation was supported by Grant CA 18029, awarded by the National Cancer Institute, DHHS. Dr. Thomas is the recipient of Research Career Award AI 02425 from the National Institute of Allergy and Infectious Diseases.

340

toward a better survival for recipients of syngeneic marrow and a worse survival for recipients of partially matched marrow, these differences are not statistically significant.

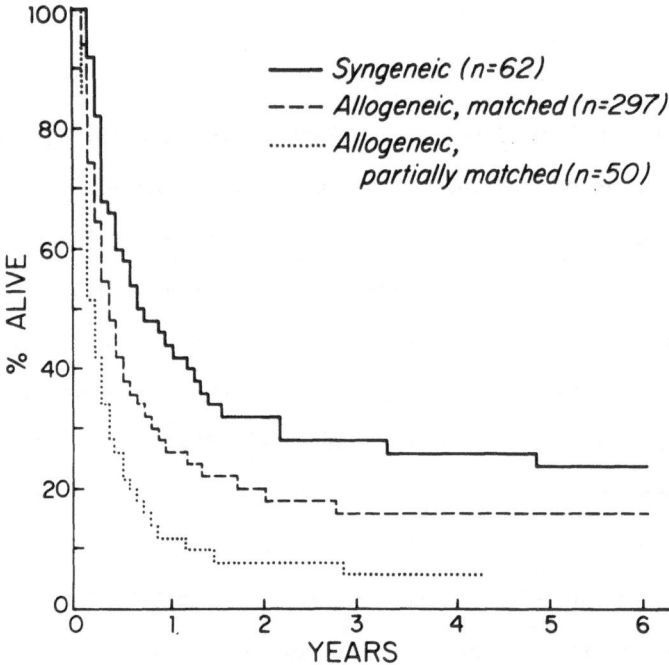

Figure 1. Kaplan-Meier product limit estimates of survival of patients with acute leukemia transplanted from syngeneic, allogeneic or partially matched donors.

An important question is whether or not a partially matched marrow graft might be associated with a lower probability of recurrence of leukemia due to an "allogeneic effect" or a "graft-versus-leukemia effect." Figure 2 shows an analysis of the probability of being in remission for the three groups of recipients as presented in Figure 1. This type of analysis censors patients who die of nonleukemic causes and permits an inspection of the rate of recurrence of leukemia. It is obvious from the figure that the rates of recurrence of leukemia are the same.

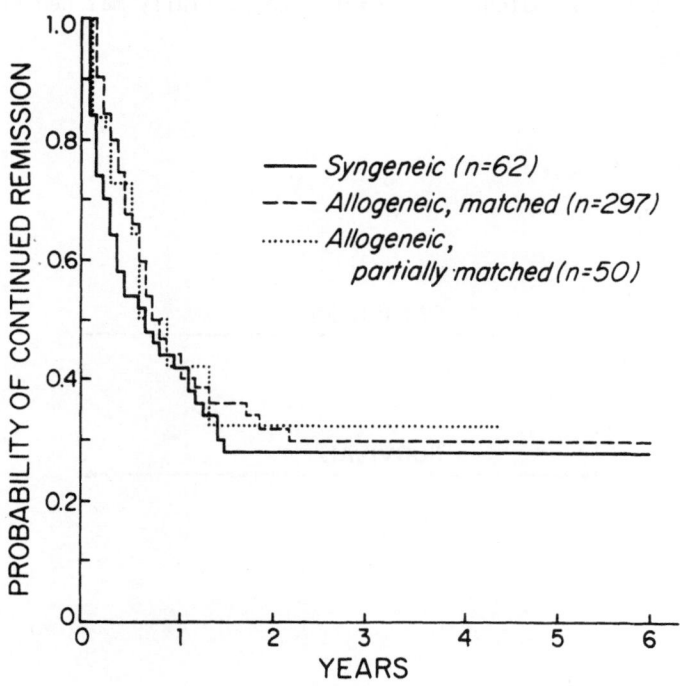

Figure 2. Kaplan-Meier product limit estimates of the probability of being in remission for patients transplanted for acute leukemia in relapse using syngeneic, allogeneic, or partially matched marrow donors.

We have transplanted 75 patients with acute nonlymphoblastic leukemia in first remission using HLA-identical donors with a minimum follow-up now greater than 3 years (4). The long-term survival and apparent cure is approximately 50% and the Kaplan-Meier analysis of recurrence of leukemia shows a probability of 0.22. Thirteen patients with acute nonlymphoblastic leukemia in first remission have been transplanted from a partially matched donor and followed for a minimum period of more than one year. Figure 3 shows that six of these patients

342

are surviving from 1 to 5 years. Figure 3 also shows that the probability of a recurrence of leukemia is 0.31. Although the number of
patients given partially matched grafts is small, it is evident that,
as yet, the results for matched as compared to partially matched grafts
are not different.

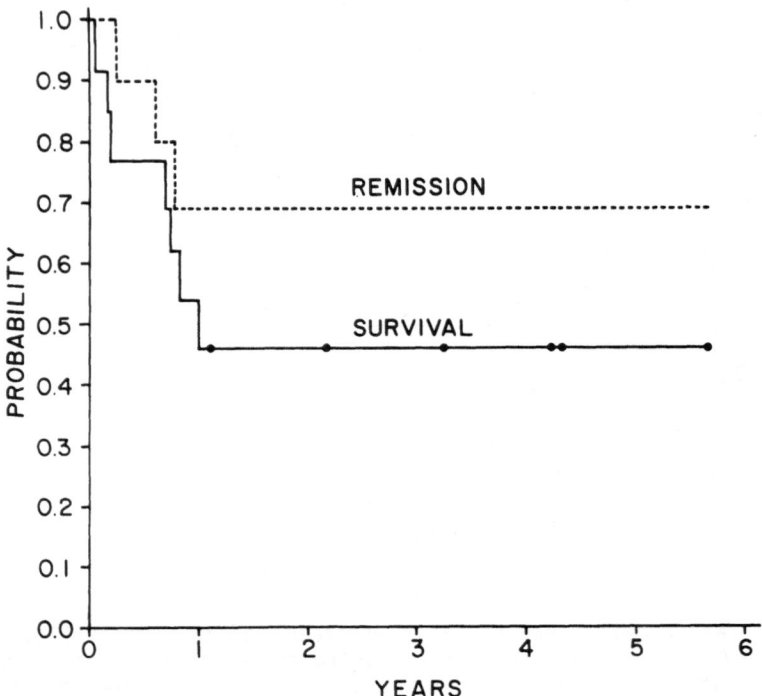

Figure 3.   Kaplan-Meier product limit estimates for 13 patients with
acute nonlymphoblastic leukemia transplanted in first remission using
partially matched donors.   The solid line indicates the probability of
survival with the dots indicating the 6 patients living in remission.
The dashed line shows the probability of being in remission.

We have now carried out more than 100 marrow grafts for patients
with acute leukemia using a partially matched donor (5).   These studies
involve several different categories of acute leukemia in several different stages of the disease.   Furthermore, the degree of mismatch, the

loci involved in the mismatch, and the family relationship between the donor and the recipient are different. These multiple subcategories make a precise analysis difficult. A proportional hazards regression analysis of the Cox type is currently underway in an attempt to sort out these multiple factors. As yet, there is no indication that a particular type and degree of mismatch or a particular family relationship differs significantly from any other.

With regard to graft-versus-host disease, our experience with more than 500 patients transplanted for leukemia using HLA-identical sibling donors shows that 37% suffered grade II or greater acute graft-versus-host disease. For recipients of partially matched grafts the incidence of grade II or more severe graft-versus-host disease is 59% for a one-locus mismatch and 56% for a two-locus mismatch. It appears that in this setting, a partially matched graft is almost as good as a fully matched transplant.

We have transplanted only two patients using a donor with one haplotype mismatched at all three loci. Both patients died of acute graft-versus-host disease.

Powles et al have reported 35 patients treated for acute leukemia using partially matched family member marrow graft donors (6). Cyclosporine was given to all patients after grafting. At the time of the report 11 patients were alive at least 6 months after grafting. Four patients suffered a recurrence of leukemia and died between 227 and 629 days after grafting.

The possibility of using unrelated donors who are phenotypically _A-identical with the patient is now attracting considerable attention. We reported such a transplant in a patient with acute lymphoblastic leukemia that was successful, but the leukemia recurred 17 months later and the patient died of leukemia (7). Although other transplant centers have now carried out transplants using unrelated donors, there is not enough experience to know whether or not marrow from an unrelated donor might have an "allogeneic effect" which would assist in eradication of residual leukemic cells.

CONCLUSION

The experience to date indicates that partially matched family members and, perhaps, phenotypically HLA-identical unrelated donors can result in successful marrow grafts associated with a spectrum of graft-versus-host disease resembling that observed following an HLA-identical transplant. The effect of different degrees of mismatching is still under investigation. There is no evidence, as yet, that partially incompatible or compatible unrelated donors will convey an advantage in terms of eradicating residual leukemic cells.

REFERENCES

1. Clift RA, Hansen JA, Thomas ED, Buckner CD, Sanders JE, Mickelson EM, Storb R, Johnson FL, Singer JW and Goodell BW: Marrow transplantation from donors other than HLA-identical siblings. Transplantation 28: 235-242, 1979.
2. Hansen JA, Clift RA, Mickelson EM, Nisperos B and Thomas ED: Marrow transplantation from donors other than HLA identical siblings. Hum. Immunol. 1: 31-40, 1981.
3. Hansen JA, Clift RA, Beatty PG, Mickelson EM, Nisperos B, Martin PJ and Thomas ED: Marrow transplantation from donors other than HLA genotypically identical siblings. In: Recent Advances in Bone Marrow Transplantation. New York: Alan R. Liss, Inc., in press.
4. Thomas ED: Marrow transplantation for malignant diseases (Karnofsky lecture). J. Clin. Oncol. 1: 517-531, 1983.
5. Beatty PG, Clift RA, Hansen JA, Mickelson EM, Nisperos B and Thomas ED: Marrow transplantation from donors other than HLA genotypically identical siblings. Proceedings: American Society of Clinical Oncology, Vol 2:178, 1983.

6. Powles RL, Kay HEM, Clink HM, Barrett A, Depledge MH, Sloan J, Lumley H, Lawler SD, Morgenstern GR, McElwain TJ, Dady PJ, Jameson B, Watson JG, Leigh M, Hedley D, Filshie J and Robinson B: Mismatched family donors for bone-marrow transplantation as treatment for acute leukaemia. Lancet i: 612-615, 1983.
7. Hansen JA, Clift RA, Thomas ED, Buckner CD, Storb R, Giblett ER: Transplantation of marrow from an unrelated donor to a patient with acute leukemia. N. Engl. J. Med. 303: 565-567, 1980.

INTENSIVE POST-REMISSION INDUCTION CHEMOTHERAPY FOR ACUTE MYELOGENOUS LEUKEMIA IN CHILDREN AND ADULTS

H.J. WEINSTEIN
R.J. MAYER
F.S. CORAL
H.E. GRIER
R.D. GELBER
D.S. ROSENTHAL
B.M. CAMITTA
E. FREI, III

Major progress in the treatment of AML has occurred during the past decade.[1,2] The higher complete remission rates for patients with AML can be attributed to advances in the application of chemotherapy, better supportive care, and carefully designed clinical trials. The median duration of complete remission and the percentage of patients surviving for 5 or more years has steadily improved. This has resulted from post-remission induction chemotherapy or chemoradiotherapy and transplantation of bone marrow from histocompatible donors.[3-10] The intensity and duration of the post-remission induction chemotherapy as well as the merits of marrow transplantation versus chemotherapy for the treatment of patients with AML in first remission have been the focus of recent clinical investigations.[11-13]

In 1976, we initiated an AML program with the acronym VAPA, which featured 14 months of intensive post-remission induction chemotherapy in an effort to improve remission duration for children and adults (less than age 50) with AML. The VAPA protocol was designed to circumvent two obstacles to cure: (1) inadequate leukemia cytoreduction, and (2) the selection and emergence of drug-resistant leukemia cells. We have previously reported encouraging results, especially in children, with this approach.[14,15]

In 1980 we began a second clinical trial for children and adults (less than age 60) with AML. The design of the second generation study (DFCI-80035) was based upon the findings of the VAPA protocol and included an intensification

of ara-c during remission induction, three drug early post-
remission induction intensification, and CNS prophylaxis with
intrathecal cytosine arabinoside for patients less than 18
years of age. In this report we update the VAPA protocol and
provide preliminary results from the second AML clinical trial.

MATERIAL AND METHODS
    Patients
    One hundred and seven consecutive previously untreated
patients less than 50 years of age were entered into VAPA
between February 1976 and May 1980. One hundred and eleven
patients less than 60 years of age were entered into DFCI-80035
between June 1980 and August 1983. The latter study was closed
to adult entry after January, 1983. The diagnosis of AML was
based on morphological examination of bone marrow and histochemical studies.
    Treatment
    In the VAPA study, remission was induced with two courses
of vincristine, doxorubicin, prednisolone, and cytosine
arabinoside. Patients achieving complete remission were
treated with intensive sequential chemotherapy for 14 months.
Central nervous system prophylaxis was not included but
surveillance lumbar punctures were performed throughout
remission. Details of the VAPA protocol have been published.[14]
    Remission with DFCI-80035 was induced with two courses of
daunorubicin and cytosine arabinoside. (Table 1) Patients
achieving complete remission were treated with intensive
sequential chemotherapy for 12 months. (Table 2) Central
nervous system prophylaxis with intrathecal cytosine arabinoside
began during induction and continued throughout the course of
treatment for patients < 18 years of age.

Table 1

DFCI 80035: INDUCTION OF REMISSION

DRUG	DOSAGE	ROUTE	COURSE I*	COURSE II
Daunorubicin	45 mg/m^2/day	IV	Days 1,2,3	Days 1,2
Ara-c	200 mg/m^2/day	Cont. IV Infusion	Days 1 thru 7	Days 1 thru 5

IV Denotes Intravenous

* Bone marrow aspiration and biopsy were performed 14 days
  after initiation of Course I. If the marrow was hypo-
  plastic with < 5 percent blasts, Course II was delayed
  until subsequent marrow aspirate (1 week later) documented
  repopulation with leukemia or remission. If the Day 14
  marrow had more than 5 percent blasts and > 25 percent
  cellularity, Course II was initiated without delay.
  Cytosine arabinoside, 40 mg/m^2, intrathecal, on Day 1 of
  Course I and II for patients less than 18 years of age.

Table 2

DFCI 80035: INTENSIVE SEQUENTIAL MAINTENANCE THERAPY

SEQUENCE I	SEQUENCE II	SEQUENCE III
Daunorubicin 65 mg/m^2 Day 1, IV	Daunorubicin 45 mg/m^2 Day 1, IV	Ara-c 200 mg/m^2 Days 1 - 5, cont. IV or SQ infusion, Day 1, 40 mg/m^2, IT, every other course for pts. < 18 yrs.
Ara-c, 200 mg/m^2 Days 1 - 5, cont. IV or SQ infusion (40 mg/m^2 IT Day 1,5 for pts. < 18 yrs.)	Azacytidine, 150 mg/m^2 Days 1 - 5, cont. IV infusion Ara-c, 40 mg/m^2, IT Day 1 every other course for pts. < 18 yrs.	
Thioguanine 100 mg/m^2 Days 1 - 5, orally q 12 hours		Thioguanine, 100 mg/m^2 Days 1 - 5, orally q 12 hours
Given 4 times at 3-4 week intervals	Given 4 times at 4 week intervals	Given 4 times at 3 - 4 week intervals

Cont. (continuous), IT (intrathecal)

Modification (Sept. 1981) for pts < 18 years of age - Daunorubicin dose reduced during Sequence I to 45 mg/m^2 and during
Sequence II to 30 mg/m^2- Sequence II reduced to 3 courses.

Statistical Analysis

The duration of survival was measured from the time of initial therapy, while the duration of remission extended from the time bone marrow remission was confirmed. Kaplan-Meier analyses were performed for survival and continuous complete remission (CCR) estimates. Remission deaths were counted as relapses.

RESULTS

Induction of Remission

The results of remission induction therapy are presented in Table 3. Rates of complete remission were similar for children and adults and did not differ significantly according to FAB subtype (data not shown). The remission induction dose of ara-c was increased from 100 $mg/m^2/d$ in VAPA to 200 $mg/m^2/d$ in the DFCI-80035 protocol, but this did not significantly influence the rate of complete remission nor the number of induction courses necessary to achieve a complete remission.

Duration of Remission

Pediatric (< 18 years of age):

In the VAPA study, twenty of 45 children who entered remission relapsed. Eight of these 20 relapses were initially detected in the central nervous system (CNS). The monocytic subtype (FAB-M5) was associated with a high risk for primary CNS relapse. The median follow-up for children in CCR is 5 years (range 3 1/2 - 7 1/3 yrs). Twenty-six patients completed therapy and twenty remain in CCR.

There were 39 children who entered remission with 80-035 therapy and five patients have died in remission and 10 have relapsed (Table 3). In contrast to VAPA, only 2 of the 10 relapses occurred in the CNS. The median follow-up of children in CCR is 22 months (range, 4+ - 37+ mos), and the two year CCR probability is 54%.

Figure 1 shows Kaplan-Meier plots of the probability of remaining in CCR for the pediatric and adult patients on the VAPA protocol. The curves in Figure 1 are not statistically significantly different at this time.

Adult (VAPA, 18-50 yrs), (80035, 18-60 yrs):

In the VAPA study there have been 2 deaths in remission and 16 relapses among the 30 adults who were complete responders. The median follow-up of adults in CCR is 3 9/12 yrs (range, 3 1/3 - 6 1/6 yrs), and 9 of the 15 patients who completed therapy remain in CCR.

There were 48 (81%) adults who entered remission with 80035 therapy and there have been 9 deaths in remission and 20 relapses (Table 3). The median follow-up of patients in CCR is 15+ mos (range, 6+ - 32+ mos), and the 2 year CCR probability is 31%. There were 9 adults greater than 50 yrs of age entered into the 80035 protocol, 5 of whom died in remission.

Table 3

RESULTS OF THERAPY FOR VAPA AND DFCI-80035 (AUGUST 1983)

	VAPA 0-17 yr	80035 0-17 yr	VAPA 18-50 yr	80035 18-60 yr
No. Entered	61	52	46	59
No. Complete Remission	45(74%)	39(75%)	30(65%)	48(81%)
Deaths in Remission	0	5	2	9
Total Relapses	20	10	15	20
CNS	8	2	1	0
Bone Marrow	11	7	13	20
Myeloblastoma, other	1	1	1	0
Probability of CCR				
@ 2 yrs	.56	.54	.56	.31
@ 5 yrs	.50	-	.29	-

Survival

Figure 2 shows Kaplan-Meier plots of the probability of survival for all the pediatric and adult patients on the VAPA protocol.

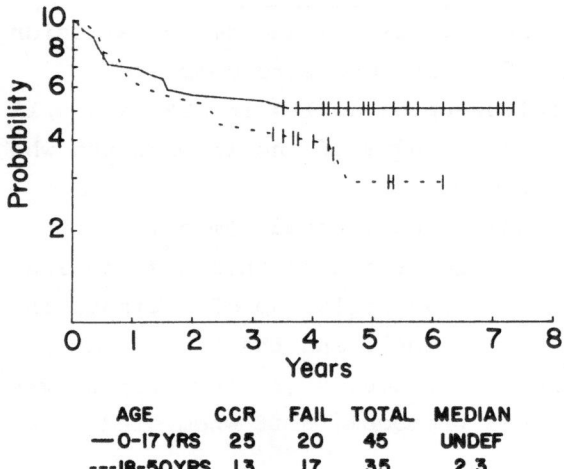

FIGURE 1. Kaplan-Meier analysis of continuous complete remission (CCR) - VAPA.

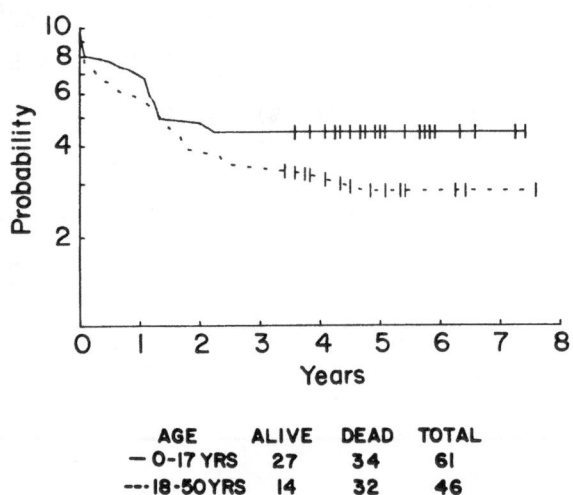

FIGURE 2. Kaplan-Meier analysis of survival for ALL patients entered on VAPA.

Toxicity

The major toxicities during the intensive post-remission induction chemotherapy phase were related to fever or infection associated with granulocytopenia, and cardiomyopathy secondary to anthracycline (adriamycin or daunorubicin) therapy. Four children and eight adults died in complete remission from infection or hemorrhage secondary to hematologic toxicity. A fifth child died from bronchiolitis 8 months after cessation of therapy and an adult suffered a fatal myocardial infarction during therapy.

During the initial year of the 80035 study, four children developed congestive heart failure (CHF) at cumulative daunorubicin doses ranging from 530 to 665 mg/m^2/d. The cumulative daunorubicin dose was subsequently reduced to 495 mg/m^2 and no additional cases of congestive heart failure have been observed. In the adult population one patient developed CHF.

There was often slow hematopoietic recovery following the daunorubicin and azacytidine courses (Sequence II). The interval between courses averaged 4-6 weeks (range, 3 - 9 weeks), and approximately one-third of patients received less than 3 courses of Sequence II.

DISCUSSION

The VAPA and 80035 protocols were designed to improve the duration of remission and overall survival for children and adults (less than 60 yrs of age) with AML. Both protocols included twelve to fourteen months of intensive sequential post-remission induction chemotherapy.

For adults between 18 and 50 years of age treated with VAPA the median relapse-free survival was 27 months and the 5 year CCR probability is 29 percent. In the pediatric age group, the probability of CCR is 50 percent at 5 years. Only two children relapsed between 2 and 7 years in remission. Follow-up of the VAPA study has demonstrated long-term relapse-free survival after therapy was stopped in the pediatric population but a continued risk of relapse in the adult age group.

The second generation AML clinical trial (80035) was designed to 1) increase the complete remission rate by doubling the remission induction dose of cytosine arabinoside, 2) increa the duration of hematologic remission by adding thioguanine to early and late intensification (Sequence I and III of 80035), and 3) reduce the incidence of primary CNS relapse in children by prophylactic administration of intrathecal cytosine arabinoside.

Our efforts to increase overall survival by a further intensification of therapy in the 80035 protocol led to an increased percentage of deaths in complete remission and no improvement in overall survival compared to the VAPA study. Prophylactic administration of intrathecal ara-c for patients less than 18 years reduced the incidence of primary CNS relapse but this did not result in an increase in overall relapse-free survival.

The results of VAPA and 80035 therapy for children with AML are superior to those obtained by using other chemotherapeutic regimens.[6,16] The only other therapy that appears to achieve comparable durations of remission for young patients with AML is supralethal chemoradiotherapy followed by bone marrow transplantation performed early in first remission. This approach is currently limited to patients with a histocompatible donor. Results of current transplant studies project 50-60% leukemia-free survival for young patients with AML transplanted in first remission.[9,17,18]

For adults between 18 and 60 years of age, the results of VAPA and 80035 are comparable to other chemotherapeutic regimens employing intensive consolidation with or without maintenance therapy.[2,3,19,20] It appears that approximately 25% of adult patients with AML who enter remission will achieve long-term relapse-free survival with intensive chemotherapy regimens. Results of current transplant studies project 30 to 50 percent survival for patients > 18 years of age with AML transplanted in first remission.[8,10] Marrow transplantation is currently limited to patients < 50 years of age with histocompatible donors.

Future progress awaits a careful examination of factors that affect duration of remission, better application of chemotherapeutic modalities, and prevention of transplant related complications such as graft-versus-host disease and interstitial pneumonia.

REFERENCES

1. Gale RPL. 1979. Advances in the treatment of acute
    myelogenous leukemia. N Engl J Med 300, 1189-1199.
2. Lister TA and Rohatiner A. 1982. The treatment of acute
    myelogenous leukemia in adults. Seminars in Hematology
    19, 172-192.
3. Clarkson BD, Dowling MO, Gee TS et al. 1975. Treatment of
    acute leukemia in adults. Cancer 36, 775-795.
4. Rai K, Holland J, Glidewell O et al. 1981. Treatment of
    acute myelocytic leukemia. A study by Cancer and
    Leukemia Group B. Blood 58, 1203-1212.
5. Lampkin B, Woods W, Strauss et al. 1983. Current status
    of the biology and treatment of acute non-lymphocytic
    leukemia in children (Report from the ANLL Strategy
    Group of the Children's Cancer Study Group). Blood 61,
    215-227.
6. Dahl G, Kalwinsky D, Murphy S et al. 1982. Cytokinetically
    based induction chemotherapy and splenectomy for childhood
    acute nonlymphocytic leukemia. Blood 60, 856-863.
7. Peterson B, Bloomfield C. 1981. Long-term disease free
    survival in acute nonlymphocytic leukemia. Blood 57,
    1144-1147.
8. Thomas ED, Clift R, Buckner C. 1982. Marrow transplantation
    for patients with acute nonlymphoblastic leukemia who
    achieve a first remission. Cancer Treatment Reports 66,
    1463-1466.
9. Kersey J, Ramsay N, Kim T et al. 1982. Allogeneic bone
    marrow transplantation in acute nonlymphocytic leukemia:
    A pilot study. Blood 60, 400-403.
10. Gale R, Kay H, Rimm A et al. 1982. Bone-marrow transplant-
    ation for acute leukemia in first remission. Lancet,
    1006-1008.
11. Champlin R, Zighelboim J, Ho W et al. 1983. Treatment of
    acute myelogenous leukemia (AML) - Bone marrow transplant-
    ation (BMT) versus consolidation chemotherapy. Proceedings
    Amer Soc. of Clin Oncol, abstract C-701, p. 180.
12. Appelbaum F, Cheever M, Fefer A et al. 1982. A prospective
    study of the value of maintenance therapy or bone marrow
    transplantation in adult acute nonlymphoblastic leukemia
    (ANL). Blood 60, p. 163a (abstract).
13. Sauter C, Barrelet L, Berchtold W et al. 1982. No
    advantage of maintenance treatment (M7) in acute myelo-
    genous leukemia after intensive early consolidation (EC).
    Proc Amer Soc Clin Oncol, abstract (C-497).
14. Weinstein H, Mayer R, Rosenthal D et al. 1980. Treatment
    of acute myelogenous leukemia in children and adults.
    N Engl J Med 303, 473-478.
15. Weinstein H, Mayer R, Rosenthal D et al. 1983. Chemotherapy
    for acute myelogenous leukemia in children and adults:
    VAPA update. Blood 62, 315-319.
16. Baehner R, Bernstein I, Sather H et al. 1979. Improved
    remission induction rate with D-ZAPO but unimproved
    remission duration with addition of immunotherapy to
    chemotherapy in previously untreated children with ANLL.
    Med Pediatr Oncol 7, 127.

17. Thomas ED. 1983. Marrow transplant for acute nonlympho-
    blastic leukemia in first remission: A follow-up.
    N Engl J Med 308, 1539-1540.
18. Forman S, Spruce W, Farbstein M et al. 1983. Bone marrow
    ablation followed by allogeneic marrow grafting during
    first complete remission of acute nonlymphocytic leukemia.
    Blood 61, 439-442.
19. Gale R, Foon F, Cline M et al. 1981. Intensive chemotherapy
    for acute myelogenous leukemia. Ann Intern Med 94, 753-
    757.
20. Preisler H, Rustum Y, Henderson E et al. 1979. Treatment
    of acute nonlymphocytic leukemia: Use of anthracycline-
    cytosine arabinoside induction therapy and a comparison
    of two maintenance regimens. Blood 53, 455-464.

REMISSION DURATION IN ACUTE NONLYMPHOCYTIC LEUKEMIA: PRACTICAL AND
THEORETICAL CONSIDERATIONS

H.D. Preisler, A. Raza, N. Azarnia, G. Browman

INTRODUCTION

As increasing numbers of patients with acute nonlymphocytic
leukemia (ANLL) have entered complete remission (CR) the major interest
of investigators has shifted from remission induction therapy to the
appropriate nature of therapy once a patient enters complete remission.
The purpose of this paper is to review studies carried out at Roswell
Park and at collaborating institutions which may shed some light on the
effects of different kinds of chemotherapy on remission duration and on
the factors which determine remission duration.

Post Induction Regimens Employed at Roswell Park: None to 5 years of
Maintenance Therapy to 4 Courses of Intensive Consolidation Therapy

From 1975 to the present time, 3 different treatment protocols
have been employed. While all have utilized cytosine arabinoside
(araC)/ anthracycline remission induction therapy (1-3), the therapy
administered to patients who entered CR has undergone a profound
change. The treatment regimens are described in Figure I. Protocol
950501 provided for 2 courses of modest consolidation therapy (white
blood cell count and platelet count nadirs of approximately 1000/ul and
50-70,000/ul respectively for <1 week's time) followed by 5 years of
maintenance therapy. Protocol 970701 (utilized at RPMI and the Ontario
Cancer Foundation) provided for 3 courses of intensive consolidation
chemotherapy (WBC and platelet nadirs of <500/ul and <30,000/ul
respectively for 7-10 days) followed by 3 years of maintenance therapy
while Protocol P 998028 utilized at RPMI, OCF, University of Chicago,
and Tufts New England Medical Center) provides for 4 courses of
intensive consolidation therapy and no further therapy (WBC and
platelet counts to <500/ul and <20,000/ul for 10-14 days).

The remission duration curves for these 3 successive studies are
provided in Figure II together with a curve for 18 patients who
received either only maintenance therapy after entering CR or who
received no therapy at all. Inspection of these curves demonstrates
that as the aggressiveness of the consolidation regimen increases there
appears to be an increase in the median duration of remission (MDR) and
in the percent of patients in remission at 4 years. The MDR for the no
consolidation patients was 7 months, for P950501 it was 16 months,
while for P70701 and P998028 it was 25 and 27 months respectively.
The percent of patients in CR at 4 yrs for the "no consolidation" is
9%, while for P950501 and P970701 it is 18% and 30% respectively.
P998028 has been in use for too short a period of time to give a
reliable 4 year projection.

Inspection of the curves in Figure II suggests that when the
conventional approach to therapy is employed, relapses begin almost
immediately after CR is induced and is a continuous process. For the

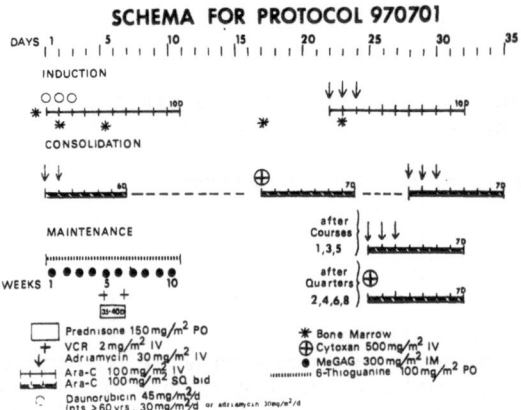

Figures I a - c: Chemotherapeutic Regimens
Figure Ia: Protocol 950501

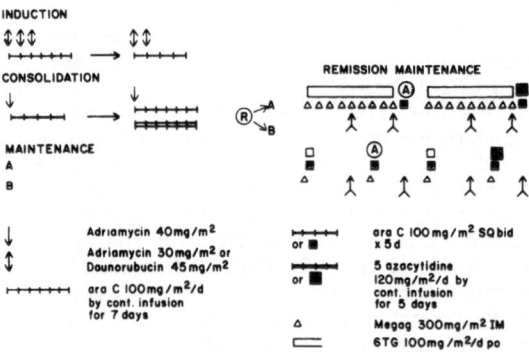

Figure Ib: Protocol 970701

SCHEMA FOR PROTOCOL P998028

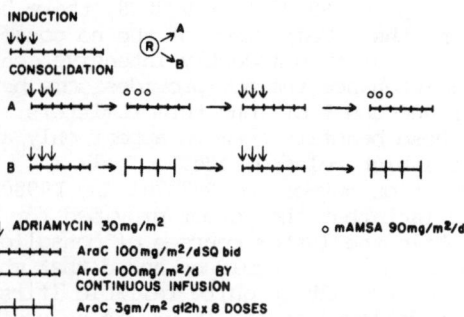

Figure Ic: Protocol 998028

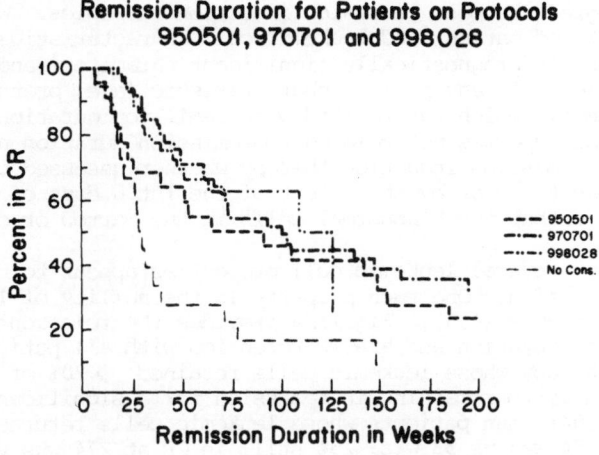

Figure II: Remission Durations
          The final fall in each curve indicates the last relapse
          The curve for the "no consolidation" patients should be
          extended paralled to the abscissa through week # 200

no consolidation patients and the patients treated on P950501 there
were 10 relapses in the 1st 5 months among 39 patients at risk. In
contrast, among the over 100 patients at risk who received intensive
consolidation chemotherapy on P979701 or 998028, there has been only 1
relapse in the 1st 5 months. Comparison of the no consolidation and
P950501 curves suggests that even modestly intensive consolidation
therapy followed by maintenance therapy provides some benefit in terms
of increasing the MDR and the % of long-term remitters. Of interest is
the suggestion that these benefits seem to appear only after at 6
months after an initial high relapse rate.

The remission duration curves for P970701 and P998028 appear to be
identical despite the fact that the former provided for 3 years of
maintenance therapy while the latter courses of consolidation therapy
are completed by 4-6 months. It should be noted that while the early
portion of the curve for P998028 is quite reliable (first 1-1½ yrs), too
few patients have been followed beyond 1½ yrs to be confident about the
configuration of the curve beyond that point.

Identification of Factors which are of Prognostic Significance with Respect to Remission Duration

When all ANLL patients are considered together aggressive
consolidation chemotherapy or allogeneic bone marrow transplantation
appear to offer advantages over conventional maintenance therapy.
Consideration of the fact that 20% of patients receiving maintenance
therapy are still in remission at 5 years suggests that this latter
subset of patients should not be exposed to the life threatening risks
of these two aggressive post remission induction therapies. We have
studied a variety of patient and leukemic cell characteristics in our
attempts to identify prognostically significant parameters and have not
been unable to identify any patient characteristic (age, pretherapy LDH
or fibrinogen level) which was related with remission duration.
Leukemic cell FAB type was not related to remission duration nor was
the response to remission induction therapy whether assessed by the
number of courses to CR or by the effect of the 1st 6 days of
chemotherapy on either the % abnormal cells in the marrow or on marrow
cellularity.

In contrast, several leukemic cell properties appear to be related
to length of remission. One such property is the ability of leukemic
cells to retain araCTP (4,5). Fig IIIa provides the relationship
between remission duration and araCTP retention with all patients
regardless of therapy whose leukemic cells retained > 20% of the
araCTP formed in vitro remaining in remission for a significantly
longer time (p=.04) than patients whose leukemic cells returned araCTP
less well (MDR 154 wks vs 53 wks; 25% still in CR at 274 wks vs 126 wks
respectively). Fig III b-d which provide these data by protocol,
suggest that as consolidation therapy becomes more aggressive, the
prognostic significance of araCTP retention declines. When patients
from P950501 and P970701 are compared, the curves for relapse rate
during the 1st 2 years of remission for patients with araCTP retention
>20% are virtually identical while aggressive consolidation therapy of
P970701 appears to benefit patients who leukemic cells retained araCTP
poorly. There have been too few relapses to date to assess the actual
relationship between araCTP metabolism and remission duration for
P998028.

The ability of leukemic cells to produce clusters or colonies in
vitro also appears to be related to remission duration (6). Fig IV a-c
provides these data for pooled P970701 and P998028 patients and for

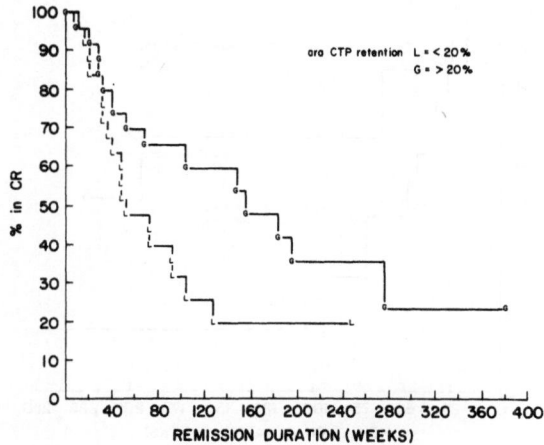

Figures III a - d: Relationship Between Remission Duration and
Leukemic Cell Retention of AraCTP
Figure III a: Pooled data for patients treated on P950501,
P970701, and P998028

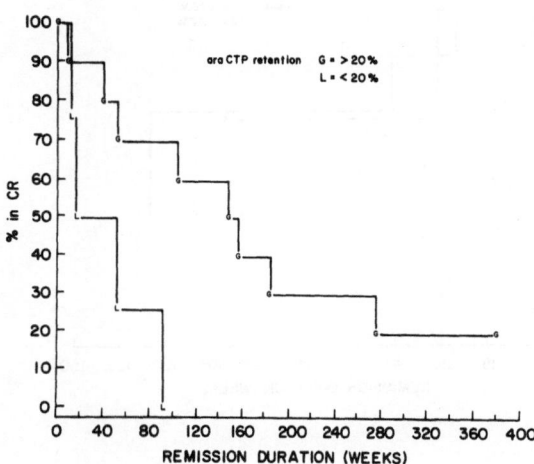

Figure III b: Data for patients treated on P950501

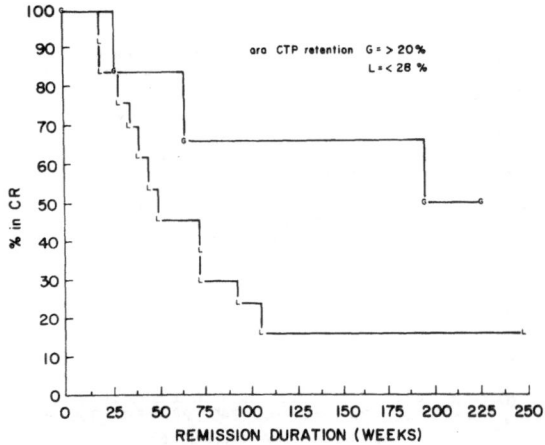

Figure IIIc: Data for patients treated on P970701 (note error in figure L = 20%)

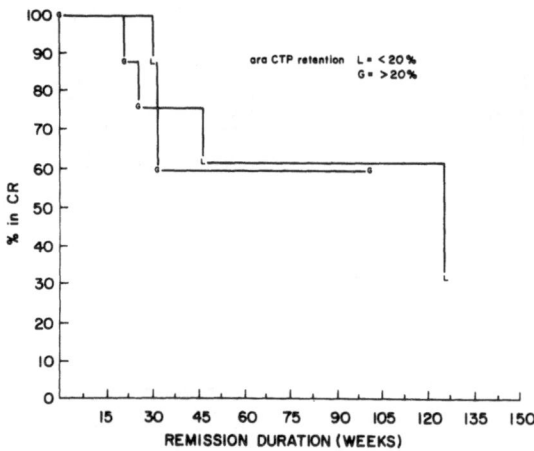

Figure IIId: Data for patients being treated on P998023

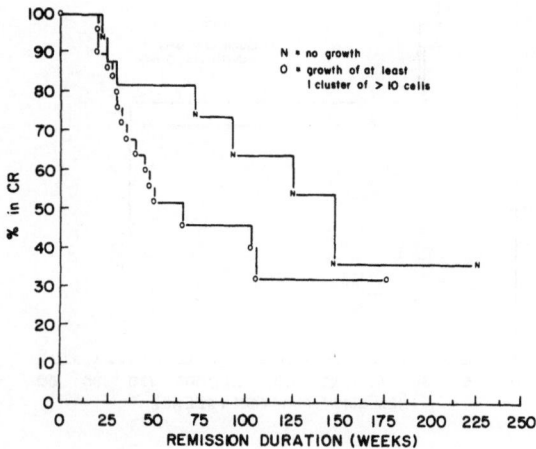

Figures IV a - c: Relationship Between Leukemic Cell Growth
                  Characteristics in Vitro and Remission Duration
Figure IVa: Pooled data for patients treated on P970701 and
            P998028

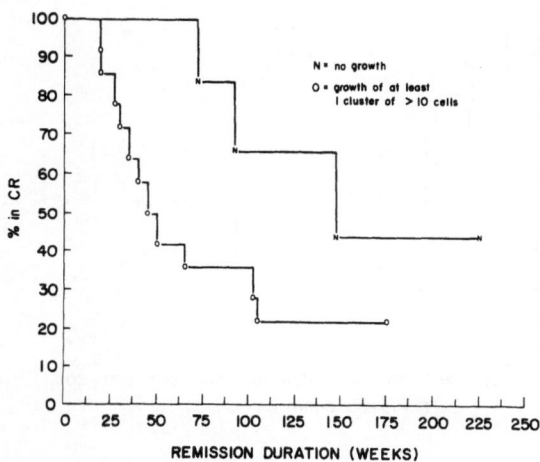

Figure IVb: Data for patients treated on P970701

366

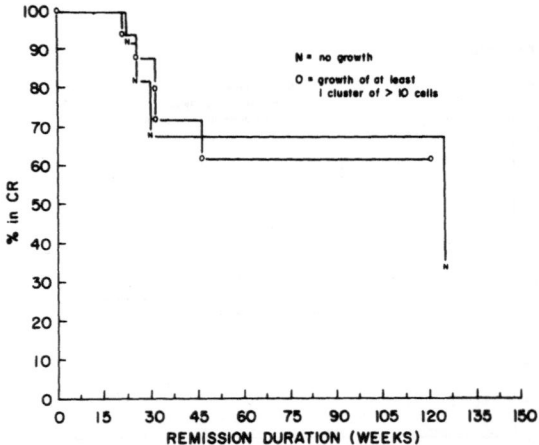

Figure IVc: Data for patients treated on P998028

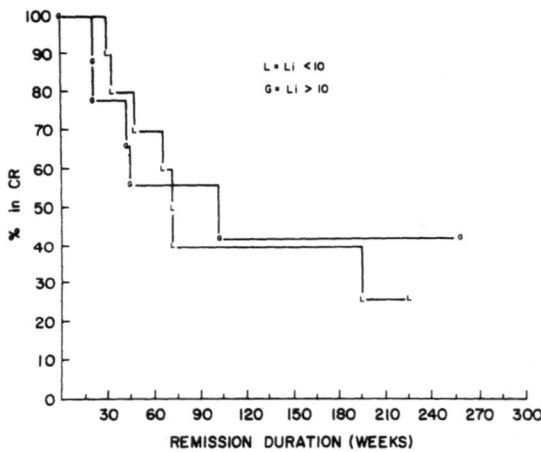

Figures V a - b: Relationship between Leukemic cell [3]HTdR
                 Labeling Index (Li) and Remission Duration
Figure Va: Patients treated on P970701

patients treated on each protocol. For the pooled patients, the MDR for the 21 patients whose cells failed to clone in vitro was 147 weeks while for patients whose marrow cells produced at least one cluster consisting of >10 cells the MDR was 66 weeks (p=.18). As with the araCTP measurement, this parameter appears to have lost its potential prognostic significance for patients treated on the current protocol (P998028).

Figure V a,b provide data relating the pretherapy ^{3}HTdR labelling index (Li) and remission duration for patients treated in P970701 and P998028. There was no difference in remission duration between patients whose leukemic cell Li was high or low for patients treated on P970701 while a trend may be emerging for patients treated on P998028 with lower Li being associated with longer remission durations.

Figure VI presents the data relating cytogenetic type (7,8) to remission duration. For the 89 patients studied (Fig IVa), the NN group had an apparent advantage over patients in whom any abnormal clones were detected (MDR 129 vs 73 weeks respectively) (p=.287). For the comparison of NN vs NA this difference approached a level of statistical significance (p=.09) (Fig VIb). Fig VIc-e demonstrate that the relationship between cytogenetic studies and remission duration was protocol dependent in that no relationship existed for patients treated on P970701 while it was statistically significant for the NN vs NA and NN vs AA comparison for P998028 treated patients. This analysis was performed using conventional methods and patients with abnormal clones were pooled into one or two groups (NA vs AA). As more detailed analyses are performed differences in the prognostic significance of different cytogenetic abnormalities undoubtedly will be recognized. For example, the presence of a Ph^1 chromosome confers an extremely poor prognosis in ANLL with respect to both the outcome of remission induction therapy and remission duration because it is associated with drug resistant leukemia (9). Cytogenetic studies after a patient enters remission also appears to be useful for establishing a patient's prognosis since in our experience patients who are in an apparent complete remisison but in whom even a single abnormal metaphase is detected appear to relapse quite promptly.

Taken together these data are of interest for they demonstrate, as might have been expected, that the properties of the leukemic cells per se play a role in determining the duration of remission. The prognostic significance of the various leukemic cell properties appear to be dependent on the therapy being administered. This is understandable in the sense that as therapy becomes more aggressive some leukemic cell properties will decline in significance while as therapy becomes shorter in duration other properties may increase in significance. The disconcerting aspects of these studies are the fact that when the pooled data are considered (Fig IIIa, IVa, VIa) it seems that there is essentially no difference in the percent of patients in long term remissions between the good and poor prognostic categories. It is possible that these negative tentative conclusions are incorrect and that with longer follow-up time for the individual protocols or that by the use of multivariate analysis patient groups with quite different long-term prognoses may be identifiable. On the other hand the phenomenon of early relapse may be different than late relapse with the latter being unaffected by factors which are prognostic for the former (and hence early relapse may be overcome by strategies which do not effect the late relapse component).

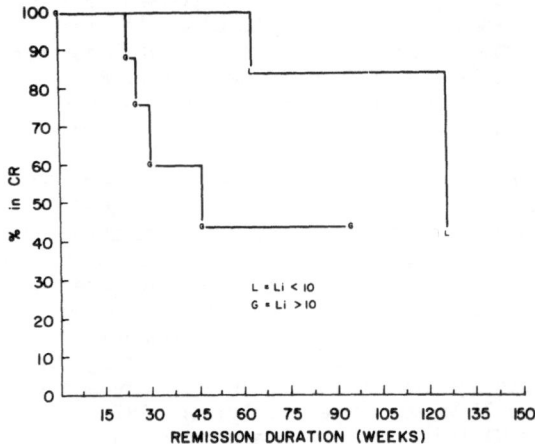

Figure Vb: Patients treated on P998028

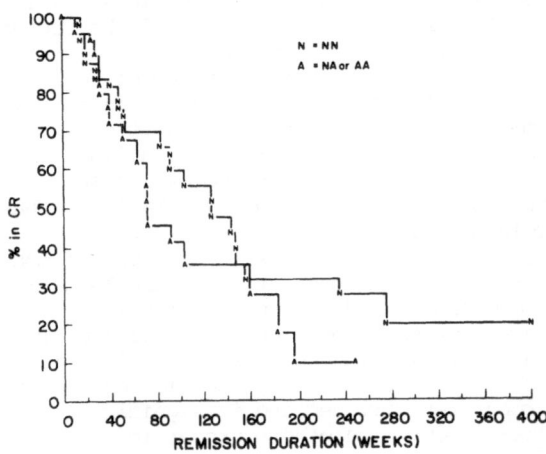

Figures VI a - e: Relationship Between Pretherapy Marrow
                  Cytogenetic Type and Remission Duration
Figure VIa: Pooled data for patients treated on P970701 and
            P998028 with respect to patients in whom only
            normal metaphases were detected vs patients in
            whom any abnormal clones were detected

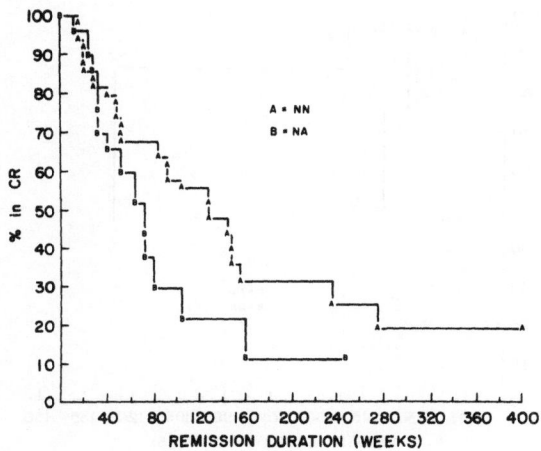

Figure VIb: Similar to "a" above but the comparison as between
patients with only normal metaphases and those
whose marrow cells contained both normal and abnormal
metaphases

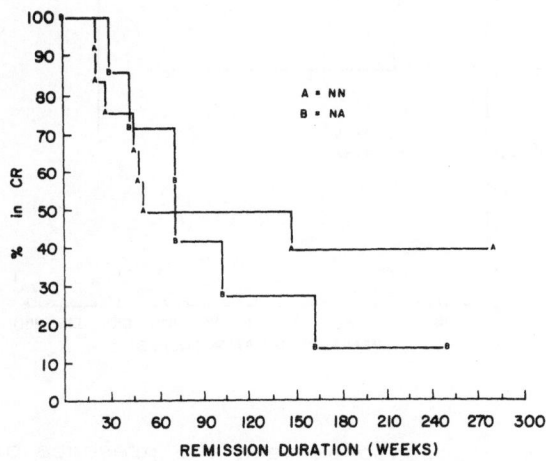

Figure VIc: Data for relationship between cytogenetic type and
remission duration for patients treated on P970701

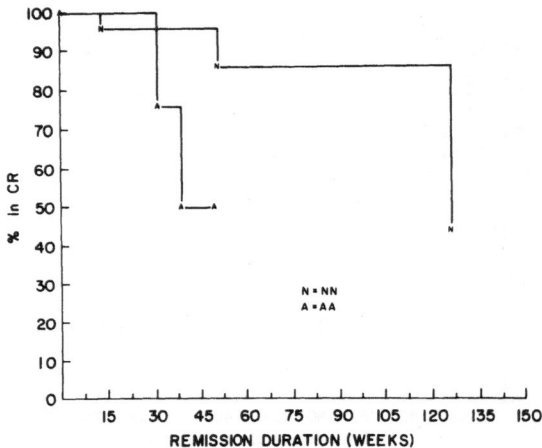

Figure VId: Relationship between the presence of only normal and mixed normal and abnormal metaphases and remission duration for patients treated on P998028) **p** = .04)

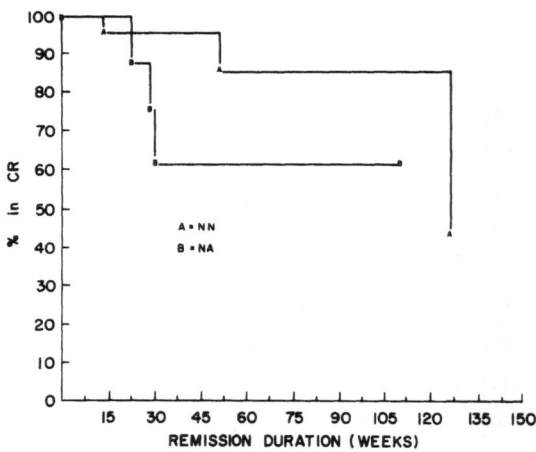

Figure VIe: Relationship between the presence of normal and only abnormal metaphases and remission duration and remission duration for patients treated on **P998028** (p = .04)

Detailed Analysis of RPMI Protocols

The remission duration data provided in Figure II are presented in a conventional manner in that data from all patients who received even one dose of consolidation/maintenance therapy are represented on the curves. This manner of data representation is appropriate if one only wants to evaluate a regimen "overall" - i.e. in terms of its "tolerability" and antileukemic efficacy. However "tolerability" depends in part on the promised benefits of therapy in that both patients and physicians are more willing to receive and administer toxic therapy if a "cure" is promised. This is well illustrated by the large numbers of patients who seek allogeneic marrow transplantation and the large numbers of investigators who are setting up transplant units despite the fact that 50% of patients transplanted in 1st remission expire in remission (10). Therefore it is also important to evaluate the antileukemic efficacy of the regimens per se, a process which can be performed only if one also analyzes the remission durations of patients who actually received the prescribed therapy excluding from analysis of those patients who were not given the therapy for reasons other than leukemic relapse or failure of the marrow to recover from the effects of chemotherapy.

The P998028 remission duration curve actually represents the clinical course of 3 different groups of patients: those treated as prescribed by the protocol, those who received fewer than 4 consolidations for reasons other than leukemic relapse or failure of the marrow to recover after a course of therapy, and those patients who received the proper number of courses but who had significant dosage de-escalations ($>$ 25%) or whose therapy was delayed ($>$ 2 weeks after the peripheral blood counts returned to normal) for reasons other than failure of the peripheral blood counts to return to normal after the previous course of therapy. These two groups of protocol violators include patients who had infections during prior courses of therapy, patients or physicians who decided the risk of therapy wasn't commensurate with the potential benefit, etc. The data presented in Fig VIIa compares the remission durations of patients who received only 1 or 2 courses of consolidation therapy with patients who received all 4 courses. Similarily Fig VIIb compares the remission durations for non-violators with that of patients who had a dosage reduction or significant delay in 1 or more courses of therapy. In each situation the patients who were treated with less than the prescribed therapy did significantly worse than those that received the prescribed therapy. Hence, while the data in Figure II for P998028 are quite good they are actually misleading with respect to the actual antileukemic efficacy of the regimen. It should be emphasized that the failure of patients to be treated as prescribed by the protocol was, as far as we could tell, in no way related to early recurrent leukemia.

A slightly different but in some ways similar observation is provided in Fig VIIc. Protocol 970701 provided for the araC of consolidation course #3 to be given by continuous infusion. For approximately half of the patients the araC was given subcutaneously twice a day instead. The remission durations of these two groups of patients are clearly different. The difference is consistent with the differences in plasma araC levels when the drug is administered by these two different routes (11). Hence, what appeared at the time to be a minor protocol violation apparently produced marked negative effects.

In reviewing reports in the literature to evaluate the effects of "consolidation" and "maintenance" therapy one cannot depend upon the authors descriptions since one man's "consolidation therapy" may be another man's "maintenance therapy"(12,13). "Consolidation therapy" should mean courses of therapy designed to produce a significant reduction in residual leukemic cell numbers. "Maintenance therapy" should be defined as therapy whose goal is to prevent the regrowth of leukemic cells. Given the nature of the currently available chemotherapeutic agents "consolidation therapy" should be associated with pancytopenia. The depth and duration of which should vary with the aggressiveness of the regimen. The depth and duration of pancytopenia produced by a course of therapy, however, is not necessarily an indication of the therapeutic efficacy of the regimen since agents with poor antileukemic effectiveness may nevertheless produce severe pancytopenia. On the other hand, maintenance therapy should be associated with minimal degrees of pancytopenia. Clearly the line between non-aggressive "consolidation therapy" and "maintenance therapy" is rather indistinct. To evaluate and compare different regimens, information must be provided by the authors regarding the length and duration of cytopenias produced by therapy, how many times and how frequently these were produced together with the nature of the drugs administered so one can evaluate the potential antileukemic efficacy of the therapy. Needless to say, information on patient compliance is also essential. Unfortunately this information is rarely provided.

Leukemic relapse is assumed to be due to the regrowth of leukemic cells because of resistance to the therapy being administered. While this statement may be generally correct it is an over simplification since resistance to the therapy being administered is not necessarily synonymous with leukemic cell resistance to the chemotherapeutic agents (14). The effect of chemotherapy is the net result of two opposing phenomena: The reduction in leukemic cell mass produced by the chemotherapy and the regrowth of leukemic cells between courses of therapy. Hence, leukemic relapse can occur in patients whose disease is drug sensitive if the doses of drugs which are administered are too low since sub-optimal killing of leukemic cells will occur. This fact provides the best rationale for employing intensive consolidation therapy. Since we know that one or two courses of remission induction therapy are required for a CR to be induced (with a 2 or more log reduction in leukemic cell mass) why should one believe that "consolidation therapy" which is less aggressive than this will produce a significant reduction in residual leukemic cell mass when such less aggressive therapy fails to produce enough reduction in leukemic cell mass to produce a CR. Inadequate therapy may also be administered even if dosage reductions are not effected since it is possible that repeated courses of chemotherapeutic agents may result in progressively lower plasma drug levels and thus ineffective therapy (15). Furthermore, if the time interval between courses of therapy is too great, regrowth of leukemic cells in the non-therapy interval will negate much or all of the effects of chemotherapy.

The frequency of relapse resulting from actual leukemic cell drug resistance is unknown. This fact makes it unwise to study patients in 1st relapse with the assumption that any regimen which induces a CR is by definition non-cross resistant with the regimen with which the patient had been treated in the past. Responses to new regimens in this situation could be associated with a cross-resistant regimen if relapse had occurred for any of the reasons discussed above other than leukemic cell resistance to the agents which had been administered.

Theoretical Considerations. The Phenomenon of Leukemic Relapse

A review of 697 patients who entered remission on CALGB protocols between 1974 and 1979 and who received conventional maintenance therapy demonstrated a median duration of remission of 13 months with 20% of patients remaining in remission at 6 years (16). There are several points of particular interest. There is no evidence of a "plateau" even at 6 years and if the curve is extended only 1% of patients would be expected to be in remission at 10 years. The remission duration curve has 2 different slopes: A high early relapse rate of (slope of the relapse curve on semilog paper = 0.54 ± 0.3) from the time the patient enters CR until year 2 and then a much lower relapse rate of 0.2 ± .02 extending from year two to at least year 6. Several implications can be drawn from this curve. Unfortunately there is no evidence of cure being assoicated with conventional therapy and therefore, the frequently reported "plateaus" may simply be a reflection of the small numbers of patients who have been followed in remission for more than 4 years. The two component aspect of the curve is of special interest since it suggests that early and late leukemic relapses may be distinct biological phenomena. This observation is compatible with the inferences drawn from our studies of leukemic cell prognostic factors. It is also likely that the 2nd relapse component is probably also operative early in remission but it is masked by the high early relapse rate. Additionally the existence of very gradual late relapse rate makes the interpretation of the efficacy of intensive consolidation therapies (either chemotherapy or transplantation) quite difficult since a therapy which supresses only the 1st and rapid early relapse component and which does not affect the 2nd component of the relapse curve might appear to be curative since the slow rate of relapse during the 2nd portion of the curve would require hundreds of patients to be recognized.

It would seem logical that the early relapse phase would be due to regrowth of the same cells which were present at diagnosis; relapse due to the overgrowth of drug resistant cells, regrowth of drug sensitive cells because cytotoxic therapy has had too little effect in the marrow. Very little is known about the 2nd component of the curve. Late relapses could in fact be not relapses but rather new leukemias in are already predisposed patients who received carcinogenic agents during the therapy of their earlier leukemia. The precedent has already been established for the occurrences of new leukemias in recipients of bone marrow allografts (17). Among our relapsed patients, it appears that late relapses are more frequently associated with an extramedullary site than are early relapses (Table I). It is

TABLE I

SITE OF INITIAL RELAPSE IN ANLL

Years in Remission	Site of Relapse
1 year	BM-23; CNS-1
1-2 years	BM-13; CNS-2
2-3 years	BM- 7; CNS-4
3-4 years	BM- 2
4 years	BM- 1; skin-2

.1 patients entered CR before 1980

possible that at least some late relapses begin in sanctuary sites which subsequently involve the hematopoietic system. In the few patients that we've seen with primary relapse in the skin, electron beam therapy has been quite effective. It would seem logical that solitary relapse in the skin should be treated with this therapeutic modality followed by several courses in intensive consolidation therapy to deal with potential seeding of the marrow by the leukemia cutis cells.

Since the overall incidence of CNS relapse is low prophylactic therapy is probably not indicated (except perhaps in FAB M5). We currently perform lumbar punctures when a patient enters CR and then yearly thereafter. We have detected two early CNS relapses and treated these vigorously with intra-Ommaya therapy and systemically administered high dose araC therapy. Both patients have been off all therapy for several years with no evidence of recurrent leukemia. In fact, the use of high dose araC in consolidation chemotherapy could serve as CNS prophylaxis as well since the high CSF araC levels which are produced are therapeutically effective (18).

Finally, the slow late relapse component could be due to a process which is akin to blastic transformation of CML. We have treated several patients for ANLL which evolved from a preleukemic state. In some, the ANLL disappeared and the previously existent preleukemic state reappeared. It is possible that in some patients with "spontaneous" ANLL chemotherapy simply supresses the new leukemic clones and re-establishes a currently unrecognizable "preleukemic" state. Such a state could be characterized by the apparently normal differentiation of the abnormal cells. In time "blastic transformation" could occur with a loss of the ability of the abnormal cells to differentiation. The biological and therapeutic implications of this state would be different from that in which the appearance of a truly new leukemia is the cause of relapse.

Comments on Therapeutic Strategy for Patients who Enter CR

The data presented here demonstrate that when conventional maintenance therapy is utilized there is no evidence at present of leukemic cure. Whether the same is true when intensive consolidation therapy is employed is unknown. A good case can be made for the use of such intensive consolidations and for the administrations of full doses of therapy 1 week after the peripheral blood counts to return to normal since compromises in dosages or time of administration or in the number of courses were all associated with early relapse. Theoretically, non-cross resistant drug combinations should be employed. The optimal number of courses which should be administered is unknown but it seem that most patients require at least 4 courses of therapy.

Much has been made of the alleged superiority of allogeneic bone marrow transplantation in 1st remission over chemotherapy. When examined closely the following can be said of marrow allografts: for patients under 20 years of age allografting in 1st remission using HLA compatible marrow appears to be superior to conventional chemotherapy. On the other hand there is no apparent advantage to allograft patients less than 20 y.o. as compared to the administration of aggressive chemotherapy since the 1st 3 year curves are essentially identical (12,19,20). With respect to older patients between 30 and 50 y.o. conventional maintenance therapy provides a 3 times longer median duration of survival and at least equivalent 5 year survival (10,16,21).

A neglected aspect of the usual comparisons made between transplantation and chemotherapy relates to the fact that "apples and oranges" are being compared since the aggressiveness of transplantation is at least an order of magnitude greater than that of the chemotherapeutic regimens currently in use. Inspection of the survival curves of patients allografted in 1st remission demonstrates that 25% of patients < 20 y.o. die from toxicity, 50% of patients between 20 and 30 y.o. die, and 70% of patients between 30 and 50 years of age die from the therapy. Clearly there is no chemotherapeutic regimen in use which produces remission mortality rate which even approaches that of the transplant regimens. Unless the efficacy of chemotherapeutic regimens of comparable aggressiveness to transplantation are evaluated no conclusions can be drawn regarding the relative efficacy of these two treatment modalities. Hence the statements regarding the superiority of transplantation over chemotherapy per se are at present without foundation and the only statement which at present can be made is that as noted above, for patients < 20 y.o. transplantation appears to be superior to conventional chemotherapy.

NN = marrow contains only normal metaphases using conventional methods
NA = marrow contains both normal and abnormal metaphases of a clonal nature
AA = marrow contains only abnormal clones
See references 7 and 8 for precise definitions

REFERENCES

1. Preisler, H.D., Bjornsson, S., Henderson, E.S., et al: Treatment of Acute Nonlymphocytic Leukemia: Use of Anthracycline/Cytosine Arabinoside Induction Therapy and a Comparison of Two Maintenance Regimens. Blood 53(3):455-464, 1979.

2. Preisler, H.D., Bjornsson, S., Henderson, E.S., Hyrniuk, W. and Higby, D.: Remission Induction in Acute Nonlymphocytic Leukemia: Comparison of a 7-Day and 10-Day Infusion of Cytosine Arabinoside in Combination with Adriamycin. Med Ped Onc, 7:269-275, 1979.

3. Preisler, H.D., Brecher, M., Browman, G., Early, A.P., Walker, I.R., Raza, A., and Freeman, A: The Treatment of Acute Myelocytic Leukemia in Patients 30 Years of Age and Younger. Am J Hemat 13(3):189-198, 1982.

4. Rustum, Y.M. and Preisler, H.D.: Correlation Between Leukemic Cell Retention of 1-B-D Arabinosylcytosine-5'-Triphosphate and Response to Therapy. Cancer Res 39:42-49, 1979.

5. Preisler, H.D., Rustum, Y., Priore, R.: Relationship Between Leukemic Cell Metabolism of Cytosine Arabinoside and the Outcome of Chemotherapy for Acute Nonlymphocytic Leukemia. Submitted to Journal of Clinical Oncology, October, 1983.

6. Preisler, H.D., Azarnia, N., Marinello, M.J.: Growth of Leukemic Cells in Vitro: Relationship to Patient and Leukemic Cell Characteristics and to Outcome of Therapy. Cancer Res, in press, 1983.

7. Sakurai, M. & Sandberg, A.: Prognosis of Acute Myeloblastic Leukemia - Chromosomal Correlation. Blood 41:93-104.

8. Preisler, H.D., Reese, P.A., Marinello, M.J. Pothier, L: Adverse Effects of Aneuploidy on the Outcome of Remission Induction Therapy for Acute Nonlymphocytic Leukemia: Analysis of Types of Treatment Failure. Br J of Haemat 53(3):459-466, 1983.

9. Raza, A., Minowada, J., Barcos, M., Rakowski, I., and Preisler, H.D.: Ph[1] Positive Acute Leukemia. Submitted to Journal of Clinical Oncology, July, 1983.

10. Thomas, E.D.: Marrow Transplantation for Malignant Diseases. Journal of Clinical Oncology 1:517-531, 1983.

11. Slevin, M.L., Prall, E.M., Aherne, G.W., et al: The Pharmacokinetics of Cytosine Arabinoside in the Plasma and Cerebrospinal Fluid During Conventional and High-Dose Therapy. Med Ped Oncol Suppl 1:157-166, 1982.

12. Preisler, H.D.: Therapy for Patients With Acute Myelocytic Leukemia Who Enter Remission: Bone Marrow Transplantation or Chemotherapy? Cancer Treat Rep 66(7):1467-1473, 1982.

13. Preisler, H.D.: Evaluation of Consolidation Chemotherapy. Cancer Treat Rep 67:203-204, 1983.

14. Preisler, H.D.: Treatment Failure in AML. Blood Cells 8:585-602, 1982.

15. Gessner, T., Robert, J., Bolanowska, W., Hoern, B., Durand, M., Preisler, H.D. and Rustum, Y.M.: Effects of Prior Therapy on Plasma Levels of Adriamycin During Subsequent Therapy. J Med 12:183-193, 1981.

16. Preisler, H., Anderson, K., Rai, K., Cuttner, J., and Yates, J: Comparison of Survival of Patients (PTS) with Acute Nonlymphocytic Leukemia (ANLL) Receiving Maintenance Chemotherapy (CHEMO RX) or Marrow Transplantation (TX) in 1st Remission. Abstracts of ASCO, May 22-24, 1983, San Diego, CA.

17. Fialkow, P.J., Thomas, E.D., Bryant, J.I., et al: Leukaemic Transformation of Engrafted Human Marrow Cells in Vivo. Lancet 1:251–255, 1971.
18. Early, A.P., Preisler, H.D., Slocum, S., and Rustum, Y.M.: A Pilot Study of High Dose 1-B-arabinofuranosylcytosine for Acute Leukemia and Refractory Lymphoma: Clinical Response and Pharmacology. Cancer Res 42:1587–1594, 1982.
19. Mayer, R.J., Weinstein, H.J., Coral, F.S., et al: The Role of Intensive Postinduction Chemotherapy in the Management of Patients with Acute Myelogenous Leukemia. Cancer Treat Rep 66:1455–1462, 1982.
20. Weinstein, H.J., Mayer, R.J., Rosenthal, D.S., et al: Chemotherapy of Acute Myelogeneous Leukemia in Children and Adults: VAPA update. Blood 62:315–319, 1983.
21. Preisler, H.D. Bone Marrow Transplantation for Adults Over 30 years of Age with Acute Nonlymphocytic Leukemia (ANLL). Recent Results in Cancer Research, Chpt 24, 127–128, 1983.

rant Support – CA 5034, Intergroup Grant CA 28734-02

he authors would like to greatfully acknowledge the contributions of the ouse officers and nurses at their Institutions without whose assistance hese studies would not have been possible. We would also like to cknowledge the contribution of the many private physicians who referred atients to our Institutions or who used these protocols as a guide in reating their patients.

MARROW TRANSPLANTATION VERSUS CHEMOTHERAPY FOR ACUTE LEUKEMIA

E. DONNALL THOMAS, M.D.

It has long been recognized that a prospective study would be necessary in order to compare the results of therpay of acute leukemia by
chemotherapy to the results of therapy including bone marrow transplantation. Such a study was started with patients with newly diagnosed
acute nonlymphoblastic leukemia more than 6 years ago (1). Patients
under the age of 18 were not included in this study because they were
being entered in a Children's Cancer Study Group protocol. Patients
over the age of 50 were excluded because of our previous experience
indicating that older patients had a poor survival on very intensive
combination chemotherapy and because patients over the age of 50 were
excluded from marrow transplantation. One hundred eleven patients between the ages of 18 and 50 were treated with daunorubicin (70 mg/m^2 on
days 1-3) and cytosine arabinoside (100 mg/m^2 intravenously every 12
hours on days 1-9) along with 6-thioguanine and prednisone on days 1-9
and vincristine on days 1 and 9. Ninety patients (81%) achieved complete remission. Patients who did not have HLA-identical siblings were
continued on chemotherapy including two consolidation treatments and
intensification therapy at 6 and 12 months. Patients with HLA-identical siblings were offered marrow transplants after preparation with
cyclophosphamide, 60 mg/kg on each of 2 days, and 200 rad total body
irradiation on each of 6 days. Prognostic parameters, including age,
were equivalent in the two groups. Forty-five patients did not have
suitable donors and were treated with combination chemotherapy. Forty-
five patients did have HLA-identical siblings and were offered marrow
transplantation. Two patients who had matched siblings relapsed before

This investigation was supported by Grant CA 18029, awarded by the National Cancer Institute, DHHS. Dr. Thomas is the recipient of Research
Career Award AI 02425 from the National Institute of Allergy and Infectious Diseases.

transplant could be carried out and were transplanted in relapse. One died at day 100 and the other is living in remission 4 years after transplantation. Eleven patients with matched siblings declined transplants and were treated with chemotherapy. Ten of these patients subsequently died of leukemia and one continues in complete remission after 3 years.

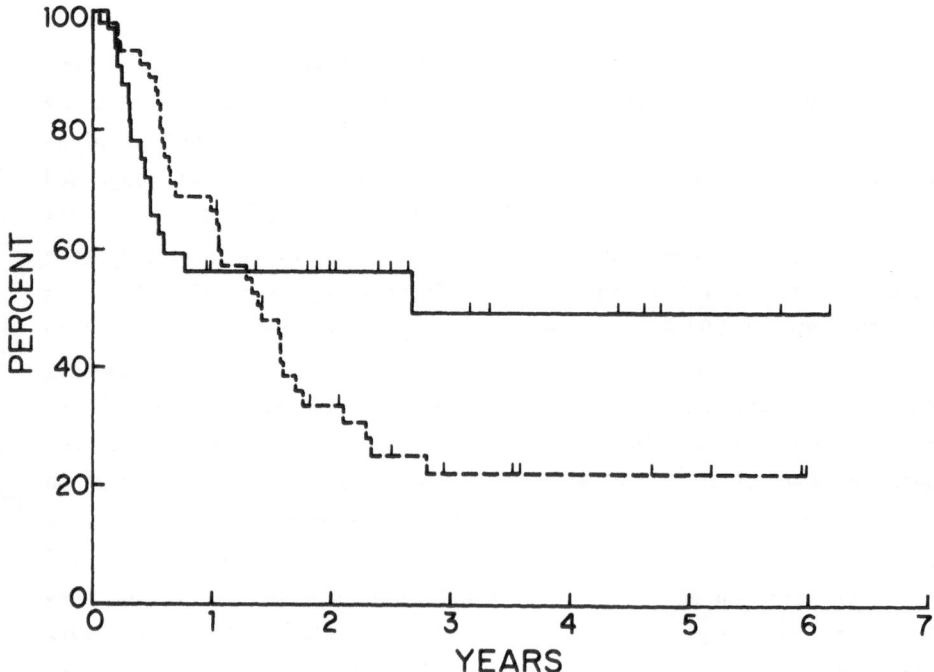

Figure 1. Kaplan-Meier product limit estimates of survival of patients treated with chemotherapy (dashed line) or with chemoradiotherapy and marrow grafting (solid line).

Figure 1 shows the actuarial analysis of survival for these two groups of patients. Thirty-three of 45 chemotherapy patients have died and 15 of 32 marrow transplant patients have died (p = 0.03). Figure 2 is an actuarial analysis of disease-free survival for the two groups (p = 0.006). Two of the patients treated with chemotherapy relapsed but are still living. It should be noted that all but two of the failures in the chemotherapy group were due to recurrence of leukemia while relapse of leukemia was seen in only four of the patients treated with

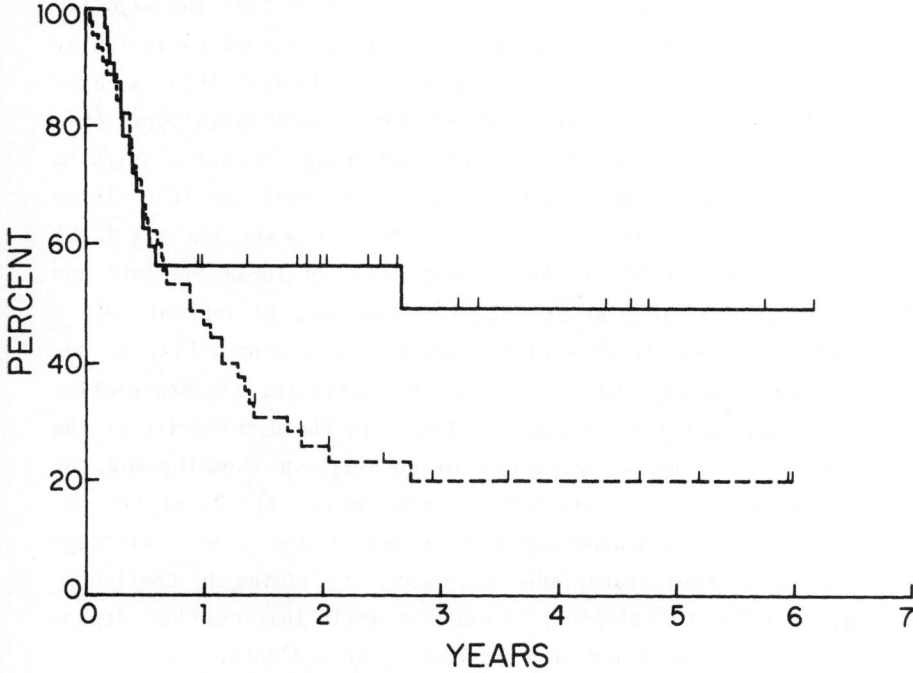

Figure 2. Kaplan-Meier product limit estimates of disease-free survival of patients treated with chemotherapy (dashed line) or with chemoradiotherapy and marrow grafting (solid line).

marrow transplantation. The causes of failure in the marrow transplant
group were related to interstitial pneumonia, opportunistic infections,
and graft-versus-host disease. This study and two similar comparisons
of chemotherapy with marrow grafting (2, 3) demonstrate clearly that
intensive chemoradiotherapy plus marrow grafting is by far the most
effective method of eliminating residual leukemic cells in patients
with acute nonlymphoblastic leukemia in remission. These three studies
also demonstrate a significant improvement in long-term survival with
marrow grafting, but one other reported comparison, with a relatively
short follow-up time, shows no differences in survival between patients
treated with chemotherapy and those given marrow grafts (4).

The eradication of minimal residual disease for patients with
acute lymphoblastic leukemia (ALL) who have relapsed at least once has
proved to be very difficult. Patients with ALL treated with combina-

tion chemotherapy who relapse are, in general, destined to die of recurrent leukemia. Several studies have demonstrated that the majority of these patients can be put into a second or subsequent remission by combination chemotherapy, but long-term survival is less than 5%, usually in patients who have relapsed after chemotherapy was stopped (5). We reported our initial studies of chemoradiotherapy in marrow grafting in 26 patients with ALL in second or subsequent remission (6). These patients have all been followed for more than 5 years and six (23%) appear to have been cured of the disease (7). In these patients and those in our subsequent studies (8, 9), recurrence of leukemia was a major problem with actuarial analyses indicating a probability of relapse for approximately two-thirds of the patients. A prospective study in one hospital (10) demonstrated clearly the superiority of the marrow grafting regimen as compared to combination chemotherapy for children with ALL who had relapsed at least once. All 21 of the patients treated with chemotherapy have relapsed and died. Although eight of the 24 marrow transplant recipients are living in continuous remission, 12 patients relapsed, indicating again that residual leukemic cells were not eliminated in the majority of patients.

Several marrow transplant teams are carrying out studies of poor-prognosis patients with ALL treated with marrow grafting in the first remission but, as yet, the number of patients is small and the follow-up interval is short.

As indicated by the above studies and by a much longer follow-up (now greater than 12 years) of earlier patients transplanted for acute leukemia in relapse who continue to be disese-free, leukemic cells can be eradicated in some patients (11). The mechanism, however, is not clear. The major assumption is that the "last" leukemic cell may be killed by the intensive chemoradiotherapy given before marrow grafting. The exponential cell kill by irradiation and by some chemotherapeutic agents such as alkylating agents (12, 13) as well as some in vivo experiments in animals (14) suggests that it may not be possible to kill the "last" leukemic cell by these modalities. We have reported a reduced rate of relapse of leukemia and an improved survival in patients who develop graft-versus-host disease, demonstrating the graft-versus-leukemia effect (15). Further, agents used to prevent or treat graft-versus-host disease (such as methotrexate and cyclophosphamide) might have an unexpectedly beneficial effect if only a few leukemic cells are left in the patient following marrow grafting. In one of our current protocols, we are attempting to create mild graft-versus-host disease in patients transplanted for ALL in relapse in an effort to take advantage of the graft-versus-leukemia effect. Several marrow transplant teams are investigating other preparative regimens designed to kill more of the residual leukemic cells by methods such as fractionated irradiation (16), high-dose cytosine arabinoside (17), and additional chemotherapy following marrow grafting (18). The results of these studies may prove to be particularly informative for all efforts to destroy residual leukemic cells whether with or without marrow transplantation.

REFERENCES

1. Appelbaum FR, Cheever MA, Fefer A, Greenberg PD, Glucksberg H, Buckner CD, Thomas ED. 1982. A prospective study of the value of maintenance therapy or bone marrow transplantation (BMT) in adult acute nonlymphoblastic leukemia (ANL). Blood 60 (suppl 1): 163a (abstract).
2. Powles RL, Morgenstern G, Clink HM, Hedley D, Bandini G, Lumley H, Watson JG, Lawson D, Spence D, Barrett A, Jameson B, Lawler S, Kay HEM, McElwain TJ. 1980. The place of bone-marrow transplantation in acute myelogenous leukaemia. Lancet i: 1047-1050.
3. Kersey JH, Ramsay NKC, Kim T, McGlave P, Krivit W, Levitt S, Filipovich A, Woods W, O'Leary M, Coccia P, Nesbit ME. 1982. Allogeneic bone marrow transplantation in acute nonlymphocytic leukemia: A pilot study. Blood 60: 400-403.
4. Gale RP for the Transplantation Biology Unit. 1981. A prospective controlled trial of bone marrow transplantation vs. chemotherapy in acute myelogenous leukemia. Blood 58 (suppl. 1): 173a (abstract #604).
5. Mauer AM. 1978. Treatment of acute leukaemia in children. Chapter 2 in: Clinics in Haematology, volume 7, edited by Simone JV. London, W.B. Saunders Co., Inc., pp. 245-258.
6. Thomas ED, Sanders JE, Flournoy N, Johnson FL, Buckner CD, Clift RA, Fefer A, Goodell BW, Storb R, Weiden PL. 1979. Marrow transplantation for patients with acute lymphoblastic leukemia in remission. Blood 54: 468-476.
7. Thomas ED, Sanders JE, Flournoy N, Johnson FL, Buckner CD, Clift RA, Fefer A, Goodell BW, Storb R, Weiden PL. 1983, in press. Marrow transplantation for patients with acute lymphoblastic leukemia: A long-term follow-up. Blood.
8. Clift RA, Buckner CD, Thomas ED, Sanders JE, Stewart PS, McGuffin R, Hersman J, Sullivan KM, Sale GE, Storb R. 1982. Allogeneic marrow transplantation for acute lymphoblastic leukemia in remission using fractionated total body irradiation. Leuk Res 6: 409-412.

9. Clift RA, Buckner CD, Thomas ED, Sanders JE, Stewart PS, Sullivan KM, McGuffin R, Hersman J, Sale GE, Storb R. 1982. Allogeneic marrow transplantation using fractionated total body irradiation in patients with acute lymphoblastic leukemia in relapse. Leuk Res 6: 401-407.

10. Johnson FL, Thomas ED, Clark BS, Chard RL, Hartmann JR, Storb R. 1981. A comparison of marrow transplantation to chemotherapy for children with acute lymphoblastic leukemia in second or subsequent remission. N Engl J Med 305: 846-851.

11. Thomas ED, Flournoy N, Buckner CD, Clift RA, Fefer A, Neiman PE, Storb R. 1977. Cure of leukemia by marrow transplantation. Leuk Res 1: 67-70.

12. Skipper HE, Perry S. 1970. Kinetics of normal and leukemic leukocyte populations and relevance to chemotherapy. Cancer Res 30: 1883-1897.

13. Bruce WR, Meeker BE, Valeriote FA. 1966. Comparison of the sensitivity of normal hematopoietic and transplanted lymphoma colony-forming cells to chemotherapeutic agents administered in vivo. J Natl Cancer Inst 37: 233-245.

14. Burchenal JH, Oettgen HF, Holmberg EAD, Hemphill SC, Reppert JA. 1960. Effect of total-body irradiation on the transplantability of mouse leukemias. Cancer Res 20: 425-430.

15. Weiden PL, Sullivan KM, Flournoy N, Storb R, Thomas ED, the Seattle Marrow Transplant Team. 1981. Antileukemic effect of chronic graft-versus-host disease. Contribution to improved survival after allogeneic marrow transplantation. N Engl J Med 304: 1529-1533.

16. Dinsmore R, Kirkpatrick D, Flomenberg N, Gulati S, Kapoor N, Shank B, Reid A, Groshen S, O'Reilly RJ. 1983. Allogeneic bone marrow transplantation for patients with acute lymphoblastic leukemia. Blood 62: 381-388.

17. Coccia PF, Strandjord SE, Gordon EM, Novak LF, Shina DC, Lazarus HM, Herzig RH. 1983. High dose cytosine arabinoside (Ara-C) and fractionated total body irradiation (F-TBI) as preparation for bone marrow transplantation (BMT) for childhood acute leukemia in remission--A preliminary report. Proceedings, American Society of Clinical Oncology, 19th Annual Meeting, May 22-24, 1983, San Diego, California, p. 175 (abstract #C-680).

18. Woods WG, Nesbit ME, Ramsay NKC, Krivit W, Kim TH, Goldman A, McGlave PB, Kersey JH. 1983. Intensive therapy followed by bone marrow transplantation for patients with acute lymphocytic leukemia in second or subsequent remission: Determination of prognostic factors (a report from the University of Minnesota Bone Marrow Transplantation Team). Blood 61: 1182-1189.

RESIDUAL REFLECTIONS ON THE DETECTION AND TREATMENT OF LEUKEMIA.

D.W. VAN BEKKUM

The many excellent and inspiring papers and posters presented at this conference focussed on three main subjects:

Markers of leukemic clonogenic cells to be used to lower the detection level of tumor cells among a population of normal hemopoietic cells.

Methods of purging of bone marrow, i.e. the removal of the (small proportion of) leukemic cells from remission bone marrow, for the purpose of reinfusing autologous marrow following ablation therapy. In this category of papers also fall those that describe attempts to selectively inactivate or remove T-lymphocytes from normal donor bone marrow as an approach to the prevention of GvH disease.

All forms of treatment of leukemias in various stages of the disease, among which consolidation treatment and maintenance treatment directed at residual disease.

The following represents a few selected reflections on each of the three topics. It is by no means an attempt to review the proceedings of this meeting.

1. THE SEARCH FOR SENSITIVE MARKERS OF LEUKEMIC CELLS

Using the conventional light microscopical inspection of stained cytological preparations of bone marrow aspirations, the level of detection is generally not much better than 5%. When the percentage of blast cells is below that value the patient is considered to be in marrow remission. Some participants expressed the opinion that when a remission had lasted less than two months, it should retrospectively not be interpreted as a remission, but rather as a treatment failure.

A variety of markers, biochemical, immunological and cytogenetic, are being studied in all stages of the disease. With most of these markers the detection limits ranged between 1 and 10%. Some speakers predicted that in the near future their favourite markers might lower that limit to 0.1%, but none ventured to reach below that value.

That leaves at best an unidentifiable amount of 10^9 leukemic cells in the patient, meaning that 9 logs out of the 12 logs representing a fully leukemic marrow will continue to escape observation. (Figure 1.)

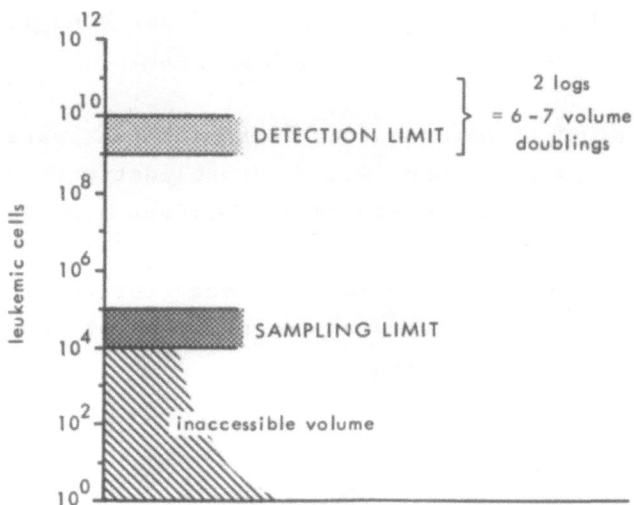

FIGURE 1. The range above the detection limit is where the tumor cell load can be quantified.

Even if the unexpected would occur and allow us to detect the last single leukemic cell in a marrow sample, there would remain an inaccessible residuum of between 10^4 and 10^5 leukemic cells as a result of the sampling limit: one bone marrow aspirate representing about 0.005% of the total bone marrow cell mass.

Such considerations lead to the first conclusion:

FOR UNRAVELING THE BIOLOGY OF MINIMAL RESIDUAL LEUKEMIA WE HAVE TO DEPEND VERY HEAVILY ON ANIMAL MODELS OF LEUKEMIA. WITHOUT A STRONG SUPPORT FROM THAT SEGMENT OF RESEARCH, THERE CAN BE NO DEVELOPMENT OF NEW RATIONAL APPROACHES TO THE TREATMENT OF RESIDUAL DISEASE.

That conclusion does not imply, however, that further efforts to develop useful markers for detecting tumor loads of between 10^9 to 10^{11} cells are not very important. Firstly, the significance of these new parameters of tumor load quantifications for evaluating the efficacy of remission induction and for earlier detection of relapse might lead to improved treatment schedules. Secondly, more sensitive tumor cell probes are essential for improving our knowledge on the regrowth rate after treatment, in the tumor cell load range of 10^9 - 10^{11} cells. This range represents 2 logs or 6-7 tumor volume doublings.

It is known from observations on solid tumors, e.g. mammary carcinoma, that accurate knowledge of the growth rate of a tumor has important implications for prognosis, early detection strategies and the selection of treatment. The introduction of regular mammographic screening procedures with methods that pick up tumors as small as 0.5 cm in diameter has provided a good insight in the range of volume doubling times for tumors over the range of 0.5 cm to about 4 cm diameter (1). From those data and by assuming an exponential growth rate from the one cell stage until the stage of detection, extrapolations can be made to estimate the length of the latency period.

This is at least one entry into the black box of tumor development below the detection limit. On doing so, it is necessary to adhere to relatively simple hypotheses, such as the clonogenic theory of carcinogenesis which implies that most tumors are initiated in a single cell and that the progeny of that cell eventually constitutes the tumor. It is true that suggestions have been forthcoming from different areas that minimal residual tumor burdens may be subject to other regulating mechanisms of growth and may perhaps smoulder for prolonged periods of time. But such suggestive observations have to be tested against the results based on calculations derived from the measurable part of the biological history of the tumor in conjunction with knowledge derived from experimental and human tumor biology.

In the case of leukemia there is a lot of reliable epidemiological data from populations exposed to ionizing radiation as a single dose or to a number of dose fractions over a limited period of time. From the Japanese Atomic Bomb data it has been derived that the shortest latent period for leukemia is about six years and the longest about twenty years (2).

The expansion from a single cell to obvious marrow involvement (10^{12} cells) requires 40 volume doublings, so that the derived minimum doubling time is two months and the maximum six months (Table 1). If it is assumed that the rate of regrowth is similar to the initial growth rate, as has been demonstrated for many experimental tumors, the remission duration corresponding to various therapeutic logs cell kill and to various doubling times can be calculated (Table 1.)

RADIATION INDUCED LEUKEMIA

Latency *   6-10 years   peaks at 10 years
             From 1 cell - 10^{12} cell = 40 doublings

6 y. latent period corresponds with 2 mo. doubling time.
10 y. latent period corresponds with 3 mo. doubling time.
20 y. latent period corresponds with 6 mo. doubling time.

CALCULATED RATE OF REGROWTH FOLLOWING
REMISSION INDUCTION OF CLINICAL LEUKEMIA
USING TWO DIFFERENT DOUBLING TIMES

Log kill	doubling time	remission duration
2	2 mo.	14 mo.
	6 mo.	42 mo.
6	2	40
	6	120
11	2	74 = 6 y.
	6	242 = 20 y.

TABLE 1.

A (limited) therapeutic effect of 2 logs cell kill
would result in a minimal duration of remission of 14
months if the leukemia doubling time is two months; on the
other hand late relapses would be expected to occur at 42
months for leukemias with a doubling time of six months.
With a treatment regimen that cures a certain proportion of
patients (about 11 logs kill), the relapses of the
fastest growing tumors would appear after six years and
those of the slowest growing leukemias would occur as late
as twenty years after treatment.
    There are now several treatment regimens that show
about 15% disease-free survival beyond five years and it
seems that very few, if any relapses, occur beyond that
time. In many patients, however, the same treatment
results in early relapses and in some a remission cannot be

induced at all. This means either that the range of doubling times is much larger than two to six months, in particular that there are many leukemias with doubling times shorter than two months, or that the differences in sensitivity to drugs are of more importance than differences in growth rate, or that the both notions apply. For a remission duration of 2-6 months following a uniform cell kill of 11 logs, doubling times of 2-6 days would be required and that does not seem to be in accordance with existing information on leukemia. From this exercise with figures two conclusions seem to emerge:

CONCLUSION 2
THE EXTENSION OF THE LIMITS OF LEUKEMIC CELL DETECTION TO AT LEAST 2 LOGS (6-7 DOUBLING TIMES) IS WORTH WHILE AND SUCH TECHNIQUES SHOULD BE MORE FULLY EXPLOITED TO DEFINE REGROWTH RATES OF LEUKEMIAS.

CONCLUSION 3
VARIATIONS IN RESPONSES TO TREATMENT CANNOT BE EXPLAINED ON THE BASIS OF DIFFERENCES IN DOUBLING TIMES (REGROWTH RATES) ONLY. IT IS MORE LIKELY THAT DIFFERENCES IN SENSITIVITY TO DRUGS APPLY TO INDIVIDUAL LEUKEMIAS AND THIS WOULD JUSTIFY INCREASED EFFORTS IN THE SEARCH FOR ASSAYS PREDICTIVE OF DRUG SENSITIVITY.

2. METHODS OF PURGING THE BONE MARROW

Purging of remission bone marrow in vitro aims at removing or inactivating all leukemic clonogenic cells from the bone marrow graft and to use it for rescuing the patient following ablative anti-leukemic treatment.

The use of cryopreserved autologous bone marrow seems to provide several advantages over allogeneic grafts. The number of candidate patients to be given intensive treatment can be considerably enlarged. Although the first groups of patients treated with one haplotype mismatched marrow as presented at this congress had about the same 2-4 years survival as MHC matched bone marrow recipients, autologous bone marrow grafts are expected to give much less complications. In addition, the age of the patients presently being limited to 30 or 40 years in many centers, could be considerably extended. Obviously, with autologous marrow grafts the presumed anti-leukemic effect of allografts will be absent, but presently there is no reliable estimate of the magnitude of this possible disadvantage.

In the past couple of years an impressive number of quite sophisticated methods has been devised for the selective elimination of leukemic cells from marrow. Selectivity implies that the treatment of marrow in vitro should spare the majority of the pluripotential hemopoietic stem cells (PHSC). The approaches are based on physical differences in density and velocity, size and shape of the cells; immunological, based on differences in surface antigens and pharmacological, based on differences in sensitivity to the action of a variety of cytotoxic drugs. In some cases these principles are combined, like in binding a toxin such as ricin to an antibody. One cannot but marvel at the sophisticated ways in which the new tools of cell recognition are being applied. Some of these methods are also under study for the selective elimination of T-lymphocytes from allogeneic marrow grafts, as the notion has now been widely accepted that T-lymphocytes are primarily responsible for the acute GvH reaction.

Several authors have demonstrated that their purging method is quite effective in leukemic models in rats or mice, others have employed mixtures of human bone marrow with human tumor cells, that could be quantitatively analysed before and after purging by suitable colony assays. However, all these elegant systems cannot be extrapolated to the situation of remission marrow with any degree of certainty, since the properties of the leukemic clonogenic cells, if at all known, are different between different forms of leukemia. The results of a number of phase I studies were presented, all comprising relatively small numbers of patients and insufficient follow-up time. Upon critical questioning the investigators admitted that their clinical data did so far not prove a benificial effect of their purging procedure and were still in the stage of phase I testing. They also stated that a controlled clinical trial with one arm receiving non-purged marrow was not an acceptable procedure in view of the unavoidable reintroduction of marrow containing an unknown proportion of leukemic cells. Three objections can be made against this position.

The first is that only comparative studies initially between purged and non-purged grafts and later between grafts purged by various methods will permit a systematic development of tumor cell separation in the field of autologous bone marrow transplantation. Secondly, even with allogeneic bone marrow grafts relapses occur. In the case of autologous marrow transplants it is impossible to distinguish between relapses stemming from the patients marrow in situ and those originating from the reinfused cells. The only way to determine the efficacy of the purging is therefore to compare the incidence of relapses between properly paired groups of patients given purged and non-purged marrow. And lastly, several patients have now been reported to survive for more than two years following rescue with unaltered autologous bone marrow. It should be kept in mind that the autologous transplant does not represent more than 1% of the bone marrow mass, so that a 2 log reduction of whatever the proportion of residual leukemic cells be in the graft is achieved in any case. Furthermore, it is likely that cryopreservation of the marrow causes losses of clonogenic leukemic cells and that leukemic cells may get lost during their circulation so that effective homing and outgrowth is not attained.

In contrast to the procedures required for inactivation of T-lymphocytes where the ratio of unwanted to wanted cells (PHSC) in bone marrow aspirates is approximately 20, the ratio leukemic cells to PHSC in remission marrow is expected to be lower than 1 in most cases.

A problem of purging of leukemic cells from autologous marrow grafts is that leukemias are so heterogeneous. Once a dependable method has been worked out for one leukemia phenotype, it is by no means certain that this will similarly apply to other cases of leukemias.

On the other hand it was shown at this conference that the PHSC has an uniform appearance even when different species are compared (3). From both rat and mouse bone marrow a nearly complete purification of PHSC has been achieved. Cell suspensions containing between 70 and 100 per cent of PHSC as measured both by spleen colony assay as well as by protection of lethally irradiated animals have been obtained with a yield of over 50% of the original PHSC population (4). In principle, the technology is now available to obtain similarly pure PHSC from human marrow, because the physical characteristics of the stem cells are accurately known and because the formation of a mixed colony in tissue culture from single cells can be developed to be used as an alternative for the spleen colony assay in rodents. Once the technique for high grade and high yield purification of PHSC has been worked out for human bone marrow it may be applied to the marrow of all patients in contrast to techniques that focus on the selective removal of leukemic cells.

Figure 2 illustrates the advantage of isolating a relatively frequently occurring cell with a unique and uniform identity over the removal of a cell type of low frequency and greatly varying properties in attempts to purge the marrow of the latter cells.

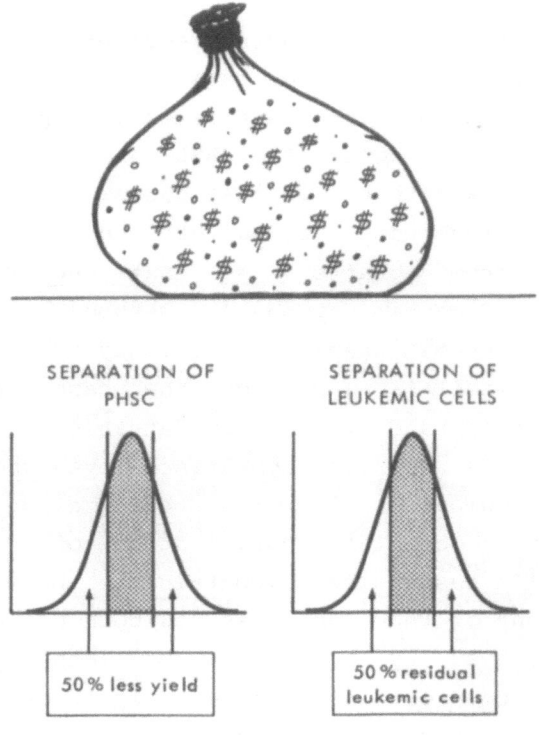

FIGURE 2. Upper part: It is easier to pick half of all the dollars out of this bag containing a lot of mixed currency than to remove the few Dutch guilders that you can hardly identify.
Lower part: Even a "uniform" cell type shows some variation in its characteristics. The central part of the area under the curve (shaded) represents the most uniform proportion of that population.

CONCLUSION 4: FOR PURPOSES OF USING AUTOLOGOUS REMISSION MARROW FOR RETRANSPLANTATION IT IS PROBABLY MORE PROFITABLE TO PREPARE PURIFIED AUTOLOGOUS PHSC SUSPENSIONS THAN TO FURTHER PERFECTION TECHNIQUES OF PURGING DIRECTED AT THE LEUKEMIC CELLS.

3. THE TREATMENT OF MINIMAL RESIDUAL LEUKEMIA

While most investigators agreed that presently available chemotherapy of childhood leukemia offers better chances for long term survival or even definitive cure than bone marrow transplantation, there was also agreement that bone marrow transplantation may be offered to those cases that respond poorly and for certain childhood leukemias with a bad prognosis. For adult leukemia the long term prognosis of treatment with chemotherapy is still considerably below the results now available for bone marrow transplantation in 1st remission. For patients over 30-40 years old the risks of allogeneic bone marrow transplantation are such that chemotherapy remains the option of choice, but this will change drastically if these patients could be treated with autologous marrow. The dilemma for the younger adults, caused by the fact that the duration of the remission is unpredictable so that a bone marrow transplant with fatal outcome could reduce the life span of some patients by one or more years, was solved by some clinicians by transplanting early in first relapse. Others, however, thought that such a strategy was not feasible under the conditions of their practice. This dilemma could, of course, also be eliminated if the risks of bone marrow transplantation were to be drastically decreased by employing autologous marrow or by further improvements in the prevention of GvHD following allogeneic marrow. A most promising approach to the latter achievement is the selective inactivation of T-lymphocytes from the graft. However, preclinical experiments with dogs and monkeys have clearly shown that elimination of T-lymphocytes decreases the rate of engraftment (5, 6). The experience from a number of different centers with Cyclosporin A given just before and for a prolonged period post-transplantation of allogeneic marrow is associated with accelerated marrow recoveries. It seems therefore that the use of T lymphocyte deprived grafts should be combined with Cyclosporin A medication.

The consensus of the meeting was that ablative therapy with bone marrow rescue, be it allogeneic or autologous, will be employed in the treatment of increasing numbers of patients in the years to come. The steadily improving results of bone marrow transplantation have stimulated the exploration of this modality for other malignancies such as lymphomas and disseminated solid tumors. It must have been gratifying for the organizers of this conference that so many distinguished leukemia researchers are now engaged in the optimalisation of autologous bone marrow transplantation, the revival of this principle having orginated nearly 10 years ago from the Rotterdam/Rijswijk transplant team.

REFERENCES

1. Kusama S, Spratt JS Jr, Donegan WI, Watson FR, Cunningham C. 1972. The gross rates of growth of human mammary carcinoma. Cancer 30, 594.
2. Sources and effects of ionizing radiation. 1977. United Nations Scientific Committee of the Effects of Radiation. United Nations, New York.
3. Dicke KA, Van Noord MJ, Maat B, Schaefer UW, Van Bekkum DW. 1973. Attempts at morphological identification of the haemopoietic stem cell in primates and rodents. Haemopoietic Stem Cells. Ciba Foundation Symposium 13. Elsevier, Excerpta Medica, North Holland, Amsterdam.
4. Visser JWM. 1983. This meeting.
5. Vriesendorp HM, Klapwijk WM, Heidt PJ, Hogeweg B, Zurcher C, Van Bekkum DW. 1982. Factors controlling the engraftment of transplanted dog bone marrow cells. Tissue Antigens 20, 63.
6. Wagemaker G, Heidt PJ, Merchav S, Van Bekkum DW. 1982. Abrogation of histocompatibility barriers to bone marrow transplantation in rhesus monkeys. Experimental Hematology Today 1982. Karger, Basel, 111.

INDEX OF SUBJECTS